The Business of Massage Therapy

The Business of Massage Therapy

Building a Successful Career

JESSICA ABEGG, LMT, MBA, MSIB

PEARSON

Boston Columbus Indianapolis New York San Francisco Upper Saddle River
Amsterdam Cape Town Dubai London Madrid Milan Munich Paris Montreal Toronto
Delhi Mexico City Sao Paulo Sydney Hong Kong Seoul Singapore Taipei Tokyo

Library of Congress Cataloging-in-Publication Data

Abegg, Jessica.
The business of massage therapy : building a successful career / Jessica Abegg. — 1st ed.
p. ; cm.
Includes bibliographical references and index.
ISBN-13: 978-0-13-505361-4
ISBN-10: 0-13-505361-7
1. Massage therapy—Practice. 2. Massage therapy—Vocational guidance. I. Title.
[DNLM: 1. Massage. 2. Professional Practice—organization & administration. 3. Vocational Guidance. WB 537]
RM722.A24 2012
615.8'22068--dc22

2010029629

Notice: The author and the publisher of this volume have taken care that the information and technical recommendations contained herein are based on research and expert consultation, and are accurate and compatible with the standards generally accepted at the time of publication. Nevertheless, as new information becomes available, changes in clinical and technical practices become necessary. The reader is advised to carefully consult manufacturers' instructions and information material for all supplies and equipment before use, and to consult with a healthcare professional as necessary. This advice is especially important when using new supplies or equipment for clinical purposes. The author and publisher disclaim all responsibility for any liability, loss, injury, or damage incurred as a consequence, directly or indirectly, of the use and application of any of the contents of this volume.

Publisher: Julie Levin Alexander
Publisher's Assistant: Regina Bruno
Editor-in-Chief: Mark Cohen
Executive Editor: John Goucher
Assistant Editor: Nicole Ragonese
Editorial Assistant: Rosalie Hawley
Director of Marketing: David Gesell
Executive Marketing Manager: Katrin Beacom
Marketing Specialist: Michael Sirinides
Managing Production Editor: Patrick Walsh
Production Liaison: Christina Zingone
Production Editor: Michelle Gardner, Laserwords Maine
Senior Media Editor: Amy Peltier
Media Project Manager: Lorena Cerisano
Manufacturing Manager: Ilene Sanford
Manufacturing Buyer: Pat Brown/Alan Fischer
Creative Director: Jayne Conte
Cover Designer: Bruce Kenselaar
Cover Visual Research and Permissions: Rita Wenning
Image Specialist: Annette Linder
Composition: Laserwords Maine
Printing and Binding: R.R. Donnelley/Willard
Cover Printer: Coral Graphics
Cover Image: Subbotina Anna/shutterstock

10 9 8 7 6 5 4 3 2 1

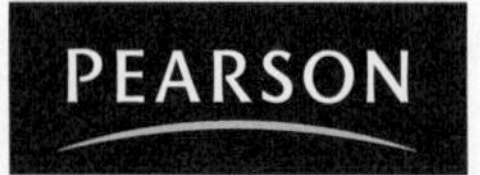

www.pearsonhighered.com

ISBN-13: 978-0-13-505361-4
ISBN-10: 0-13-505361-7

Dedication

For my fabulous husband Bill and my beloved son Liam; may the path before you both shine with limitless love and joyful successes. I am blessed and grateful to have a family so loving, supportive, and playfully fun.

Brief Contents

Preface

Welcome to the wonderful world of massage! As a massage therapist, you are joining a worldwide network of healers, and are positioned for a challenging and rewarding career. The potential for success in massage is limitless, and now is one of the best times to be in practice. Demand for massage is surging, and opportunities are everywhere. No matter where you are with your massage career or where you want to go, this book was written to help you on your path.

The last decade has seen a revolution in the massage industry, and rapid growth has provided unprecedented opportunities for practitioners.[1] Both supply and demand for massage therapists have exploded. There are as many reasons attracting individuals to this ancient profession as there are working practitioners. Regardless of the ultimate reasons motivating you personally, or the direction you want your career to take, it has become imperative to sharpen your professional and business skills in order to develop a thriving practice and achieve economic independence.

At the same time that the massage industry has experienced massive growth, it has also seen a record increase in turnover among its practitioners. Many massage schools estimate the "failure rate" of new therapists to be as high as 90 percent, defining this failure as students who are no longer practicing massage within one year of graduation.[2] In such a rewarding and flexible career, such statistics can be at once surprising and discouraging.

At the risk of overgeneralizing, many enter the profession because they are drawn to the qualitative aspects of service, independence, and healing. Many who chose a career in the holistic health care field often find they dislike or distrust the business aspects, and either ignore them or reject them altogether. A common misperception is that those practitioners with the best technical skills are automatically successful. However, many soon find that without the balance of quantitative business skills, massage skills alone will not get them very far. Many soon give up and leave their fledgling massage career for more secure employment.

While technical skills and innate talent are incredibly important, they are not enough to sustain a career in massage therapy. Some individuals find self promotion difficult, or experience a disconnect between their personal integrity and the unsavory practices often associated with business in the media. Many find the marketing aspects of job seeking to be challenging, while others view the managerial and administrative aspects of running their own practice to be just as intimidating and overwhelming. Unfortunately, many leave the massage profession altogether. This book was written with all these individuals in mind. It aims to bridge the gap between your natural healing capacity and the success that awaits you. In the process, you may even find an entrepreneurial spirit you did not even realize you possess.

HOW TO USE THIS BOOK

Rather than a stuffy, inaccessible textbook that typically gathers dust on the shelf, *The Business of Massage Therapy* is meant to be an interactive exploration and resource guide. Contained within its pages you will find useful exercises, functional suggestions, helpful resources, case studies, and action steps to help you on your way. It can be approached linearly and read from cover to cover, or accessed for specific concerns or specific areas you would like to work on. It may be beneficial to read it through once to gain familiarity, and then return to the sections that seem most helpful to your particular situation. However you approach the book, take your time and engage the material with an interactive mentality. Relax as you read, and allow yourself to fully absorb the information. Take time to complete the exercises in the book, allowing yourself space for self-exploration. Like anything else in life, this book will only be as useful as you make it.

Organizing your thoughts in a tangible way can be a large part of your success. Throughout the book you will see little tips on "Getting Organized." It is highly recommended that you create your own *The Business of Massage Therapy* notebook: a 2- or 3-inch binder from your local office supply store should work just fine. To help you get and stay organized, you may find it helpful to get section dividers for each chapter. As you go through the chapters and do the exercises in the book, you will be able to organize your work, collect materials and resources, and see the results of all your hard work. If you collect business cards or brochures from other therapists, keep them in your notebook as well. If you learn of marketing techniques you would like to emulate, keep samples of them in this notebook for later. This will allow you to gauge your development, and it is always fun to look back on your starting point as you advance on your path. As your career and/or business grow, both your notebook and *The Business of Massage Therapy* will be good references for you.

As you read, you will see a lot of pictures and symbols. These indicate additional tips, ideas, and activities for you to engage in throughout the book. Keep your eye out for the following icons:

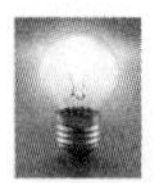

Bright Ideas

Inspiration: Ideas, anecdotes, and quotes to help motivate you.

Getting Organized

Organization: Fun ways to help plan, structure, and keep your business in order.

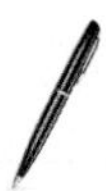

Put It in Writing

Pen to paper: Fun exercises, quizzes, and activities to get you engaged in your business.

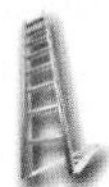

First Steps

Getting started: Small steps to help you try something new.

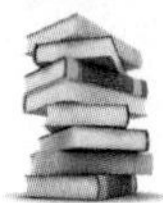

Helpful Resources

A little help here?: Books, magazines, or online resources to help you out.

Pitfalls

Things to look out for: Common mistakes to avoid with your career and/or practice.

Although written from a massage therapist's point of view, this book contains concepts, business practices, and resources applicable to anyone in a healing profession. Thus, acupuncturists, counselors, homeopaths, aromatherapists, and wellness practitioners of all kinds will find assistance within these pages. Just as you are assisting your clients on their own paths to optimal health, this book strives to aid you on your path to optimal professionalism, an optimal practice, and an optimal financial achievement. Wishing you all the success on your journey!

Acknowledgments

Thank you to my husband, Bill, who has been my recoverer of documents, my proofreader, my Dell Whisperer, and my best friend all these years. Thank you for your unwavering enthusiasm, support, and for always smiling and saying "that is a fabulous idea," no matter how many times it wasn't. You are my Mosty.

Thank you to my amazing immediate family: To my sister, Rachel, who has never faltered in being the best sister and friend I have ever known. To my mother, Gina, who gave me the enthusiasm and support to say yes to the world, to always be compassionate, and to try everything life has to offer. To my father, Chenia, who gave me an insatiable love of learning, an appreciation for solitude and stillness, and a profound respect for others' experiences and beliefs. Thanks to all my myriad friends and family who have never failed to provide support, laughter, insight and perspective over the years. My cup runneth over!

Thank you to all the therapists and helping professionals who have shared their wisdom and experiences with me, and who devote their lives to being of beneficial service: May your practices and careers continue to flourish.

Thank you to all my amazing clients over the years for honoring me with the chance to work together. I count among my blessings all the people who have crossed my table and worked for health and balance in their own lives.

Thank you to Mark Cohen, John Goucher and Nicole Ragonese at Pearson and Michelle Gardner of Laserwords Maine for all your explanations, process ministering, and support. I could not have asked for better editors! Thank you to Alison Sullenberger-Keiser for connecting me with Pearson, and for meeting me on my way to Beijing to sign everything before leaving the country!

Thanks also to Nisarat and Suchin Sirimaharaj and the entire Sirimaharaj family for welcoming me into their home with such open arms, and for tucking me into their beautiful corner of Thailand for a magical place to start writing this book.

Reviewers

Michelle Bequeaith, LMT
Capri College of Massage Therapy
Davenport, Iowa

Lucinda Castro
Long Beach, California

Beverley Giroud, LMT
Desert Institute of the Healing Arts
Tucson, Arizona

Holly Huzar, LMT
Center for Natural Wellness School of Massage Therapy
Albany, New York

Tom Johnston, MEd, LMP
Body Mind Academy
Kirkland, Washington

Cecile Martin
Bodyworks Massage Institute
Evansville, Indiana

Kathy Peltier
Irene's Myomassology Institute
Southfield, Michigan

Lou Peters, LMT, CNMT
American Institute of Alternative Medicine
Columbus, Ohio

Chris Rider, LMT, BS
Carlson College of Massage Therapy
Anamosa, Iowa

Carol Rifflard, LMT, BS, MEd
Keiser University
Port St. Lucie, Florida

Michelle K. Tenpenny, LMT, BA
Kaskasia College
Centralia, Illinois

About the Author

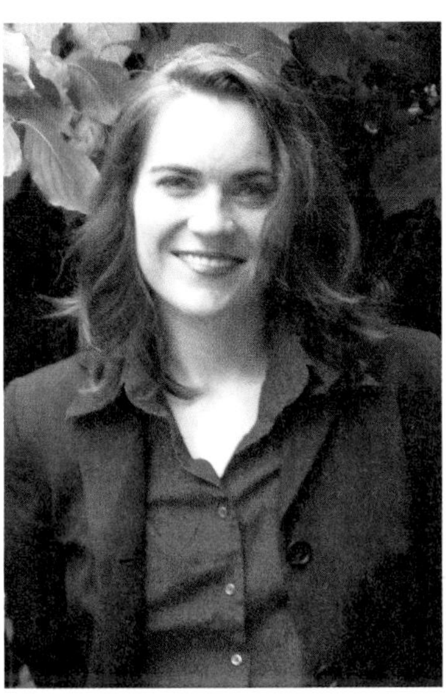

Jessica Abegg is a licensed massage therapist, business owner, business coach, workplace wellness trainer, and writer. With over ten years of private practice, she knows the ins and outs of starting a massage business from scratch. She has coached many small business owners across industries along the path to their own success. She is the owner of the holistic business coaching service. Massaging Success (www.massagingsuccess.com), and Sanctuary Massage & Wellness (www.sanctuarymassage.net) in Denver, Colorado. She has also founded several other service businesses over the years. Jessica serves on the committee for the National Certification Board for Therapeutic Massage and Bodywork. Jessica received her MBA and MS in International Business from the University of Colorado.

An itinerant gypsy with an insatiable passion for learning holistic wellness, Jessica has traveled to over 30 countries to study, experience, and live different cultural approaches to health and healing. In her leisure time, Jessica enjoys reading, writing poetry, personal finance, yoga, hiking, and spending time with her family. She lives with her husband and son in Denver, Colorado.

Contents

APPENDICES

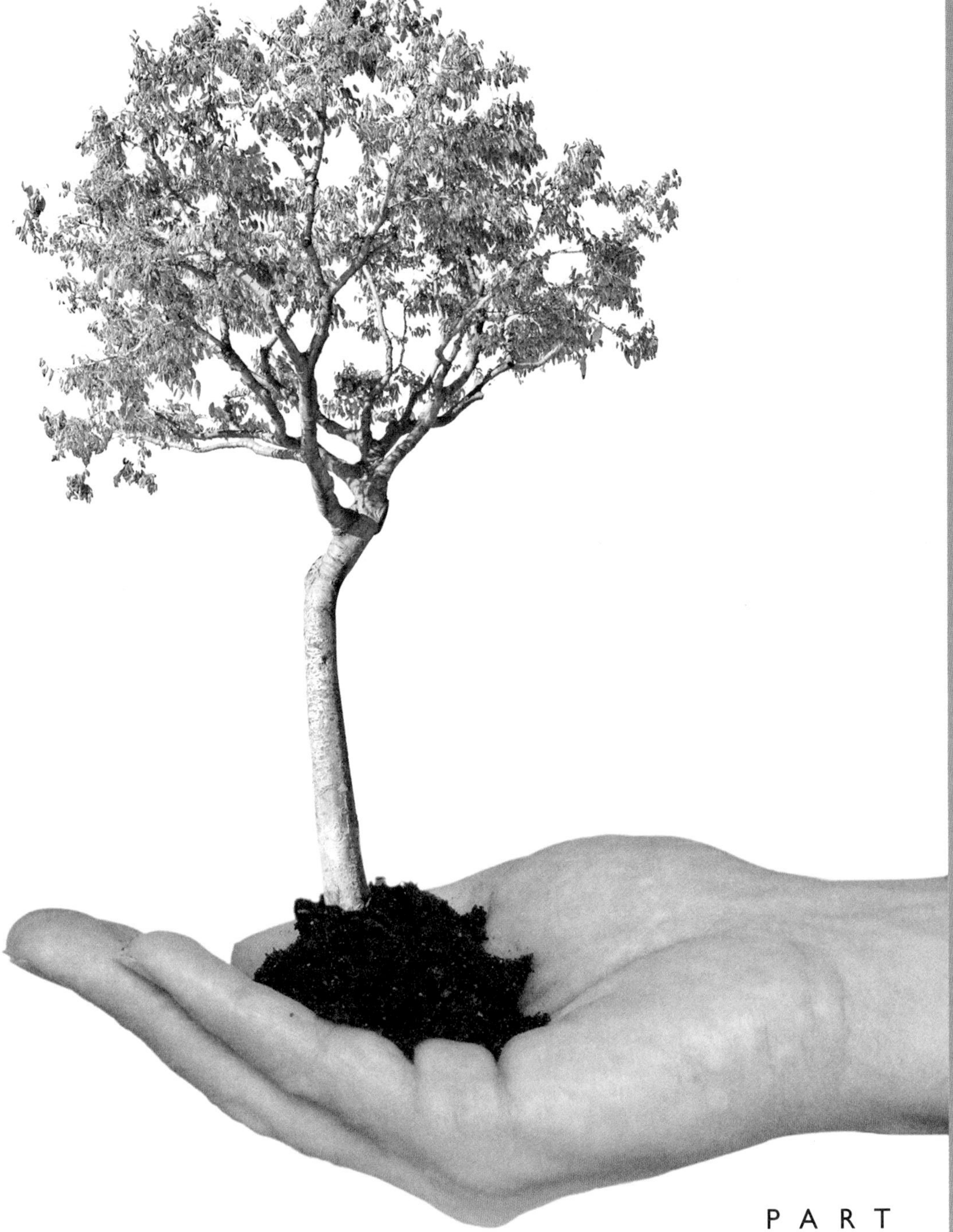

PART

1

Thriving Professional Development for the Massage Therapist

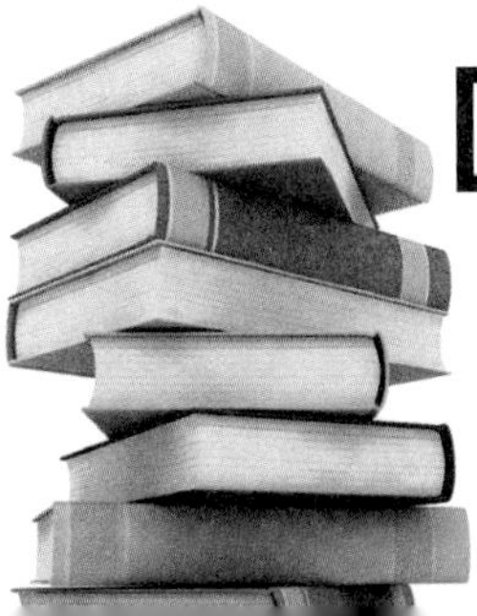

CHAPTER 1

Is a Massage Therapy Career Right for You?

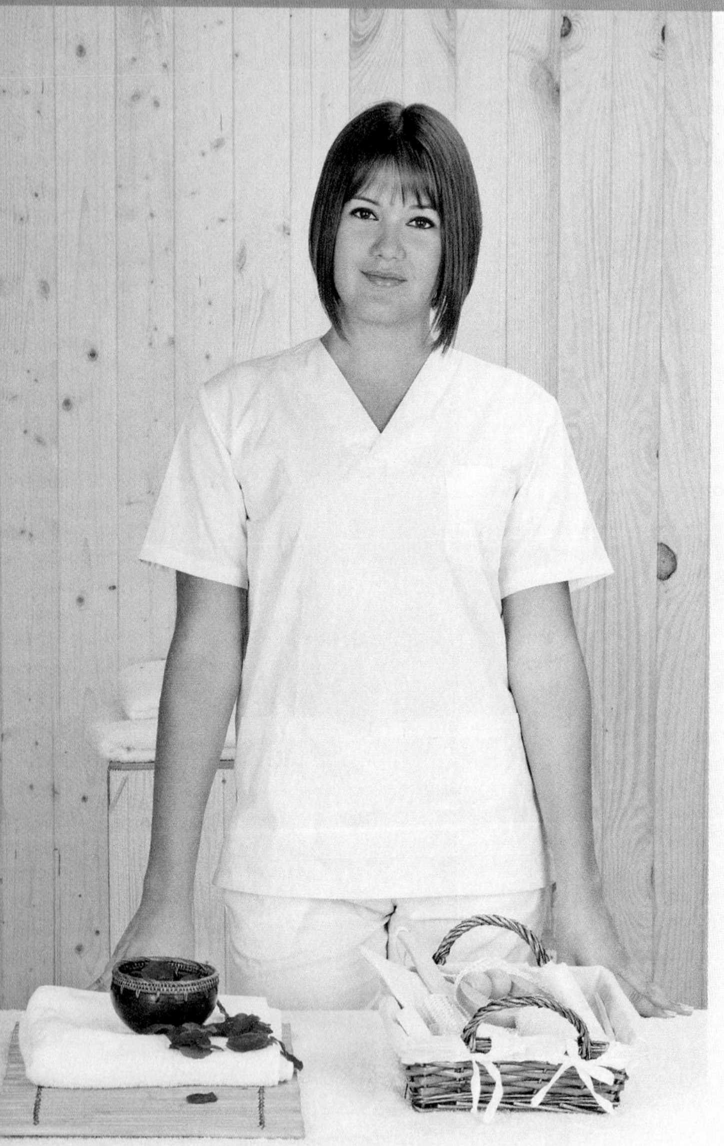

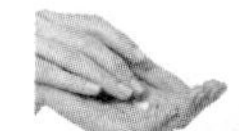

CHAPTER OUTLINE

LEARNING OBJECTIVES

1. Explore the massage therapy career
2. Define helping professions and identify characteristics of a helping professional
3. Examine the importance of balance
4. Evaluate a massage career in the context of one's life
5. Explore aspects of a massage therapy employee, and aspects of an entrepreneur
6. Contrast the benefits and drawbacks of employment and business ownership
7. Define an elevator pitch and its importance to your career

KEY TERMS

allopathic *7*
balance *10*
boundaries *5*
craniosacral therapy *9*
deep-tissue massage *9*
determination *11*
elevator pitch *11*
entrepreneur *11*
healthy touch *5*
helping professional *4*
hot stone massage *9*
massage therapy *4*
myofascial release *9*
neuromuscular therapy *9*
passion *11*
pre/post-natal massage *9*
promotion *11*
reflexology *9*
shiatsu *9*
sports massage *9*
Swedish massage *9*

A CAREER IN MASSAGE THERAPY

Not until we experience it is it more than just words. After we experience it, there is no need for words.

—Milton Trager

Massage therapy is an umbrella term that refers to various types and modalities of soft tissue manipulation. Massage is an ancient art that has been practiced in many cultures throughout history. Massage can offer a rich and gratifying career, and can give you the opportunity to do work that is meaningful, important, and helpful to others. In a fast-paced, stress-filled world, providing a safe space for others to relax and heal can add real value to your community, and can enrich your own life. There is no "right" way to pursue a career in massage therapy, and part of the allure is the blank canvas that such a career presents. Massage therapists can work in luxury day spas, at destination resorts, for chiropractors, with AIDS patients, in wellness centers, or create their own practice. You can own a day spa with forty therapists, or see your own clients from a home office. There are as many career paths as there are massage therapists, and your possibilities are endless.

Just as there are many options to pursue within a massage career, there are many motivations propelling people into the world of massage. Whatever form your career ultimately takes, it is important to know yourself before pursuing any path. Perhaps you are drawn toward helping others, perhaps you like the portability of skills that you can apply virtually anywhere, or perhaps it is the flexibility of hours that attracts you. Many therapists have experienced the powerful healing benefits of massage on their own bodies and want to share that experience with others. What are some of the aspects attracting you?

The mind cannot forget what the hands have learned.

—Jon Zahourek

WHAT ARE THE QUALITIES OF A HELPING PROFESSIONAL?

A **helping professional** is a practitioner that works with a body's natural restorative and curative properties to optimize that body's health. Helping professionals promote health and address challenges in another person's physical, emotional, psychological, or spiritual being. Examples of healing professionals include doctors, counselors, ministers, social workers, and of course, massage therapists.

It takes a special kind of person to be a helping professional, and when you become a massage therapist, you are being entrusted with a unique and personal aspect of the well-being of another human. At its essence, massage is the exchange of energies, and you communicate volumes with your touch. Clients must be able to trust you if they are going to get on your table, and enduring trust must be established for them to return for subsequent treatments. Part of that trust comes from intentional behavior and part of that trust comes from your innate character. Before anyone else will trust you with his or her body, it is imperative that you trust and know yourself well. Do you see yourself as a helper or a healer? Take a moment to ask yourself the following questions on the next page and explore your answers. Grab a pen and paper and tally up your scores. Keep in mind that there are no "right" answers to these questions, only areas of yourself to explore.

PITFALLS

A Quiz Is a Quiz

Although it can help you illuminate aspects of your character that either lend themselves to massage or do not, a quiz isn't the definitive authority on your career prospects. This is an important thing to keep in mind throughout all of the exercises and quizzes in the book. Don't be discouraged if your score is low, but rather think of ways you can improve your score and get started doing so. Not all helping professionals are strong in every area, but work hard at honing their healing capacity over time.

A VERY BRIEF OVERVIEW OF MASSAGE HISTORY

Whether you are a massage student or a professional therapist who has picked up *The Business of Massage Therapy* for a little professional development, chances are good that you will have already been exposed to the information in the next few sections. However, in order to know where we are

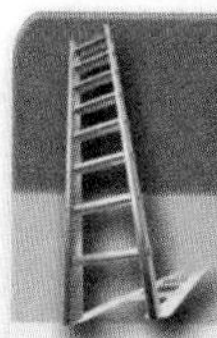

FIRST STEPS

Seek out a practicing massage therapist and learn more about the profession. What have been some challenges the therapist has faced? What does he or she love about doing massage?

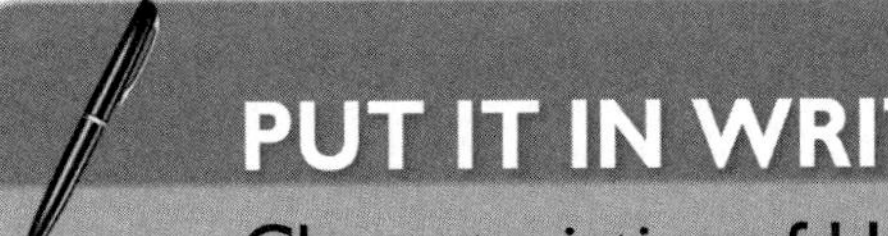

PUT IT IN WRITING

Characteristics of Helping Professionals: An Exploration

1. *Are you comfortable touching and being touched?* Some people naturally gravitate toward physical contact, while others are very protective of their physical space.
   ____ a. No one leaves without a hug!
   ____ b. Although I don't mind giving or receiving hugs or other forms of touch, I respect if others don't care to be touched.
   ____ c. I only touch people I'm very close to; anything else is inappropriate.
   ____ d. I get very uncomfortable when someone else touches me; I never initiate personal contact.
2. *Did your family use* ***healthy touch****?* Some families are very tactile, and physical connection is a natural characteristic. While not essential, familiarity with healthy touch can be helpful.
   ____ a. Back rubs and bear hugs were part of my everyday life growing up.
   ____ b. My family was fairly tactile, and touch was always comfortable, although not excessive.
   ____ c. My family was very reserved about touch; we relied more on verbal communication.
   ____ d. Physical touch was strictly taboo in my family.
3. *Are you comfortable in your own body?* Are you judgmental of your own or others' bodies? Clients come in all shapes and sizes, and it's important to explore your own hang-ups around body image.
   ____ a. I abhor changing in locker rooms. I don't want anyone to see me, and I don't want to see them. I can't stand the body I'm in!
   ____ b. I wouldn't mind losing a few pounds, but all in all I'm pretty comfortable in my own skin.
   ____ c. Check me out! Have you ever seen anyone this beautiful?!
   ____ d. As soon as I lose 20 pounds, things will be fine. And maybe a little plastic surgery.
4. *Do you have good physical stamina?* Depending on your client load and your technique, massage can be incredibly demanding on your body. Not everyone can physically handle the demands.
   ____ a. I am tireless and can go all day. Bring it on!
   ____ b. I get winded pretty easily, and need a lot of rest after any activity.
   ____ c. I haven't been very active lately, so my endurance isn't as good as it has been. I'm sure that would improve with practice.
   ____ d. I'm tired just reading this book.
5. *Are you good at conversation?* For many people, massage is therapy in more ways than one. Clients may open up to you about a myriad of personal issues. Are you comfortable with that role?
   ____ a. Shut up already!
   ____ b. People often come to me with their troubles—I'm very comfortable with people sharing if they want to.
   ____ c. The doctor is in! Tell me all about it!
   ____ d. I know that everyone has their problems, but it's none of my business. I don't want to pry.
6. *Are you good at silence?* Some clients need massage to be a calm and peaceful mental escape, and it is just as important to be comfortable in silence as it is in conversation. A good therapist is able to "read" the needs of their clients when it comes to balancing with silence.
   ____ a. Somebody say something! This silence is killing me.
   ____ b. I fully respect the importance of stillness and silence in the healing process, and always welcome it in my sessions.
   ____ c. Nobody say a word—it's completely inappropriate to talk during a massage and chatter undermines the healing work that I am doing.
   ____ d. If my client doesn't want to talk, that's fine by me.
7. *Do you have healthy* ***boundaries****?* While empathy is incredibly important, it is also important to maintain boundaries with your clients. Maintaining professional distance from the emotional and physical struggles of clients is necessary.
   ____ a. I am usually very good about professional boundaries, but sometimes the lines are vague to me.
   ____ b. There's nothing wrong with dating or having a sexual relationship with a client. What's the problem?
   ____ c. When someone shares his strong feelings with me, I find myself feeling what he describes, often for some time afterward. When someone else has a headache, I often get one, too.
   ____ d. My relationships with friends and family are characterized by clear boundaries: mutual respect, equal giving and receiving, and autonomy.
8. *Are you willing to invest the time and money for school, continued education, equipment, and supporting supplies?* There are many costs involved with becoming a massage therapist, as well as ongoing costs to sustain licensure, group membership, and a strong practice. Are you willing to commit to the financial investment?
   ____ a. I know it will be a hardship at first, but with hard work, professionalism, persistence, flexibility, and a little luck, it will pay off.
   ____ b. I didn't realize it would cost that much. There's no way I can pay for that!
   ____ c. Once I'm done with school, I won't have to pay for anything else. What's one year?
   ____ d. The best investment I can make is in my ongoing education and continual professional development. I am comfortable with sacrifice when it comes to my own success—those costs are an investment in my career.

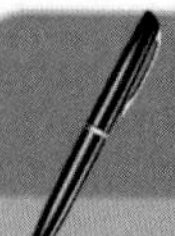

PUT IT IN WRITING

Characteristics of Helping Professionals: An Exploration (continued)

9. *Do you take good care of your body?* The physical rigors of massage will take a toll on your body if you do not take measures to care for it. Regular exercise, a healthy diet, and other aspects of self-care are important.

____ a. I don't really care about exercise or my diet. It's not that significant to me.

____ b. My health is my most important asset. I always make exercise and diet my first priorities.

____ c. Although I'd really like to, I just never seem to have enough time to work out or cook a healthy meal. I would if I could.

____ d. Although I'm not fanatical about it, I eat pretty well and exercise often. I feel good about the state of my health.

10. *Are you comfortable promoting yourself?* Whether in private practice or working for someone else, it is important to promote your skills to people in order to propel your career forward. Are you comfortable with that?

____ a. It is so hard for me to promote myself. It feels really awkward to tell others how great I am. I'd rather not do it at all, or have someone do it for me.

____ b. I'm fabulous, and the world should know about it. If I don't tell people, no one will ever know what I have to offer.

____ c. Although it can feel a little uncomfortable to "sell myself," I recognize it as being an important part of any successful practice.

____ d. The skills speak for themselves. Massage is an art, not a business, and a true artist never "sells herself."

Scoring Guide:

Now that you've completed the quiz, go back and score it.

1) a = 3 b = 4 c = 2 d = 1 6) a = 1 b = 4 c = 2 d = 3
2) a = 4 b = 3 c = 2 d = 1 7) a = 3 b = 1 c = 2 d = 4
3) a = 1 b = 3 c = 4 d = 2 8) a = 3 b = 1 c = 2 d = 4
4) a = 4 b = 2 c = 3 d = 1 9) a = 1 b = 4 c = 2 d = 3
5) a = 1 b = 4 c = 3 d = 2 10) a = 2 b = 4 c = 3 d = 1

Now add up your scores:

33–40: Healing hands indeed! You're definitely on the right career path, and will find massage to be a great fit for you. Congratulations!

26–33: Looking good! Massage could definitely be the right fit for you, though you may have a few areas to work on to make this career path more smooth. You're on your way to being a great therapist!

18–25: Could be! This might be a great time for you to think about what's drawing you to massage and to look closer at your misgivings about this career choice. What could you work on to make it easier? What things are non-negotiables?

10–17: Hmmm... are you sure you're in the right place? Massage may present real challenges for you on your career path. Take some time to look closely at the areas you may struggle with.

Regardless of where you score, go back through the quiz and examine areas where you may have had a low score. Is there something that you could work to improve?

and where we are going, it is crucial to understand and reflect upon where we come from. The following is a very brief synopsis of the history of massage therapy, current trends in the industry, as well as an overview of some of the most popular modalities currently being practiced.

Massage therapy has long been a part of human history. Recorded evidence of therapeutic massage as a popular ancient healing practice has manifested in disparate cultures and geographies, from the Mayans to the Egyptians, the Persians to the Polynesians.The oldest known book about massage therapy, the Chinese *Cong-Fu of the Toa-Tse,* hails from 3000 BCE.[1] The *Huangdi Neijing,* the seminal medical text of early China that emerged in the first century BCE, talks at length about the virtues of massage.[2] In the Western hemisphere, the Greeks and Romans were the first to record the use of massage therapy; Hippocrates (of Hippocratic Oath fame) was a steadfast supporter and promoter of the therapeutic applications of massage, and between 100 and 144 BCE Julius Ceasar received regular massage to relieve his neuralgia and epileptic seizures.[3] And just like today, massaging the original athletes and Olympic competitors was common practice among the Romans and Greeks.[4]

It is also important to remember the antiquity of other complementary and alternative medicines, the interrelated counterparts of massage. Health modalities such as acupuncture, nutrition therapy, herbal medicine, yoga, and tai chi have all long been a part of the human experience. What we consider "alternative" medicine practices are the ancient healing tradition and techniques carried on for centuries and even millennia in many cultures. Reflexology can trace its origins to ancient Egypt and China, where records of its use date to around 4000 BCE.[5] Herbal medicine has been used for more than 60,000 years, and traditional Chinese medicine and acupuncture have been practiced in Asia for over 5000 years.[6]

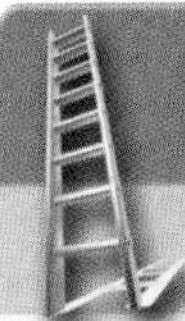

FIRST STEPS

It can be a lot of fun to trace the origins and fascinating history of massage therapy. It can also be of great interest to your clients to know that they are participating in an ancient tradition when they get a massage. Get on the Internet or head to your local library and see what you can learn about massage therapy throughout history and across cultural traditions.

The definitive heredity of the word *massage* is debatable, and many different theories have emerged. However, it is certain that the word and practice of massage have many different cultures and traditions embedded in its roots. It is a derivative of the French word *massage,* "friction or kneading." It may also originate from the Arabic word *massa,* (to touch, feel or handle), the Greek word *massin* (to knead or manipulate), the Hebrew *mashesh* (to press or squeeze), or even the Latin *massa* (dough).[7] The fact that the word bears a likeness to words from so many different traditions attests to its ancient and universal application.

Scientific massage therapy was introduced in the United States by New York physicians George and Charles Taylor. These brothers had studied massage in Sweden under the tutelage of Mathias Roth.[8] Public clinics for medical massage were opened in the United States after the Civil War by two Swedish doctors, Dr. Baron Nils Posse in Boston and Dr. Hartwig Nissen in Washington, DC.[9] In 1929, the health advocate John Harvey Kellogg (yes, of Corn Flakes fame) published *The Art of Massage.*[10] However, massage therapy fell from collective grace for many years, in part due to its association with sexual massage parlors and its rejection by the mainstream medical community at large.[11] In the 1960s, as America began to expand its global awareness due to cultural movements, the spread of international trade and travel, and expanded media availability, massage and other ancient therapies regained popularity in the United States. During this innovative, exploratory, and restless decade, interest in natural healing surged, and massage therapy was revitalized.

THE MASSAGE INDUSTRY TODAY

Knowing that massage is a dynamic, developing industry today, it shouldn't surprise you to know that the massage industry has seen significant changes in the last two decades, nor that it continues to evolve. For many years, individual massage therapists and collective massage organizations have fought for legitimacy and professional respect. It wasn't long ago that people used the term masseuse or masseur interchangeably for therapeutic and sexual work. But differentiation from the shady massage parlor has not been the only area in which professional massage therapists sought legitimacy. Being recognized as a reputable member of the medical family has also been a challenge to the massage community. The United States has traditionally relied on **allopathic,** or conventional, medicine, and only in recent years have alternative modalities gained (or regained) popularity.

In the last decade, the landscape has continued to shift. As demand grows and more people seek to join the health and wellness industry, massage therapy training facilities are springing up rapidly. Schools vary significantly in curricula and size of student body, but the obvious result of this is that far more therapists are competing in the market than ever before. The National Certification Board for Therapeutic Massage and Bodywork (NCBTMB) reports that there are nearly 90,000 nationally certified practitioners serving consumers.[12] The American Massage Therapy Association (AMTA) estimates that there are 265,000 to 300,000 practitioners in the United States.[13] Not every practicing therapist receives national certification however, and not every state requires some form of licensure to practice. When the U.S. Department of Labor did its most recent industry survey in 2010–2011, 42 states and the District of Columbia had laws that regulated massage in some way.[14] In addition, not all therapists practice full time, and many use occasional massage appointments as a way to supplement other income. Thus, it is difficult to determine an exact number of practicing therapists in the country, though estimates range from 350,000 to 450,000.[15]

Another interesting aspect of massage therapy is how and where therapists actually work. The U.S. Department of Labor reports that 60 percent of therapists are self-employed. Those that are self-employed either own their own businesses or contract out independently. It is projected that employment opportunities for massage therapists will grow 20 percent between 2006 and 2016, far above the

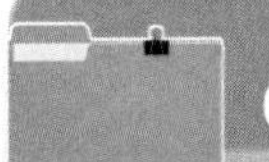

GETTING ORGANIZED

It isn't just death and taxes that you can count on—it's also the fact that regulations and laws change. Regulating bodies that govern massage are often changing licensure laws, and you always want to be on the right side of that issue! Stay abreast of changes in your area, and any time a change is made, get a paper copy and file it away in your *Business of Massage Therapy* notebook.

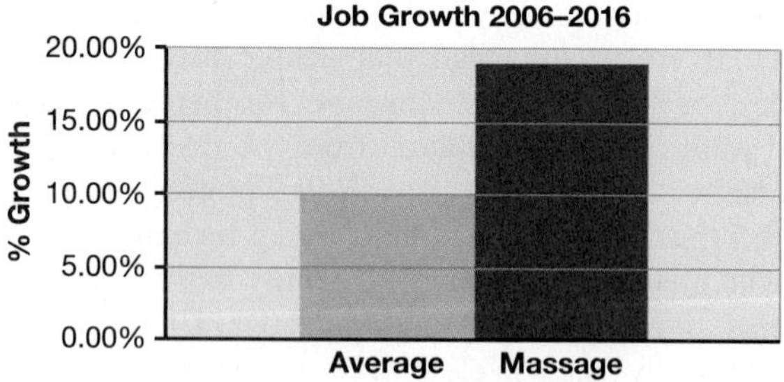

FIGURE 1-1

Projected Job Growth for Massage Therapists from 2006 to 2016.

Source: U.S. Department of Labor.

average for other industries[16] (see Figure 1-1 ■). One of the allures of massage therapy is that it is a portable skill, one that can literally be done just about anywhere. Jobs are available throughout the country and throughout the world, although, like most work, opportunities are most abundant in areas of concentrated populations.

In recent years, the economic downturn has given many spa and wellness business owners headaches, but there are many demographic trends supporting the continued growth of massage therapy. One of the most notable is the active and aging U.S. population. As you recall, many of the people who made massage popular in the 1960s are now approaching retirement, and have much more disposable income than they did 40 years ago. This doesn't just mean that you should rush out for gerontology massage courses, however—you will also be replacing many seasoned therapists who are closing the doors on their working years and leaving behind clients of all demographics. Thus, this trend has a twofold benefit for broadening your career options and potential client base: both the retiring baby boomer therapists and the clients they are leaving behind will need new skilled therapists.

As was mentioned previously, massage schools and training facilities are springing up to respond to the mounting demand in the market. Trade, vocational, and technical colleges have now added massage therapy to their academic repertoire, competing with the smaller, more traditional massage schools focused solely upon therapist training. This may seem like a discouraging fact, but keep in mind the true critical mass of massage therapists it would take to reach complete market saturation. Supply rises to meet demand, as any good economist will tell you, and data reveals that demand continues to trend upward (see Chapter 12 for more on Supply and Demand theory). In other words, there is very little chance that the increase in massage schools and new therapists will seriously dampen your career or employment prospects as a new therapist. The Associated Bodywork and Massage Professionals (ABMP) report that Americans receive 230 million massage sessions a year, establishing massage therapy as a $15 billion industry.[17] Even as economic challenges have made people think twice about services such as massage, the mainstream acceptance of massage as well as the inevitable aches and pains of the human body continue to present opportunities for the massage industry. As one sage therapist observed, "There are always enough sore muscles to go around."

KINDS OF BODYWORK

Massage today is a highly differentiated industry. Although the origins of massage therapy date back thousands of years, new techniques and modalities seem to surface every year. Some are combinations and incorporations of established techniques, while others contribute genuinely unique procedures and approaches. The ABMP places the number of existing modalities to be around 250, although that number is evergrowing.[18] This can be a cause of bewilderment to both massage therapists and massage consumers, and it becomes increasingly necessary to educate both parties. The responsibility for that, of course, is on the practitioner, and you may find that it is necessary to "educate in order to create" a following for a new modality. Figure 1-2 ■ illustrates the 10 most commonly practiced (and subsequently most readily identified by consumers) modalities.

This textbook, of course, is not a massage training manual and in no way intends to be instructive about techniques. You will have (or have had) many other classes in your training program or ongoing education that will address these modalities directly. However, because no two massage schools' curricula are identical, and because it never hurts

Common Massage Modalities
Sports Massage
Pre/Post-natal
Myofascial Release
Reflexology
Swedish
Shiatsu
Deep Tissue
Cranio-sacral
Hot Stone
Neuro-muscular

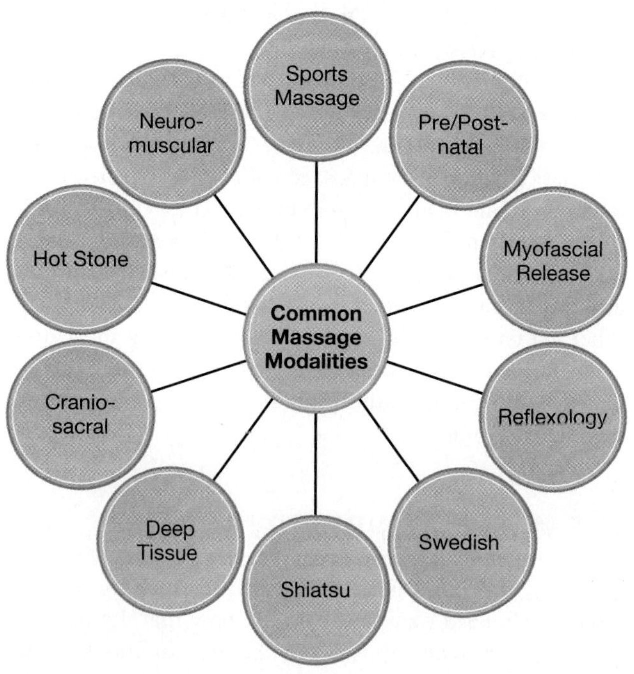

FIGURE 1-2

Common Massage Modalities.

to review the basics, take a moment to briefly examine characteristics of these top 10 techniques.

Swedish massage: Swedish massage uses kneading and gliding strokes to increase blood flow. It focuses attention on the more superficial muscles of the body, and fosters healthy oxygen flow and toxin release from muscles. Techniques include *petrissage* (a kneading motion), *effleurage* (a gliding motion), and *tapotement* (a percussive motion). Strokes are directed toward the heart. Swedish massage is generally very relaxing.

Shiatsu: Shiatsu is known as the Japanese art of finger pressure. In this technique, the therapist uses fingers, knuckles, elbows, feet, and the palm of the hand to apply pressure to a series of points along a muscle group. The goal is to restore *qi,* or proper balance. Shiatsu incorporates traction, passive stretching, and acupressure. Unlike many modalities that are performed on an elevated massage table, Shiatsu is usually administered on a mat set on the floor to facilitate the therapist's full body techniques.

Deep-tissue massage: Although some deep-tissue practitioners incorporate some Swedish massage techniques, deep-tissue massage (as the eponymous technique implies) focuses on the interior core muscles beneath the superficial ones. This is typically quite focused work, and the therapist accesses deep layers of soft tissue to release chronic adhesions, tension, and pain.

Reflexology: In this technique, pressure points on the feet and hands are stimulated with a therapist's thumb, finger and hands. Reflexologists maintain that the pressure points follow the body's energy meridians and correlate with different internal organs and muscle groups. Oil and lotion are typically not used in reflexology.

Sports massage: Sports massage has risen in popularity as recreational athleticism has grown in the United States. Sports massage focuses on muscle systems appropriate for particular sports, and can be used before, during, and after athletic events. The goal is to help the athlete reach peak performance by increasing circulation, reducing swelling, elongating muscles, reducing tension, reducing lactic acid accumulation, and preventing injuries.

Craniosacral therapy: Craniosacral is a gentle, subtle treatment technique that evaluates and corrects the craniosacral system. During a treatment, a therapist detects and corrects cerebral and spinal imbalances or impasses that could be causing physical dysfunction.

I'm not a healer and I'm not a doctor, he would say. I'm just a mechanic.

—Lauren Berry

Hot stone massage: Hot stone massage incorporates heated stones into the treatment; these stones are usually basalt, a black volcanic rock that absorbs and retains heat well. The heat facilitates a highly relaxing, stress-reducing experience for the client. The heat also assists the release of tight muscles. The stones can be used to work the muscles therapeutically, glided over the skin with a lubricant, or simply placed upon a client. The high iron content in the basalt rock helps to absorb and retain the heat, as do the microscopic air bubbles within the stones.

Neuromuscular therapy: This technique aims to balance the client's central nervous system with his/her musculoskeletal system through soft-tissue manipulation and sustained pressure applications. The therapist aims to alleviate underlying causes of chronic pain problems maintained by the central nervous system. Neuromuscular therapy can be used to eliminate trigger points, restore alignment, and relieve ischemia or nerve entrapment.

Myofascial release: Myofascial release aims to realign the body and clear up restriction in a client's fascia, the strong connective tissue that surrounds the muscle and provides structural support throughout the body. The therapist begins myofascial release treatments with a visual analysis of a client's upright body, whereby physical imbalances, such as thoracic rotations and pelvic torsions, can be observed.

Pre/post-natal massage: This technique aims to support women during their pregnancies, as well as during and after labor. It can help to alleviate discomfort, as well as reduce stress and physiological imbalances. Benefits extend to both mother and baby. Pre/post-natal massage is performed by therapists specially trained to understand the unique needs of women during the different stages of pre/post-partum; they also understand the relevant risks, contraindications, and associated specialized techniques.

STRIKING A BALANCE

There's no secret to balance. You just have to feel the waves.

—Frank Herbert, author

One mistake that many people make when embarking on a new career is that they fail to look at that career in the context of the rest of their lives. Although it will be important to devote much of your time and energy to finding a job and/or developing your practice, especially in the beginning, keep

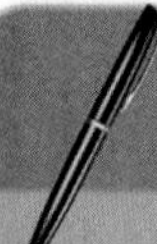

PUT IT IN WRITING

The Wheel of Life

Look at the spokes in Figure 1-3 ■. Each one represents an aspect of your life that is important to you. Choose eight of the most significant areas in your life, and fill them out on the wheel below. Some common examples are: Health, Personal Relationships, Education, Finances, Family, Spirituality, Work, Travel, Volunteer Work, Play, Home Life, Creativity, Personal Growth, Adventure, Community Involvement, and so on. Put down anything that is important to you.

Every individual will have different spokes on his or her wheel. Once you've decided upon yours, take a moment to reflect on each spoke and how developed it is in your life. If 0 is the center, and 10 is the spoke's end, evaluate each area of your life along that scale and draw a line that represents your level of satisfaction. For example, you may feel frustrated in your personal relationships or stalled in your creativity, and assign these areas a 3 out of 10. Once you've assessed each area, connect your dots on the diagram. What is the shape of your life's wheel? What will a ride be like upon your wheel as it looks today? Would the shape of your wheel be easy to throw off course? Don't worry if you aren't a perfect 10 on all (or any) of your life's spokes. This exercise is only to provide a graphic for your life, and help you see where you'd like to improve the wheel for a smoother ride.

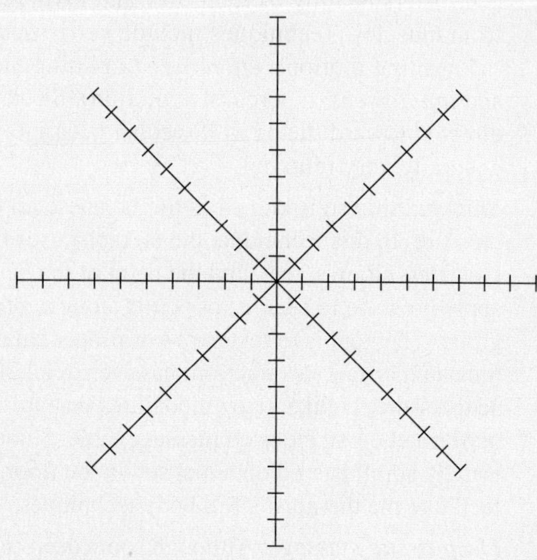

FIGURE 1-3

Finding Balance on the Wheel of Life.

in mind that there are multiple other aspects of your life that will need to be nourished. Attending to these other areas will not only help you to be a better therapist, it will help you to be a happier person. An exercise that coaches often use when working with jobseekers and new business owners is the Wheel of Life exercise. This will help you assess your current state of equilibrium between the different areas of your life.

GETTING ORGANIZED

Once you've finished your Wheel of Life and reflected on your state of balance, put the exercise in your *Business of Massage Therapy* notebook. As you advance in your career, you can come back to it and see how far you've come. You can also re-do this exercise occasionally, and see how your wheel evolves over time.

Balance is the ability to evenly distribute one's energy to the things he or she values, while maintaining physical, emotional, and mental equanimity.

WORKING FOR THE MAN (OR WOMAN) AND WORKING FOR YOURSELF

As a massage therapist, there are so many options for how to fashion your career. The first part of this book is devoted to professional development and the second part toward entrepreneurship and self-employment. Many massage therapists will be both employees and business owners at different points in their careers, and both are fabulous options. But not every massage therapist is meant to be a business owner, and not every therapist will thrive as an employee. Although the subject of entrepreneurship will be discussed in depth in the second part of the book, it is helpful to examine both paths in any conversation about career strategies for the massage therapist. In Chapter 2, you will learn more about the distinction between employees, independent contractors, and people who rent space in an established business, but for now, just think in terms of working with others and working on your own.

As you will see in the next chapter, an employee is someone who is hired to perform a job for an individual or a company, and carries out activities and services for them. As an employee therapist, your boss or company typically assigns your schedule, provides all needed equipment, schedules your clients, and attends to the business side of operations like marketing, administration, and financial management. As an employee, you can work in a number of different settings, from doctors' offices to cruise ships, from corporate offices to farmers' markets. In many situations, the type of massage you perform will be dictated by an employer, and you may be required to wear a uniform.

Many massage therapists dream of having their own practice or of becoming small business owners. They envision freedom, control, and the ability to create their vision independently, free from the expectations and constraints of others. Massage is an excellent way to be self-employed. It is a creative, portable, and meaningful career path that inspires many new entrepreneurs. An **entrepreneur** is one who creates a new business venture and assumes the financial, personal, and professional risks involved. The word entrepreneur derives from the French words *entre* (to enter) and *prendre* (to take)[19], and applies to anyone who acts upon opportunities to create something new in the business market.

One of the most important characteristics for any entrepreneur is passion. **Passion** is the compelling excitement for, belief in, and devotion to one's chosen focus. As a massage therapist, you are selling both the benefits of massage and yourself as a practitioner. Sincere enthusiasm is the best prescription for transmitting a message and making a sale. Anyone can learn business skills, but without the passion behind it, success is hard to find. This genuine zeal for massage is what will keep you going through lean times (which just about all business owners face at one time or another) and will help you overcome innumerable challenges. Passion is hard to fake and people will know immediately if you are not genuine. Authentic enthusiasm and passion will be reflected in every aspect of your practice, from your voice mail message to your one-on-one massage sessions. It will manifest in your phone calls with clients, your networking activities, and your marketing materials. If you submerge yourself into what you are doing and offer your very best from that passion, success will likely follow.

Another key for starting a small business is **determination.** Determination keeps you committed to your goal or desired outcome regardless of any circumstances, be they external challenges or internal difficulties. It is hard work owning your own business, and a massage practice is no exception. Are you willing to consistently devote the time and energy to making your business a success? Any entrepreneur will tell you that self-employment often means working nights and weekends and putting the needs of the business above your personal life. If you want to succeed in the increasingly competitive world of massage, you must have a willingness to work hard. Not everyone is comfortable or adept at working without oversight. How well do you work without supervision? Are you good at setting deadlines and, more importantly, meeting those deadlines?

A very important element of business ownership is the ability to promote. **Promotion** is the spreading of information about products and services for a specific company or brand. Elements of promotion include word of mouth, advertising, public relations, and publicity. It is one of the primary ingredients of a strong marketing mix, a concept you will learn much more about in Chapters 11 and 12. One of the most important promotional tools in an entrepreneur's toolbox is the elevator pitch. An **elevator pitch** is a brief overview of a product or service. It's how you would sell your massage practice to someone in a limited span of time—the time it takes to ride an elevator for example. Elevator pitches are invaluable anytime you are at a party, a networking event, a book club—essentially any time you come into contact with potential clients. Successful business owners find that promotion and marketing are a never-ending endeavor. However, elevator pitches are not only for business owners; in an era of job-hopping and competitive job markets, employees can benefit from having a solid pitch of their own skills and offerings. You will explore more about elevator pitches as a great career and business building tool later in the book.

There is no exact science that dictates who will be a successful business owner and who will not be. It is also important to remember that many of the most successful businesspeople have traveled roads paved with "failures" before they reached their destination of success. As John Dewey wrote, "Failure is instructive. The person who really thinks learns quite as much from his failures as from his successes." Felicia Brown of Spalutions said, "If you never fail, you probably weren't trying very hard."[20]

It can be said, however, that successful business owners often share similar characteristics. They are self-starters and are not discouraged easily. They are willing to do whatever it takes to see their dreams come true. Are you? The following "Put It in Writing" exercise is a self-employment checklist, with scores ranging from 0 for "never or rarely" to 5 for "always." Be honest and easy with yourself as you go through the list and look at your internal inventory. And keep in mind that giving yourself a low score on some of the questions does not rule you out as an entrepreneur. Time management, goal setting, organization, and many other entrepreneurial skills can be learned, and will be explored in depth in later chapters.

If you scored low on some or many of the questions, or if your answers to the questions surprised you, do not panic. Remember, there is no right way to be a massage therapist. Contrary to popular belief, the entrepreneurial

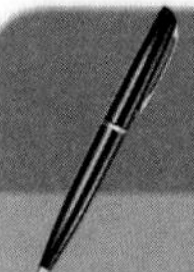

PUT IT IN WRITING

Entrepreneurial Essentials

Answer the following questions. For all answers, 0 = Never, 1 = Almost Never , 2 = Occasionally , 3 = Frequently , 4 = Almost Always, 5 = Always

1. Am I a go-getter?

   0 1 2 3 4 5

2. Am I good at time management?

   0 1 2 3 4 5

3. Am I well organized?

   0 1 2 3 4 5

4. When I set goals for myself, how often do I achieve them?

   0 1 2 3 4 5

5. It may take awhile to generate income from my massage business—am I prepared to live on less while I'm getting started?

   0 1 2 3 4 5

6. Am I good at networking and building professional relationships?

   0 1 2 3 4 5

7. How well do I handle rejection—do I recover quickly after setbacks?

   0 1 2 3 4 5

8. Do people respond positively to me? Do I have an outgoing personality?

   0 1 2 3 4 5

Now add up your scores:

32–40: Wowsa! You're busting at the seams to start a new business.

24–31: You're a bona fide entrepreneur!

16–23: Definitely a budding impresario. Keep polishing those skills!

8–15: Although you have some promise, you have a few areas to strengthen.

0–7: You've got a bit of work ahead of you to mold yourself toward creating a successful business.

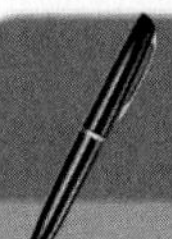

PUT IT IN WRITING

Employment Versus Entrepreneurship

Now is your chance to write out your thoughts about employment versus entrepreneurship. Let your imagine run wild with the responses to the following questions. Write your answers in the spaces provided below, or in your *The Business of Massage Therapy* notebook.

- What time commitment can I give to a new business? What potential obstacles might I face committing that time? In what ways would it be better to go work for someone else?

  ____

  ____

  ____

- What will being an employee mean for my personal or family life? How would owning my own business affect those areas?

  ____

  ____

  ____

- If I were to give a 30-second promotional "elevator pitch" about my work as an employee, what would I say? How about my pitch for my own business?

  ____

  ____

  ____

- What value will I be adding to my clients and my community when working for someone else? What value will I contribute as a business owner? How important is that to me?

  ____

  ____

  ____

- Where can I find support to get started in my own business? Is there more support for being an employee?

  ____

  ____

  ____

- What concerns or misgivings do I have about running a business? What concerns do I have about working for someone else?

  ____

  ____

  ____

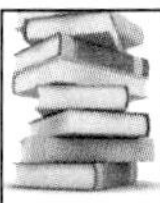

HELPFUL RESOURCES

There are a number of great resources out there to help you assess your personality and career options. Myers Briggs is a very popular personality test that helps you determine your psychological type, as well as how to better interact with other types. The official website is www.myersbrigs.org. *Callings: Finding and Following an Authentic Life* by Gregg Levoy (1998, Three Rivers Press) is a wonderful read for anyone beginning a new career, as is *What Color is Your Parachute* by Richard N. Bolles (2008, Ten Speed Press). Also, grab a copy of *How to Make One Hell of a Profit and Still Get in to Heaven* by John DeMartini (2004, Hay House Press).

spirit can be engendered with enough enthusiasm and the right business tools, and even the most independent and innovative spirit can be an incredibly successful employee. Marsha Sinetar coined the popular phrase, "Do what you love and the money will follow" in her seminal book of the same title.[21] Though there is absolute resonation and truth embedded in that sentiment, it is important to alter it slightly: do what you love *strategically* and the success will follow. Dovetail your limitless love into sound business practices and professional development, and the possibilities are endless. Passion, a positive attitude, a sense of adventure, and determination are the keys. It is no mystery that the rewards of any career are greatest when you are engaged in what you do. Presumably, if you have read this far, you have the zeal for massage and the earnest desire to learn the business, whether as an employee or an entrepreneur. The rest of this book will give you the integrated tools to go forth successfully.

COLLECTING A PAYCHECK VERSUS STRIKING OUT ON YOUR OWN: WEIGHING THE PROS AND CONS

As with most things in life, choices about employment and entrepreneurship all come with pros and cons. Of course, benefits and drawbacks are relative terms depending on an individual's goals, personality, and personal strengths.

There are many benefits and challenges to being an employee. Working for other people can require patience and flexibility, but it can also provide a lot of freedom in the rest of your life. Employees are not responsible for the day-to-day operations of a business, such as paying taxes, doing marketing, paying bills, scheduling clients, keeping business records, and so forth. Many find that they love the ability to show up, do the work they love (massage), and collect a paycheck without being responsible for anything else.

Because employees typically have far less assumption of risk than business owners, they often make significantly less money. While many people prefer to be an employee because they feel it will provide a more stable paycheck than entrepreneurship, this is not always the case in massage, where employees are often paid only when clients come through the door. Employees often have less control over the work environment, and less flexibility in schedules. Employees are also limited in their ability to promote and market their services. Being an employee is a great option for many therapists, but it is not the right choice for everyone (see Figure 1-4 ■).

While self-employment and entrepreneurship also offer wonderful benefits, it is not always an easy path to take. It involves hard work, assumption of risks, a courageous spirit, perseverance, and stamina. Self-employment is not necessarily the right direction for everyone. Though everyone's experience will differ due to skill, drive, market forces, and (let's face it) luck, there are universal pros and cons of being on your own (see Figure 1-5 ■).

FIRST STEPS

Look at these lists and see if there are things you would like to add to both columns. What are the stories you have about heard about self-employment? What are the stories you have told yourself? Are there hidden challenges you may not have considered before? If you have a friend or family member with self-employment experience, ask them what the peaks and pitfalls have been for him or her. Think of pros and cons for both sides that are not listed, and write them here.

EMPLOYEE

Pros	Cons
____________	____________
____________	____________
____________	____________
____________	____________
____________	____________
____________	____________

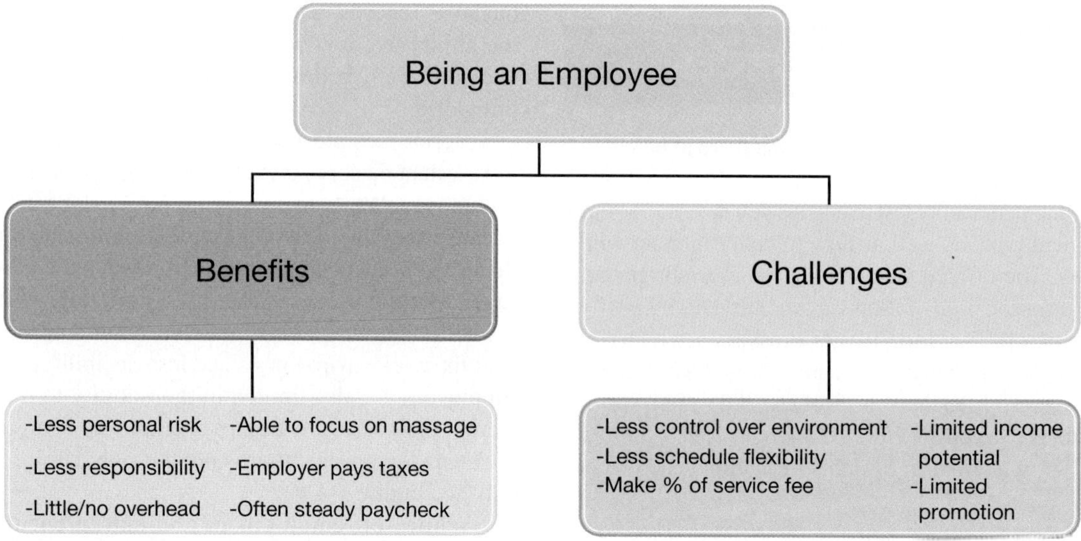

FIGURE 1-4

Some Common Pros and Cons of Working for Others.

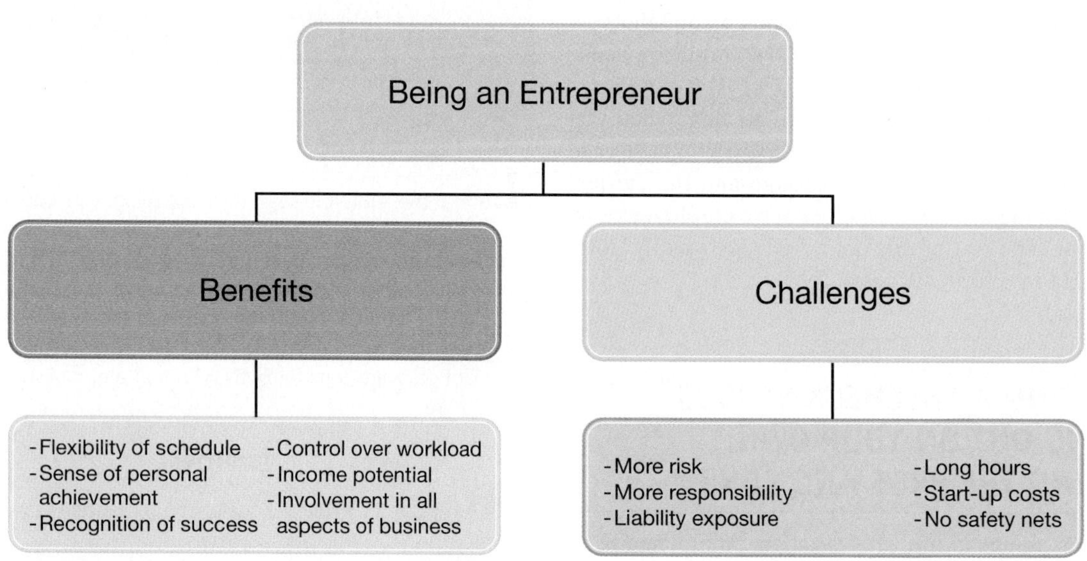

FIGURE 1-5

Some Common Pros and Cons of Working for Yourself.

CHAPTER SUMMARY BY LEARNING OBJECTIVES

1. **Explore the massage therapy career** Massage therapy has experienced massive growth and offers a multitude of career possibilities. However, with that growth has come an increase in competition. Business skills for the massage therapist are now more important that ever.
2. **Define helping professions and identify characteristics of a helping professional** Although there is no one "type" of helping professional, there are some characteristics that many helping professionals share. Helping professionals are comfortable with the physical body, both their own and those of others. They are comfortable touching and being touched, and have good professional boundaries. They are empathic without internalizing the challenges of their clients.
3. **Examine the importance of balance** Balance is the ability to evenly distribute a person's energy to the things he or she values, while maintaining physical, emotional, and mental equanimity. Balance is a very important concept for helping professionals.
4. **Evaluate a massage career in the context of one's life** Any successful therapist must consider the full context of the life into which they are incorporating massage. One must look at balance in all areas of life, and understand areas that might need improvement.
5. **Explore aspects of a massage therapy employee and aspects of an entrepreneur** Many massage therapists will be both employees and business owners at different points in their career, and both are fabulous options. But not every massage therapist is meant to be a business owner, and not every therapist will thrive as an employee. Successful employees are typically flexible and reliable. Successful business owners typically have passion, determination, and good promotion skills.
6. **Contrast the benefits and drawbacks of employment and business ownership** As with most things in life, choices about employment and entrepreneurship all come with pros and cons. An employee typically has lower expenses, less risk exposure, and less responsibility for business operations. Income can be more consistent as an employee, although this is not always guaranteed for massage therapists. Employees often have less control over schedules and work environment. There are pros and cons involved with working for oneself. Benefits include control over schedules and work conditions, self-fulfillment, and profit potential. Drawbacks include income uncertainty, long hours, initial instability, stress, and personal risk.
7. **Define an elevator pitch and its importance to your business and your career** An elevator pitch is a brief overview of a product or service. It's how you would sell your massage practice if to someone in a limited span of time—the time it takes to ride in an elevator for example.

ACTIVITIES

Discussion Questions

1. As discussed, massage has experienced a boom in popularity and acceptance over the last twenty years. Why do you think that is?
2. Massage schools reported an influx of new students during the first few years of the twenty-first century. What were some world events that might have contributed to the surge? How might those events impact the massage industry? What events occurring today do you think might have an impact on the profession?
3. Industry reports indicate high turnover rates among massage therapists, and that many therapists leave the career after only a few years. Why do you think this is? What do you think are some of the difficulties therapists face that leads to this? Can you think of some ways to avoid those difficulties?
4. Some massage therapists consider themselves to be healers, while others resist this term altogether. Do you think this is an appropriate word to describe a massage therapist? Why or why not?
5. Some characteristics of a helping professional were included in the text. Can you think of additional ones? What or whom do you think of when you hear that word?
6. Entrepreneurs were also defined. What do *you* think it takes to be a successful business owner? Do you know someone who has been a successful entrepreneur? What did he or she do that you would like to emulate?

Beyond the Classroom

1. Do some online research to learn more about the massage industry. General industry trends will be explored further in later chapters, but see what you can find out about massage in your area.
2. Find a massage therapist who has been practicing for five or more years. Ask him if you could do an informational interview with him. Offer to meet at his office, or take him out for coffee or lunch. Find out the things he has learned during his practice, and lessons he might be willing to impart to someone just starting out. What has lead to his success? Review the lists of characteristics for both helping professionals and entrepreneurs. How many of these do you think he exhibits?
3. Get a copy of a business publication, and compile a list of entrepreneurs, both current and past. What has been their path to success? Did they stumble before they got there? Do you see characteristics of yourself reflected in their stories?

Case Study

Elena

Elena had always wanted to be a massage therapist, and when she was laid off from her corporate job, she jumped at the chance to make her dream a reality. After researching schools throughout her state, she finally settled upon one that seemed to embody many of the holistic healing beliefs she already had. The school also had a great reputation and was well established in her community, and was even less expensive than some of the less reputable programs. Once in school, Elena worked hard to do well academically after being out of school for so many years; she quickly excelled and thoroughly enjoyed her massage school experience.

Elena was praised by her teachers for her natural touch and her quick adoption of the various techniques she was studying. While she excelled in class, she was slow to attract new clients. She noticed that a few of her classmates with considerably less skill were already marketing themselves and quickly building clienteles. She was turned off by the way they endorsed themselves, and felt uncomfortable promoting herself in the same way. She had faith that she was called to do massage, and that her amazing natural skill would be sufficient in developing a clientele and sustaining her practice.

Upon graduation, Elena had only a few clients, and most of them were family or friends. She could not help but feel envious that some of her friends from class had nearly full appointment calendars and were poised for self-employment due to the marketing they'd done during school. Unable to support herself with only a few clients, Elena got a job doing massage at a local spa. She promised herself it would be temporary as her practice grew through word of mouth.

Time went on, and though she did excellent bodywork, word of mouth referrals were not as plentiful as Elena had hoped. Worse still, she saw advertisements for other therapists nearly everywhere she went and the competition overwhelmed her. Though she was grateful for her job at the spa, her income was limited and the friends that she made kept leaving and being replaced by new therapists. When the spa manager announced that they had to cut commissions in order to keep operating, Elena realized that she would have to get yet another job to cover her expenses. With only so much energy, she saw fewer and fewer of her own clients, and began to feel quite burned out. Discouraged, Elena made the very difficult decision to leave her career in massage therapy after only one year in practice and returned to a corporate job similar to the one she had had before massage school.

Case Study Questions

1. What happened? Elena had so much passion for a career in massage therapy, and clearly demonstrated natural skill. Why do you think she did not succeed?
2. When other classmates worked on self-marketing and the promotion of their services, Elena viewed them as being shameless and arrogant. What do you think about that? What are your views towards self-promotion? How do you regard people who promote themselves with relative ease?
3. What did you think when the spa cut the therapists' commission to keep the doors open? How likely do you think such a situation is?
4. How typical do you think Elena's situation is?
5. If you were Elena, what would you have done differently?

CHAPTER 2

Career Strategies and Professional Development

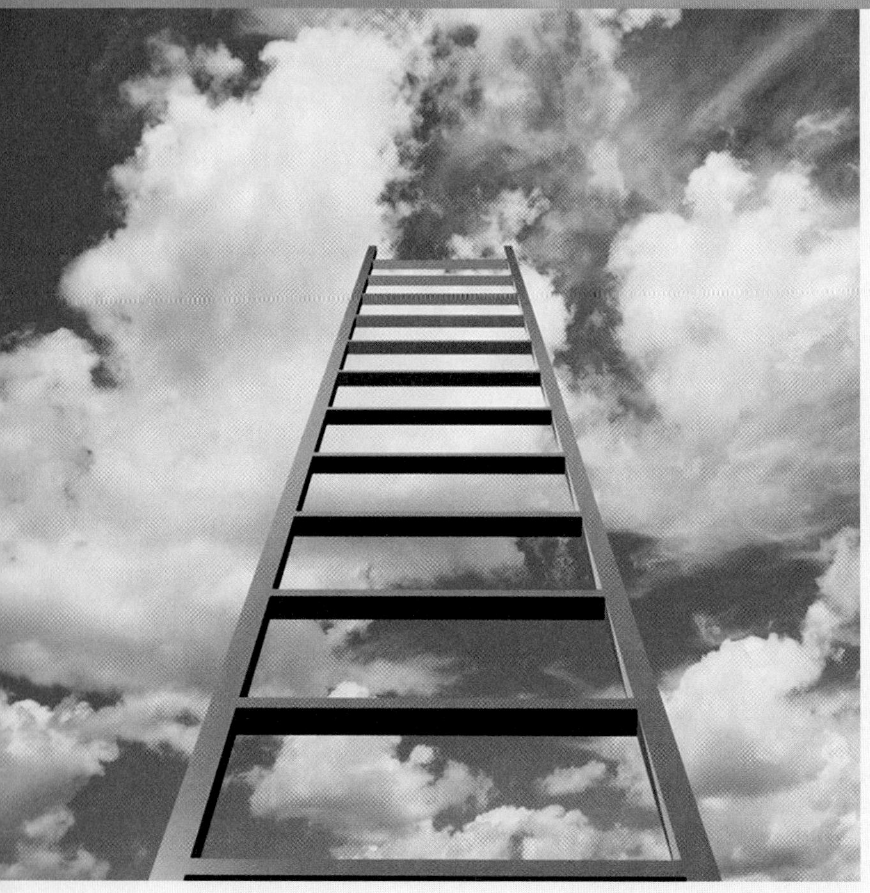

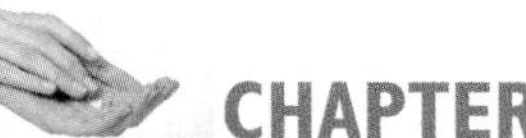

CHAPTER OUTLINE

LEARNING OBJECTIVES

1. Identify and explore options for massage careers
2. Describe employment venues
3. Contrast status of employee, independent contractor, and room renter
4. Identify ways to find jobs
5. Create a captivating cover letter and winning résumé
6. Explore interviewing and communications skills
7. Relate the concept of culture and the importance of "fit"
8. Evaluate the fine points of negotiation and examine your rights and obligations as an employee
9. Illustrate why marketing still matters as an employee
10. Explain the importance of continuing education and professional development

KEY TERMS

Choose a job you love, and you will never have to work a day in your life.

—Confucius

PLAYING THE FIELD: EXPLORE ALL YOUR OPTIONS

Later in this book you will explore all the aspects of running a massage career as an entrepreneur. But do not think for a moment that this is the only path, the best path, the most virtuous path, or anything other than what it is—just another path. As the ancient Chinese proverb observes, there are many paths to the top of the mountain. You may have no interest in your own practice, or you may find that you will work for others at many different stages of your career. Few career trajectories ever represent a straight line. It is important to understand the massage industry from all angles—as a technician, a business owner, an employee, a consumer, a critic, and a devotee. Only 65 percent of massage therapists are self-employed, leaving a vast population of therapists who need to focus on career development rather than business management.[1]

This section of the book will explore the many different avenues of a massage career, as well as help you formulate and develop a professional repertoire that will propel you forward. And remember—even if you never decide to have your own practice, learning the principles of entrepreneurship and understanding what goes in to running a business will make you a much better (and more valuable) employee.

THE MASSAGE WORLD IS YOUR OYSTER: EMPLOYMENT VENUES

The world of massage offers the individual so many directions from which to choose. Because healing takes so many forms, there are as many different career paths in massage as there are massage therapists. As you learned in Chapter 1, the massage profession is enjoying healthy growth; the U.S. Department of Labor projects that the industry will have grown 20 percent by 2016.[2] This is due to many factors, such as the increasing adoption of massage therapy by mainstream healthcare practitioners, referrals from these practitioners, and the overarching cultural acceptance of massage as a contributing factor to good health. In addition, the aging of the baby boomer generation has created a large population that has age-related massage needs and disposable income. The American Massage Therapy Association (AMTA) reports that 47 million Americans received a massage between 2007 and 2008.[3] With so much demand and so many different options, the massage world really can be your oyster. Surely you have already begun to consider different career paths in massage. Perhaps you already have an idea of where you would like to go with your career or a precise picture of what you want it to look like. Before you explore some of the opportunities before you, take a moment to examine the ideas you already have with the following "Put it in Writing" exercise.

Perhaps this exercise was not as easy as you would have liked because you don't feel you are aware of all the choices out there. Take a few moments to consider a few massage career snapshots, and see if you envision yourself pursuing one or more of these opportunities. Keep in mind that the following list is merely an overview, and that there are no

PUT IT IN WRITING

Multiple Routes

There are many different avenues for practicing massage. Take a moment to consider the following questions and write out some of the things that interest you. Pay attention to the things that you know you *don't* want to do, too.

I think it would be really fun to do massage in places like ______________________.

I am interested in a massage path where I can travel to ______________________.

It would be very meaningful for me to do massage in places like ______________________.

Some of my friends and mentors have found rewarding careers doing massage ______________________.

I think I would make a very good living doing massage ______________________.

A few career options I am definitely not interested in include ______________________.

When I think of my ideal career path, the thing that excites me most is ______________________.

When I think of my ideal career path, the thing that scares me most is ______________________.

hard-and-fast rules for what you will find in any given environment. Such is the diverse nature of the business.

Chiropractor's Office: Chiropractors often hire massage therapists to loosen and condition soft tissue before or after doing skeletal adjustments. Massage therapists offer sessions of varying length, and the focus is typically on rehabilitation and/or complementing the chiropractic treatment. Although this is not true in all states, some chiropractors often handle the insurance billing for massage on their clients, and pay therapists an hourly wage or a commission of services. Many chiropractors rent out office space to independent contractors rather than employ therapists directly. Some therapists greatly enjoy being a part of the mutual therapy program, while others have reported feeling rushed through sessions to get a large number of clients through to see the doctor.

Health Club: Clients in health clubs often seek massage modalities that support athleticism, such as sports massage, joint range of motion, and Muscle Activation Technique. Because health clubs tend to have high concentrations of health-minded individuals, therapists report building loyal clientele quickly. Others have complained of the noisy locker-room ambience or utility-based approach in health clubs. Some clubs hire therapists as employees, paying a commission on services, while other therapists rent space from the clubs for their private business.

Spas/Resorts: A recent report showed that 32 million visits were made to U.S. spas in 2007, and of those 32 million, nearly 70 percent came for a massage.[4] Clients typically come to spas and resorts to relax and be pampered; even if they get an intense therapeutic massage, they typically expect to do so in a luxurious setting. Spa therapists in the United States have reported being paid anywhere from $8 per hour to 90 percent of services (as much as $100 plus tip).[5] Typically spas provide all the materials you will need and provide all your clients. Many therapists enjoy the soothing atmosphere typical of spas, while others dislike the emphasis on pampering.

Hotel: Working for a hotel usually involves working in its spa, although many small boutique hotels that do not have the space for spas will contract with companies or individuals to do in-room massage for their guests. This will typically require you to carry your table and materials from room to room. Commission percentages vary, but tips for in-room massage can be quite good.

Where your talents and the needs of the world cross, there lies your vocation.

—Aristotle

On Site/Chair Massage: Due to the portability of a massage chair and the fact that clients need not disrobe, chair massage can be done almost anywhere—parks, offices, grocery stores, teachers' lounges, foyers, lunchrooms, patios, parties. Sessions usually last only 10 to 20 minutes and clients do not undress. Chair massage businesses will typically supply the materials, space for sessions, and clients to the therapists they hire. And self-employed massage therapists often create entire or partial private practices out of doing on-site chair massage. Usually the businesses pay to provide this service to employees, although occasionally clients will pay the therapist directly. Many therapists enjoy the change of scenery, the abbreviated sessions, and the volume of people they are able to treat, while others find all the travel and equipment set-up less attractive.

Hospital/Doctor's Office: Nearly 70 percent of hospitals hire massage therapists to manage pain and reduce stress for their inpatient and outpatient client services, as well as to help hospital employees through preventative medicine.[6] Here therapists often work with clients who are chronically ill, recovering from surgery or trauma, or have age-related conditions that are improved with massage. Hospitals typically pay by the hour, or bring therapists in as independent contractors (this often helps them minimize their liability costs). Employee benefits are often a big draw for this option (see Figure 2-1 ■).

Corporate Offices: With the growing emphasis on employee health, many companies are now hiring massage therapists as part of their wellness repertoire. Although corporations usually bring therapists in to do

Potential Opportunities for Massage
Wellness Centers
Cruise Ships
Chiropractor Offices
Spas
Health Clubs
Hospices/ Elder Care
Birthing Centers
Hospital/ Doctors' Offices
On-site/ Chair
Hotels & Resorts

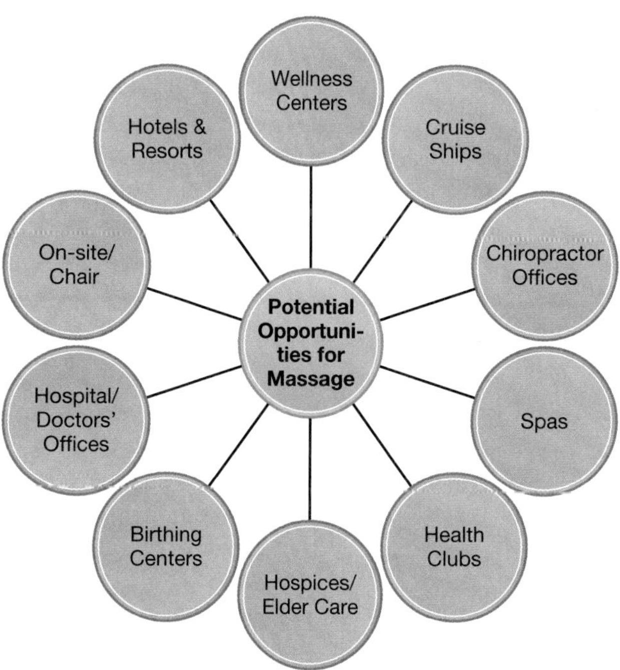

FIGURE 2-1

Some of the potential work opportunities for massage therapists.

chair massage for their employees, many businesses have rooms permanently designated for table massage and full-time therapists on staff.

Hospice: For the terminally ill and those in their last stages of life, massage is an invaluable therapy that provides pain minimization and comfort, while providing real meaning and connection to clients. Therapists working in elder care and hospice settings need to be particularly attuned and sensitive to the rapidly changing and fragile conditions of their clients; usually they need to go through hospice-specific training before working with clients.[7] Although it can be emotionally challenging to work with clients in the end-of-life stage, many therapists have found this to be an incredibly rewarding and meaningful path.

Elder Care/Retirement Community: Although still a geriatric-centric environment, elder care and retirement communities have different massage applications than hospice work. While many geriatric patients require special considerations due to susceptibility to injury and illnesses that are typically not applicable to other client populations, residents are often very healthy and active. More and more elder care facilities and retirement communities are recognizing the benefits of massage for their residents and are beginning to retain a massage therapist on staff. As with hospice care, the emotional rewards of geriatric massage can be enormous.

Wellness Centers: Many massage therapists find that working in physical proximity to other wellness practitioners can be very rewarding, collaborative, and successful. A wellness center is a facility that features different holistic modalities, such as nutrition, fitness, life coaching, prenatal care, yoga, acupuncture, hydrotherapy, massage, counseling, and any other application that supports clients' optimal health and wellness.

Sporting Events: Some companies specialize in massage for sporting events, working to prepare athletes for optimal performance and recovery after intense exertion. Sports therapists often travel to events such as marathons, triathlons, bike races, even the Olympics. Those lucky enough to secure contracts with professional sports teams may end up flushing lactic acid from the muscles of a celebrity athlete. However, the work can be very demanding physically, and may require a good deal of travel.

Cruise Ship: Those with a sense of adventure and good sea legs might consider a job on a cruise ship. You get to travel the globe, meet people from around the world, and typically get your room and board covered in the deal. However, reviews from cruise line therapists differ significantly, and reports of grueling long (11–12 hours) days, cramped quarters, working more than sightseeing, and substandard pay are very common.[8]

Airports: A wonderful new trend in travel has seen massage services cropping up in airports, where stressed travelers can benefit from seated and table massage between flights. The environment may be a bit more hustle-bustle than other settings, but many therapists enjoy minimizing the physical tolls of travel while providing an oasis amidst the stress and strain of traveling.

Because the massage industry is always evolving, there are no set standards for compensation for any of the above outlets for massage. Some employers compensate their therapists as much as 90 percent plus tips and benefits, while others pay their therapists less than 20 percent of the money charged to clients and offer no benefits. Generally speaking, it is not standard to tip for massage administered in medical settings, such as hospitals and hospice care, while tipping in day spas and cruise ships is typically expected.

As you consider different employment options, it is important to understand a few elements of pay and earnings. Typically your compensation directly connects with how much effort, resources, and work you are required to put forth. Employers who provide all of the clients, do all of the marketing, book all appointments, provide all massage materials, wash all the sheets, and handle all of the other logistics

PUT IT IN WRITING

Setting the Scene

The career options list above is not exhaustive, and surely you can think of other settings for a massage career. You can probably think of a great deal more pros and cons for each situation than was listed above as well. Brainstorm some other ideas and write them down here, using personal experience and your imagination to fill in the gaps. Pay particular attention to the environments and settings that seem to be a good match for you.

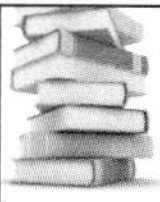

HELPFUL RESOURCES

A great way to get more information on massage job opportunities is to check with niche-specific trade associations. Organizations such as the Hospital-Based Massage Network, Sports Massage Association, On Site Massage Association, American Medical Massage Association, and many others offer members job boards and links to helpful resources. Do some online research to see what support is out there for you.

tend to pay their therapists less than employers who require you to bring or build your own clientele, provide your own table, manage your own schedule, and so on. As a general rule in business, the less risk and responsibility you assume, the less you typically are paid.

As more and more massage therapists have come into the market, and more and more corporate massage companies and spas have emerged, many therapists report that their compensation has trended down. As an employee, finding companies that provide generous commissions and benefits has become more difficult. However, don't be discouraged—there are still great paying gigs out there for massage employees, and tips can often compensate for lower pay scales. Figure out what works for you and your financial needs.

INDEPENDENT CONTRACTOR OR EMPLOYEE: WHAT AM I?

Much of the first part of this book looks at professional development from an employee's point of view. The outcome of most interviews is to be offered employment with a company, but do not automatically assume that working with a company

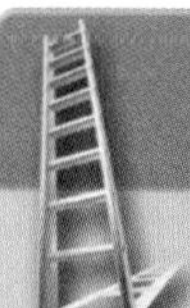

FIRST STEPS

One of the best ways to learn which environment works best for you is to actually put yourself in different ones. Talk with therapists working in different venues, and find out what they do and don't like about different settings. Call around to massage sites of interest, and tell them that you are a massage student who is currently exploring different career paths in the industry. Many employers are happy to do informational interviews with students wanting to know what it's like to work with them. (Informational interviews are discussed later in the chapter.) Some places may even offer you an internship—or a job!

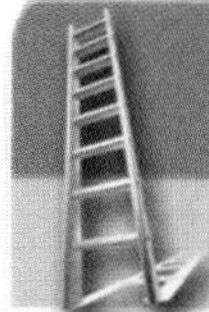

FIRST STEPS

If you ever find yourself in a situation that you fear violates labor laws, you have several options. The first, and most proactive, is to confront your boss directly (and respectfully). Although ignorance is never a defense against the law, many people simply are not versed in the labor classifications. They might even appreciate you bringing it to their attention, as it will help them to run their business better. If you feel you are not being heard, you may consider relocating, or seeking advice from a labor specialist (an attorney or a government agent).

ensures you employee status. Different business relationships exist between companies and holistic practioners, and you will need to be clear on your status category and the different classifications of work within a new organization. Just because you were offered a place in the company does not necessarily mean you are technically employed by the company, and many businesses will go through the interview process for independent contractors and room renters just as with employees. The distinctions of different business relationships are made and roles clarified by the Internal Revenue Service and the U.S. Department of Labor (2000 Publication 3518, Catalog 73164X). It is not only important to be clear on your status to be sure you are operating under the boundaries of the laws, but to make sure that any company you work with is treating you fairly and legally. A 2002 report showed that nearly 90 percent of businesses in the beauty and wellness professions were operating their employee relationships under the wrong classifications; this can be a problem for both the individual and the company.[9] Check out the Internal Revenue Service's Twenty Factors test in Appendix B, or visit the IRS and U.S. Department of Labor websites at www.irs.gov and www.dol.gov to learn more and to ensure you are properly classified in your workplace.[10]

As you may already know by now, an **employee** is someone who performs activities and services for an organization that controls what, when, and how those activities and services will be done.[11] As an employee therapist, the company assigns your schedule, provides all needed equipment, schedules your clients, and attends to the business side of operations like marketing, administration, and financial management. The employer is also responsible for deducting taxes from your salary and tips, and must provide you with a W-2 form for your taxes at the end of the year.[12] As an employee, you are covered by workers compensation and state unemployment. You may be paid an hourly wage, salary, or a commission on your services, depending upon your employee agreement. An **employee agreement** is a document that serves as a contract between a company and an employee that outlines rights and obligations of each party. There are sample agreements for employees and independent contractors in Appendix B (see Figure 2-2■).[13]

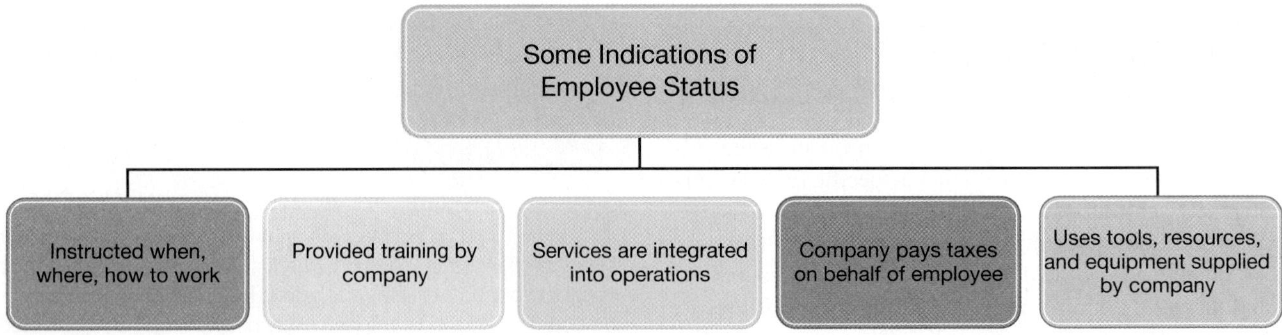

FIGURE 2-2
Indicators of employee status.

There are many upsides to working as an employee, including less responsibility and risk. Often the employer handles everything but the actual massage, freeing you to focus solely on the technical aspect of the work you so love to do. You also have no expenses associated with running a business, as the space, materials, and marketing are all handled for you by the employer. Some companies offer their employees benefits such as health insurance, retirement investment accounts, continuing education allowance, and vacation time. In companies that offer benefits, there is often a minimum requirement of hours to be met before an employee can receive them. Such benefits can add a lot of value to you and your family, and save you a lot of time and money in managing your own benefits.

One of the drawbacks of working as an employee is that you are more limited on the amount of money that you can make. Employers have been known to retain up to 90 percent of the money that clients pay for services; this goes to pay overhead costs, marketing expenses, and administrative salaries in the company. As an employee, you also have less control over your schedule and less influence over the environment in which you work. Dress codes, service standards, behaviors, and activities are all under the control of the employer.

PITFALLS

Managers of a Different Feather

As you enter the world of a working massage therapist, you may find yourself in a situation where you are being managed by someone who is not a massage therapist. This situation has been the source of frustration for some employee therapists, who find that management does not grasp the demands and unique aspects of the profession. If you find yourself with a nontherapist manager, you may be able to help sidestep aggravations or misunderstandings by having open communication about issues such as your need for breaks between clients, the importance of stocked supplies, and so forth.

When people go to work, they shouldn't have to leave their hearts at home.

—Betty Bender

Of course, not everyone working within a company is an employee. A **room renter** is a business owner who leases space within an existing company and operates his or her business out of that space. While technically an independent contractor, room renters are unique in that they build the bulk of their own business within the parameters of someone else's. Similar to booth renters in the salon world, where hairstylists and nail technicians rent actual booths or stalls, the term is often used to describe massage therapists that pay a flat rate for use of a massage room within an established business. Some chair massage therapists operate out of a booth or stall.

Room renters are responsible for booking clients, setting their own service fees, and managing all the aspects of their small business. A room renter must pay his or her own taxes and insurance. Renting space from an existing company can be very advantageous, as you can benefit from their established brand and clientele. Many companies will still go through the interview process with a room renter, although it may not be as formal an interview as for an employee. Even though room renters pay to work in a space, good company managers will still want to ensure that renters fit into their culture and are a good match for their operations (more information on company culture can be found later in this chapter and in Chapter 14). If you do elect to do booth rental in a salon, spa, wellness center, or other business, and you are selling and making commission on retail products, you are part of the supply chain of

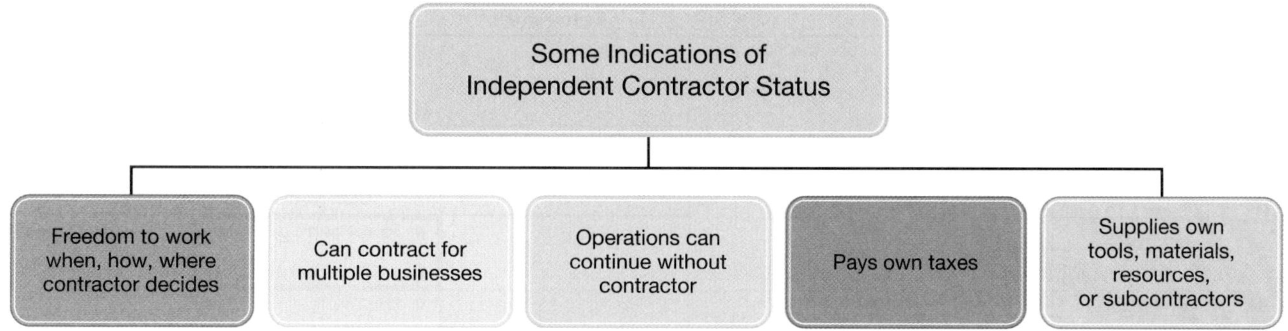

FIGURE 2-3

Indicators of employee independent contractor status.

those products and have the same liability as the company does.[14] You will learn more about supply chains and product liability in the second part of this book, but for now just be aware that renting space and running a business out of another business still carries exposure to risk.

Many massage therapists are brought in as independent contractors under the auspices of established companies. **Independent contractors** are individuals who provide services or perform activities for a company, but, like room renters, are not employees of that company (Figure 2-3■).

The IRS makes the distinction that a company only has "the right to control or direct *the result* of the work and not the means and methods of accomplishing the result" of an independent contractor.[15] In other words, a company cannot dictate the schedule, dress code, or even execution of services from an independent contractor. Independent contractors are self-employed, and thus are responsible for their own taxes, insurance, and business expenses. They often contract with more than one company at a time, or as a supplement to their own established business.[16]

Similar to a room renter, independent contractors are independent of the company or business owner. But unlike a room renter, contractors typically represent the company that hires them when providing services—they are not building their own business. In other words, an independent contractor that is hired to provide massages for a business understands that the clients "belong" to the business, and is not building his or her own private practice. Independent contractors often work with more than one business in more than one location at a time. **Form 1099** is a form from the IRS that an independent contractor receives at the end of the year from any business that has paid him or her in excess of $600 for services performed.[17] A room renter, on the other hand, may have to provide the business with a 1099 form for rents that have been paid in excess of $600[18] (see Figure 2-4■).

Independent contractors operate in the continuum between employer (of their own business) and employee (of someone else's business); while technically self-employed, they represent the interests, culture, and brand of the businesses for which they contract. Because of this, it is quite likely that you, too, will have to go through some sort of interview process to become an independent contractor with a business.

Whether you enter into a relationship with a business as an employee, room renter, or independent contractor, you are highly encouraged to create a contract (if one is not provided). This will help to clarify roles, expectations, and determine what each party is legally responsible for in the relationship. Although there are many form contracts that you can access or purchase, be certain to have a lawyer peruse anything you use, as the wording of the contract will be what safeguards and protects you in the event of a dispute or legal action.

Although much of the remainder of Part I of *The Business of Massage Therapy* will be looking through the viewfinder of the employee, it is important to be aware of the different distinctions for work relationships. Not only will this give you choices, it will help to clarify your rights and obligations in any work situation. Many therapists find that they may exist in several different work relationships at once, such as supplementing their own business by working for someone else a few days a week. As mentioned earlier, cultural fit between a therapist and a company is essential regardless of technical employee status. After all, you will be working in the same environment day after day, and every individual in the mix can affect the company's brand and its impact on clients, guests, and consumers. As such, much of the following information on professional development will be relevant and useful whichever path you take in this career or any other.

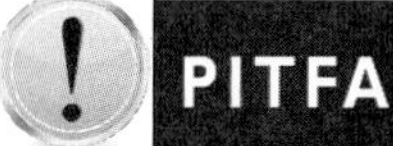

PITFALLS

Tax information is always subject to change, and you should always keep yourself abreast of any changes. Speak with a tax attorney, a tax specialist, or check the IRS website (www.irs.gov) to learn what forms and information you are responsible for as an employee or an independent contractor.

☐ CORRECTED (if checked)

PAYER'S name, street address, city, state, ZIP code, and telephone no.		1 Rents $	OMB No. 1545-0115 **2010** Form **1099-MISC**	**Miscellaneous Income**
		2 Royalties $		
		3 Other income $	**4 Federal income tax withheld** $	**Copy B** **For Recipient**
PAYER'S federal identification number	RECIPIENT'S identification number	5 Fishing boat proceeds $	6 Medical and health care payments $	
RECIPIENT'S name		7 Nonemployee compensation $	8 Substitute payments in lieu of dividends or interest $	This is important tax information and is being furnished to the Internal Revenue Service. If you are required to file a return, a negligence penalty or other sanction may be imposed on you if this income is taxable and the IRS determines that it has not been reported.
Street address (including apt. no.)		9 Payer made direct sales of $5,000 or more of consumer products to a buyer (recipient) for resale ▶ ☐	10 Crop insurance proceeds $	
City, state, and ZIP code		11	12	
Account number (see instructions)		13 Excess golden parachute payments $	14 Gross proceeds paid to an attorney $	
15a Section 409A deferrals $	**15b** Section 409A income $	16 State tax withheld $ $	17 State/Payer's state no.	18 State income $ $

Form **1099-MISC** (keep for your records) Department of the Treasury - Internal Revenue Service

FIGURE 2-4

Sample 1099 form.

Source: Internal Revenue Service, www.irs.gov.

HOW TO SCOUT OUT JOBS

Okay, now you have a handle on some of the great venues where massage careers can flourish. You have a good idea of the options of different working relationships between yourself and potential companies. So now what? With so many wonderful career options out there, how do you find the right massage job for you? There is no magic formula for landing a dream job in massage, or for any industry; however, traditional methods of employment hunting often lead to success in massage careers as well. Just as with many situations in life, one of the best ways to find a position is through the people that you know. Tap into your networks to see what opportunities exist in your local community. Talk to the people in your circles and tell them what you are looking for after graduation from massage school. You never know who might know someone who knows someone who ... you get the idea.

One of the best things to do as a student is to leverage your status as a student. Many massage schools offer job placement assistance for students and recent graduates, and if yours does, be sure to take advantage. School job boards and career placement centers can help connect you to vacancies in the setting you desire. Other students can be great resources too, as they may be able to help get you a job where they themselves are working or provide you with useful tips that they used in their own job search. Some massage schools even host career fairs. If yours does, attend as many as you can, talk to people, and gather business cards from representatives of any organizations that pique your interest. It is always a good idea to follow up with recruiters or representatives from companies that you are interested in. Send them an email or phone them to set up a time for an informational interview.

In an **informational interview,** one is seeking advice and gathering information rather than just employment. Here, a student or job seeker is gathering useful knowledge about a particular company or career while building a professional network. In an informational interview, you are the one who is asking most (or all) of the questions. This allows you to ask a potential employer all about their business or the industry. You can ask what she or he loves about the company, what challenges the industry is currently facing, where the growth opportunities lie, or any other question that is dancing through your mind. Remember, leverage that student status—it's your prerogative to be inquisitive, and people are much more lenient with students than they are with professionals. There is nothing wrong with taking notes during an interview (this is true whether the interview is professional or informational). Taking notes helps you to remember key points of the discussion and to organize your follow-up communications. However—although less formal than an employment interview, you should always treat informational interviews professionally. Dress as you would for a regular interview, be courteous and respectful, and be sensitive to the fact that the person is volunteering his or her time for your benefit. It is always a good idea to collect the business card of your interviewee, as you can then send them a follow-up thank-you card or letter.

A **thank-you card** is generally a handwritten or typed note that expresses your gratitude, highlights your interest in the company, and helps to solidify a professional relationship. Some professionals prefer the more formal thank-you letter, which is more elaborative and almost always typed. If you meet with someone and have interest in working for that person or that company in the future, indicate that in your note or letter. *Always* send follow-up thank-you cards to anyone who grants you any kind of interview: not only does it set you apart among your peers, it helps to build your professional brand (more on this topic in Chapter 6, "Networking").

There are other channels to help you find your dream jobs as well. As with other industries, more and more employers and job seekers alike are turning to the Internet to find one another. Traditional job sites such as Monster, CareerBuilder, and Craigslist often connect job candidates to great opportunities in their area. Specialty sites such as Massage Jobs.com, Spa-jobs.com, or Find Touch feature job listings for massage therapy exclusively, and can often connect you to possibilities all over the world.

Yet another way to uncover opportunities in massage therapy is to *create them yourself.* Many enterprising therapists have eked out jobs in surprising or nontraditional settings where jobs may not have existed before. By getting creative and thinking outside of the box, therapists have found jobs traveling with professional athletes, going to disaster sites with Red Cross volunteers, as part of permanent support staff for large corporations, as exclusive on-call therapists to wealthy individuals, even as in-flight therapists on some airlines or charter jets. As the massage therapy industry continues to grow, so will the possibilities.

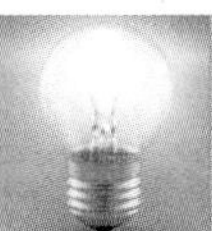

BRIGHT IDEAS

Elevator Pitch for Interviews

In Chapter 1 you heard about elevator pitches, concise synopses of who you are and what you have to offer. You're going to learn the ins and outs of these pitches and how they help business owners in Chapter 12, "More Marketing for Massage." However, elevator pitches can help you whether you are an employee, contractor, or business owner; in fact, they can be invaluable during an interview. Whether you are doing an informational interview or a formal job interview, crafting and polishing a great elevator pitch can help you catapult your career.

RÉSUMÉS REVEALED

In the hunt for the perfect massage therapy job, there should always be a few essential items in your tool kit that will help you succeed. Two of these are cover letters and résumés, your quintessential marketing package. A **cover letter** is the letter of introduction and intent that typically accompanies a résumé. Cover letters provide an overview of the information in your résumé, and compel the employer to take the time to read the rest of your information. A **résumé** is a document that demonstrates your abilities and provides a synopsis of your professional and academic credentials, as well as any relevant accomplishments and skills you may have. A cover letter complements (but does not parrot) your résumé, and is targeted to the individual and company that you are approaching. Many recruiters and employers report that they will not read a résumé if the cover letter that precedes it is not engaging or does not demonstrate a compelling reason of why you are a great candidate for the job.[19] See Appendix B for sample résumés and cover letters.

Going job hunting without a cover letter and résumé is a bit like going fishing without bait and tackle. You could sit there a very long time and never catch a thing. Cover letters and résumés are often the first point of contact between an employer and a job seeker, and are often used as a way to screen potential candidates. Even if you are introduced to an employer directly or granted an interview without a preliminary résumé submission, it is typically expected that you will still provide a cover letter and résumé as supporting documents in the consideration process. Some massage businesses may not ever ask for these, but it is always a good idea to have them ready in case they do.

Many job seeking massage therapists don't devote the necessary time to crafting a winning résumé, and this can be a big mistake. Because cover letters and résumés are often the

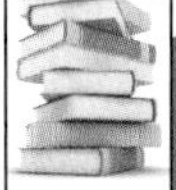

HELPFUL RESOURCES

As more and more massage companies are going corporate and public, you can often learn more about companies and career opportunities than ever before. Through business and career websites and resources such as Wetfeet, Riley Guide, Dunn & Bradstreet, and Hoover's, you can uncover information on company sizes, corporate leadership, average salaries, company culture, financial data, and much more. Some of these sites charge a fee for the information, but it can be worth it to make informed decisions on your career path.

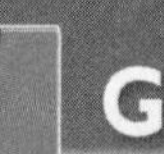

GETTING ORGANIZED

Making the Pitch

Elevator pitches are a great job search tool, and once you have one crafted it's a good idea to save it and to always have on hand for future reference. Remember, elevator pitches help inform potential employers and clients about who you are, what you have to offer, and why they should work with you above anyone else. And a good pitch will also help *you* clarify the work that you really want to do in the world (see Figure 2-5 ■).

To help you get started writing your pitch, answer the following questions.

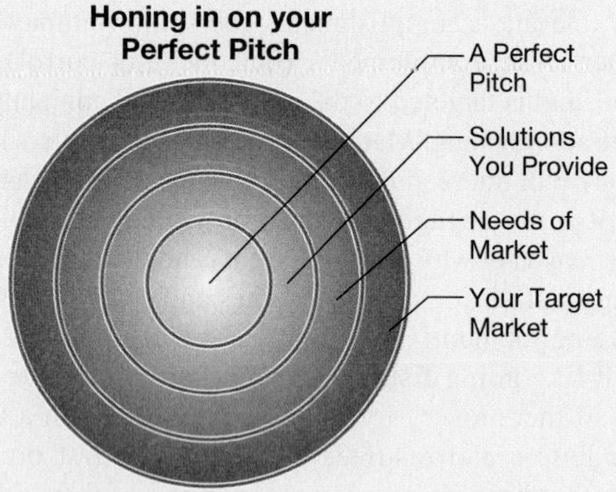

FIGURE 2-5

Crafting the perfect pitch.

1. What is the focus of my search? What do I want to do in my job/career?

____
____
____

2. Who do I most want to work with? Who will benefit the most from what I have to offer?

____

3. What are the needs of that target group? What problems do they need solved?

____
____
____

4. What am I offering that will solve that/those problems, and how will I do that?

____
____
____

5. What differentiates me from my colleagues or job competitors? Why would someone want to employ or work with me over others?

____
____
____

Now, take the answers to the questions above and create a concise 30–60 second pitch about who you are, what you offer, the need your services fill, and anything else that will demonstrate why people should work with you. Play with this pitch in front of a mirror or with a friend, and when you have something you feel good about, write it down here:

My Pitch:

____
____
____
____
____
____
____
____

Keep this and reference it any time before you go to an informational interview, a formal interview, a networking event, or a chance when you will have an opportunity to share the amazing value you and your skills offer the world. (If you feel you would still like more help with using elevator pitches in your career, take a look at Chapter 12.)

first contact you have with a potential employer, they can make or break your chances for getting a job. While you want to be true to yourself, résumés and cover letters are not the place to tap into your creative side—keep your focus on a professional presentation. While electronic résumé submissions are becoming more and more popular, if you are going to submit a hard copy of your résumé, it is recommended that you use heavier résumé paper and a high-quality printer. Small errors in appearance, grammar, spelling, or even formatting could cost you the interview. This is always true, but especially when different job market conditions make competition fierce. A **slack labor market** occurs when there are more job seekers than jobs available, and competition between job hunters can be very fierce. Slack labor markets can be good for employers, as they have very talented pools to choose from. With its massive layoffs and mounting unemployment, the recent international economic crisis is a prime example of a slack labor market. A **tight labor market** occurs when there are more jobs than there are job seekers, resulting in competition between employers to recruit and retain quality talent. Here, job seekers are in a better position, as they have many job opportunities from which to choose.[20]

PUT IT IN WRITING

Through Thick and Thin

If you have been in the working world for a few years, chances are good you have experiences in both slack and tight labor markets. Even if you haven't, you should know someone who has. Think about those experiences as you answer the following questions.

1. When you have applied for jobs in the past, was it easy or difficult for you to find a job?

   ____

2. How much do you think the external job market had to do with your challenges or success? How much responsibility do you think you had in the situations?

   ____
   ____
   ____

3. When you think about the job market now (or the one waiting for you when you get out of school), does it seem tight or slack? Why do you think this?

   ____
   ____
   ____

4. How do you think the current market will affect your job search?

   ____
   ____
   ____

5. Brainstorm a few things that you think will help you find a job, regardless of current market conditions. To get you started, these could be things like your excellent training, your winning personality, or your geographic area.

   ____
   ____
   ____
   ____

Regardless of external job market conditions, you will always want your résumé to pop and sizzle and to get the attention of potential employers. So how do you make your résumé stand out and set you apart from other job seekers? Résumés can have very different styles and functions, depending on the position you are applying for and what you want to emphasize about yourself.

Traditionally, there are four essential résumé styles: chronological, functional (skill-based), combination, or targeted[21] (Figure 2-6■). A **chronological résumé** begins by listing your work experience in sequential order, starting with your current or most recent position and working backward in time. This is a good résumé choice if you have a strong professional background in the field for which you are applying. Chronological résumés help employers get a feeling for your work history, as well as patterns of longevity with various jobs.

A **functional résumé** provides a summary of your skills rather than your specific work history and time line; this style of résumé is typically useful with individuals who are just beginning their careers, are changing professions, or have long periods out of the workforce. As the name indicates, a **combination résumé** merges the attributes of a functional résumé with a chronological résumé, typically listing skills first and professional time lines second. Combination résumés allow the job seeker to emphasize the skills that he or she feels are most relevant to the job, while still highlighting work history that employers may want to see.

Many people will use a general functional, chronological, or combination résumé for all of the jobs that they apply for, making little or no changes to the general résumé sent out. This is particularly true if they are applying for only one

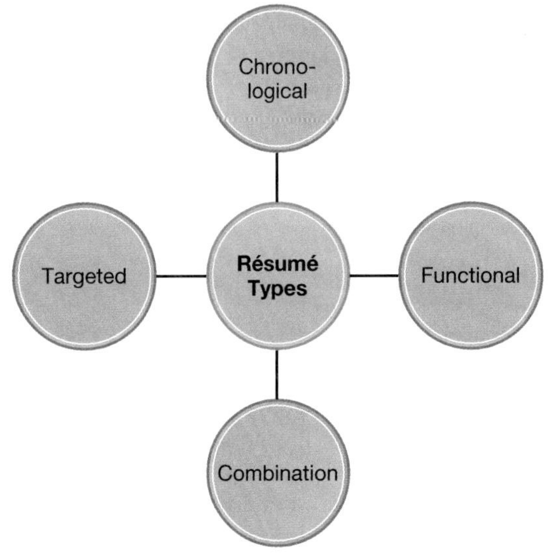

FIGURE 2-6

The most common types of résumés.

type of job where required skills and abilities are similar. For example, if you are only applying for massage jobs with chiropractors, you will probably not have to tailor your résumé much. However, some people who are applying for different types of jobs may find they will occasionally need to create a targeted résumé. **Targeted résumés** are customized for specific jobs, highlighting different strengths and skills than those emphasized in other résumés. For example, if you have sent out 10 résumés to hospitals in the area, but decide to also apply for a job at a day spa, you might send the day spa a targeted résumé that highlights your customer service experience or training with elite clientele.[22] Sample résumés and cover letters can be found in Appendix B.

So you've crafted a fantastic résumé and want to get it out there to potential employers. However, before you start distributing your résumé like candy, there are a few things you will want to do first. What was the first thing *you* did when you began considering places to work and building your list of possible employers? Chances are you hit a search engine such as Google or Yahoo and did a little research. With the increasing reliance on online information sources, chances are very high that potential employers will be running searches on you, too. Estimates vary, but the majority of employers and recruiters report that they run Google searches on job applicants as a way to do a little background and character checking.[23]

Although they may not know it, many people have been passed over for interviews because of information found on the Internet relating to them. **Digital dirt** is any information available about you online that could be viewed unfavorably by employers or other Web users. This could be related to pictures posted of you, blog postings, or even associations you are involved with. Even if the Facebook photos of your best friend's twenty-first birthday party in Vegas seem harmless enough to you, they have the potential to derail your possibilities if those photos turn off a potential employer. Remember, as an employee, you are an extension of that company's brand, and if what is presented about you online does not match what they want their image to be, they may assume that you don't match either. If you haven't already done so, it might be time to engage in a little "**narcisurfing,**" the act of searching for yourself on various search engines to see what you can find out about yourself and what your personal brand is saying about you.[24] (You'll learn more about your personal brand and the Internet in Chapters 6 and 15—"Networking" and "Leveraging the Internet").

So how is one to sweep away the digital dirt that is floating about the ether in order to get that job? Surely you shouldn't be penalized forever because you had a good time. There are several things that you can do to clean up your online image.[25] The first is to implement any available controls and security features, which most of the social networking sites now have. You can also remove your name from risqué or wild pictures that others have posted, or simply ask friends or family to take them down. If you are on sites that allow others to comment, you can block this feature or manually remove comments that could be detrimental.

But you don't have to deconstruct what's already out there; you can also build replacement information that presents a more professional picture of you, and let it work for you in mass circulation. Adding new content will bump older data down the line in search results and even on to other results pages, where few people are likely to look. If you haven't already done so, join social networks that are more geared to professional networking, such as LinkedIn, Xing, or the Latino Professional Network. You can also generate professional articles on your niche modality for sites such as EzineArticles.com, or create a blog on massage and wellness that you can update frequently. By proactively constructing the image you want to convey while tidying up any digital dirt, you will boost your chances of impressing employers, getting the interview, and landing that job!

! PITFALLS

Recruiters report that one of the quickest ways to get your résumé discarded is through typos, spelling, grammar, or punctuation errors. Even the most seasoned professionals can make mistakes, and word processors are not foolproof. Edit your résumé carefully. Repeat. Repeat again. Just when you think you're finished repeating, ask a friend to lend you a fresh set of eyes so that your résumé is as polished as it can be. All that repetition is worth it.

> *It takes twenty years to build a reputation and five minutes to ruin it. If you think about that, you'll do things differently.*
>
> —Warren Buffett

THE INTERVIEW: YOUR TIME TO SHINE

So you have created a zinger of a résumé, crafted a fabulous virtual identity, and wowed a potential employer so much that they have contacted you for an interview. An **interview** is a formal meeting that is designed to gauge the qualifications, skills, and fit of a potential employee by an employer, and vice versa. The goal of an interview is to take your two-dimensional résumé and cover letter to the next level, where you can expand on all of your great characteristics and skills, as well as the intrinsic value you will bring to any work situation.

Interviews can be conducted either in person or over the phone. For positions where employers or recruiters are screening a lot of applicants, preliminary phone interviews are common, as they help to weed out less suitable candidates from consideration. If you are asked to do a phone interview, treat it as you would a regular interview. Take the call in a private space with no interruptions or background noise. Dress as you would for a face-to-face interview. While some might think this is overkill, many career specialists advise that dressing nicely helps you to feel more confident and, in turn, project a professional image through the phone.

As with so many things in life, preparation is a key ingredient in successful interviewing. It is entirely normal to be nervous before an interview, but the more you research and prepare, the more confident you will feel in the interview. Of course you will want to know as much about the company and the position for which you are interviewing as possible. Nothing irks recruiters and employers more than people who show up for interviews knowing nothing about the company.[26] A company's website will help you to uncover clues about the organization's culture, learn about current initiatives and past successes, and give you a lot of background information you can discuss in the interview. It will also help you to formulate sophisticated questions for your interviewer that reflect that you've done your homework, and aren't just asking obvious questions that can be addressed by a cursory glance at the website.

You will want to be as fluent as possible in the industry language; if you are just coming out of school and have never worked in a professional massage environment, you will want to familiarize yourself with niche-specific lingo. For example, if you are interviewing to be a therapist in a hospital, you will want to be familiar with some medical terminology and be conversant in pathologies and contraindications. If you are looking to work in a spa setting, you might want to get familiar with the function of a vichy shower and a spirulina wrap.

FIRST STEPS

To-Do before the Interview

As you prepare for your interview, considering taking the following actions.

______ If they have one, research the company's website. This will give you many clues and conversation points for the interview.
______ If possible, speak with a current or past employee of the company. He or she may be able to give you some tips on personalities and culture.
______ Anticipate and practice responses to common interview questions. Use a mirror or get a friend to help you out.
______ Be prepared to ask questions. Doing so shows that you are interested and serious about gauging a mutual fit between yourself and the company.
______ Make a dry run to the interview location so you have a good idea of directions, traffic, drive time, and parking.
______ Get a good night's sleep the night before the interview.
______ Dress professionally and conservatively (minimal jewelry and fragrance).

As you go in for the interview, bear in mind the reality that you are always communicating on many different levels, and the bulk of that communication is nonverbal. **Nonverbal communication** is the sending and receiving of messages without any words exchanged. It can include gestures, posture, facial expressions, eye contact, and many other silent clues about what is occurring within another individual (Figure 2-7■). Studies have shown that at least 55 percent of human communication is nonverbal, giving nearly as much power to what isn't said as to what is said.[27] Your physical presentation (your clothes, hair, jewelry, style) will be immediately evident to an interviewer, and they will be "listening with their eyes" to your nonverbal communication throughout the interview.

When a potential employer sits down to interview a potential candidate, there are a few elemental questions that the employer wants answered. It's important to anticipate these questions, as well as to understand the motivation behind the questions.[28] First of all, employers will want to know if you are able to do the job. Have your education, experience, skills, and innate talents prepared you to do the work they will need you to do? Remember, even if you are making a career transition into massage therapy, there are likely skills that you bring from your last job or academic experience that transfer into this career, such as sales, teamwork, customer service, and case management.

Second, employers will want to know if they can afford you. Because there is a wide range of salary potential in the massage career, and industry standards vary significantly, employers will want to know that what they are offering will work for you. Make sure you do your research on what other therapists are making for similar jobs in the area. You can do this by asking others directly or by looking at sites such as Salary.com or PayScale, which give snapshots of salaries in your geographic area. Salary strategies and negotiations will be discussed later in this chapter.

Another important question that employers want answered is whether you will fit with the company. Will you be a good

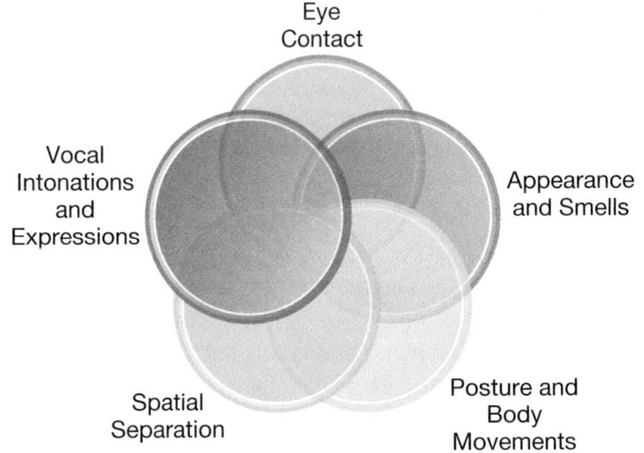

FIGURE 2-7

The ways we convey information without saying a word.

match for the rest of the team with whom you will be working? Will you be happy in their environment? Employers often invest a lot of resources into new employees through training, education, and development, and if they hire you they want you to stick around.

Behavior-based interviewing is a technique grounded in the idea that how you have acted in previous situations will indicate how you are likely to act in future ones. Behavior-based interviewing invites the interviewee to recount stories from past experiences that convey skills, knowledge, behaviors, and solutions.[29] Ideally your responses will reveal your ability to perform job functions or will demonstrate ways that you might bring value to the organization. This interviewing technique has become very popular, and many employers use it to evaluate potential candidates for open jobs. Examples of behavior-based interviewing questions include inquiries that begin with "Tell me about a time when . . . "; "Give me an example of when . . . "; "Describe for me . . . "; or "Walk me through a time when . . . ". If you hear those openers, your interviewer is likely using behavior-based techniques. You would be wise to have a few stories at the ready that will illustrate your successful behavior in past situations. And don't worry if your work history is limited. These stories could come from academic experiences, volunteer work, leadership experiences, extracurricular activities, involvement in a religious community . . . really anything that demonstrates a transferable skill.

While many people excel at speaking at length about themselves, it can be a real skill to streamline your stories into a crisp and concise delivery that will compel and satisfy the interviewer. You don't want to wax poetic about a previous job, veer off on a lot of tangents, and leave the interviewer wondering if you ever answered the initial question that was asked. As you formulate some good example stories, it may help you to keep your thoughts succinct and easily understood (and useful) to the interviewer to remember the STAR technique. A great interviewing tool, the **STAR technique** is an acronym for **S**ituation, **T**ask, **A**ction, **R**esult; it helps convey all the relevant and valuable information about you that interviewers are seeking. Not only do you explain the circumstance as asked for in the behavior-based interview question (Situation), you also describe what goal or outcome you sought to achieve (Task), the steps you took to achieve it (Action), and the eventual outcome of your actions (Result). Use this formula to guide your storytelling, and see if it helps you deliver a winning response to interview questions.

Although there are "standard" interview questions that you will likely be asked, it won't be possible to anticipate and prepare for everything an interviewer will ask. Some interviewers like to think outside of the box, and are assessing your ability to do the same. One massage recruiter peppers her "common interview questions" with out-of-the-ordinary queries such as "If you had a camera and could only take three pictures, of what would they be?" and "If you were a crayon, what color would you be and which color would you ask to the prom?" Her intent is not to throw curve balls or to stump her interviewee, but to ease the tension and gauge creativity levels.

As the interview winds down to its natural conclusion, you'll want to take a few steps to ensure your advantage in the interview process. Summarize the key points of why you think you would be a good match for the company, and ask if there are any other questions that you could answer to demonstrate or clarify that you are a great addition to the team. If the interviewer doesn't ask you to provide a sample of your massage techniques or unique touch, offer to do so. Ask when the employer hopes to make a decision, inquire about the next steps, and see if it is all right for you to follow up in a week or two. Finally, make eye contact, smile, offer your hand, and thank the interviewer sincerely for his or her time.

As helpful as it is to be prepared by anticipating questions, be mindful of your body language, and master all the other interviewing skills, don't become overly rigid with techniques or feel you have to memorize a performance. Allow the process to flow, and remember the intrinsic value that you are bringing to the table. Look at interviews as well-prepared opportunities to shine. The company would be lucky to have you, and if this one isn't a right fit, remember the abundance of other opportunities awaiting you in the massage industry.

You did it! You made it through the interview, and you did a great job. But you aren't done just yet. As you saw earlier, it is always very important to follow-up after an interview. **Follow-up** is the proactive post-interview behavior that keeps you active in the candidate selection process through assertive and professional communication. Follow-up can give you the competitive edge in the job seeking process and make you stand out from other interviewers who believe the

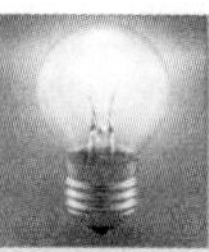

BRIGHT IDEAS

Many holistic practioners find interviews challenging because they aren't comfortable speaking candidly about their strengths, value, and accomplishments. Many therapists also struggle to highlight their individual achievements, and so focus on collective triumphs or successes. Although it's admirable to think of others and to regard efforts collectively, it is important to let yourself shine in an interview. If you really struggle to sell your greatness, you can get around this by citing or demonstrating feedback, praise, or accolades from others. Some examples are "my student clinic supervisor always said I was the most intuitive and hard-working in clinic," "my boss always regarded me as the go-to person for marketing solutions," or "as you can see on my feedback forms, I have received top ranking and consistent praise on customer service by all my clients." This might feel more comfortable than saying "I'm the absolute queen at hard work, marketing, and customer service." Besides, having supporting acclaim from another party can lend credibility to your assessment.

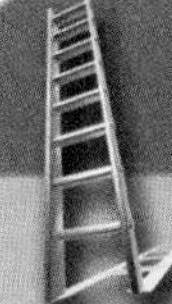

FIRST STEPS

The STAR Technique

The following is an example of a response to a common interview question using the STAR technique. After you read the sample, write out your own STAR response to one of the questions provided below.

Interviewer: Tell me about a time you had a difficult experience with a customer or client.

Interviewee: (Situation): Although I have typically had very positive experiences in customer service, there was a time when I was working as a flight attendant during a pilot strike. Flights were being cancelled and delayed, and passengers were all very upset. Some were downright hostile, and I had to deal with everyone's frustration.

(Task): My goal was to ease as much client frustration as I could. Because I believe that most people really just want to be truly heard, I made it my goal to really listen to grievances without being personally drawn in, and to do whatever I could within my power to make it better.

(Action): I know that communication is crucial to solving any challenge. While many of the other airline personnel avoided passengers, I developed a system with the other flight attendants and ground crew to provide cell phones to clients trying to reach family (at a time when not everyone had one). I also communicated with ground crew to help connect passengers to alternative transportation options, such as trains, buses, rental cars, and ride shares with other passengers.

(Result): Because my colleagues and I worked hard to be compassionate and helpful, and really listened to clients' needs, we were able to help get people where they needed to go even if we couldn't affect the flight schedules. Within a few weeks, I received a number of letters of thanks from clients who made it to a daughter's play, a job interview, or wherever they were heading. Not only did that win loyalty to my airline, it made me feel wonderful!

Now you give it a try. Choose one of the following common interview questions, and answer using the STAR technique:

- Tell me about a time you had a conflict with a coworker that was resolved successfully.
- Describe for me a time when you had too many things to do and you had to prioritize your tasks.
- Tell me about a difficult decision you've had to make in the last year.
- Give me an example of when you showed initiative and took the lead on a project or work environment.

(**S**ituation): ______________________________

____

(**T**ask): ______________________________

____

(**A**ction): ______________________________

____

(**R**esult): ______________________________

____

process ends when the interview does. Many recruiters recommend sending a thank-you letter rather than a thank-you note, particularly after a professional interview. Like a note, a **thank-you letter** allows you to recap highlights from your interview, clarify any areas you felt might be of concern to your interviewer, and to address the ways you will resolve any challenges or problems the interviewer needs fixed. Remember the notes you took during the interview? Use those to outline your letter and fill it with key conversation points from your interview. As with your resume, be sure to edit your follow-up correspondence thoroughly before sending.

You will want to send your thank-you notes and letters immediately after the interview—either the same day or the next morning. You want the employer or recruiter to get your follow-up correspondence while you are still fresh in his or her mind. Some people elect to do their follow-up in e-mail form, which is increasingly acceptable as people collectively turn away from snail mail and move into digital communications. Still, there is something about the tangible letter, and a handwritten correspondence adds that personal touch that is hard to match in an e-mail. Regardless of the medium you choose, it is essential that you follow up with the interviewer to communicate your interest in the position and to reiterate what a great addition you will be to the team. Even if you aren't truly interested in the job, a follow-up thank-you is still a good idea in establishing your professional image and personal brand. You want to leave all bridges intact. After all, it is a small world and you never know who you will meet again further down your career path.

CULTURE AND THE RIGHT FIT

Job seekers often spend a great deal of time and energy convincing potential employers that they are the right person for the job without really considering whether the employer is really the right company for them. When you start seeking jobs, one very important thing to keep in mind is that you are looking for the right work environment just as much as potential employers are looking for the right employee. As you go through the interview process, you may get so preoccupied with trying to impress the company that you forget that you are evaluating it as well. But an interview process is always a mutual exploration. Although the main apparent goal is to sell yourself and

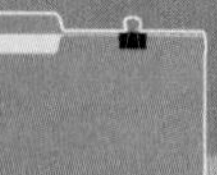

GETTING ORGANIZED

Preparing for Common Interview Questions

Although the format and content can differ somewhat, there are many common interview questions that interviewers ask. Familiarizing yourself with some of them will help you feel more confident and better prepared in your interview. Jot down a few answers to the questions below, and then come up with a few possible questions that are not on the list.

- Tell me about yourself.

  ____

  ____

- Why should we hire you?

  ____

  ____

- Why did you leave your last position?

  ____

  ____

- What are your strengths?

  ____

  ____

- What are your weaknesses?

  ____

  ____

What are some other questions that you might anticipate in the interview? Write them down here (if you get stuck, feel free to search online for common interview questions).

____

____

____

____

____

____

It is a great idea to flesh out some of your ideas for interview responses and file them away. It will help you review and brush up on your answers to common questions any time an interview comes up in the future.

get the interviewer to fall in love with you (professionally speaking of course), you are there to evaluate them as an employer. Because no matter how wonderful the company thinks you are, if you aren't going to be happy working there, it won't be a good situation for you or for the company.

As you are interviewing, keep company culture and your fit within it at the forefront of your evaluation. **Company culture** is the set of shared values, attitudes, and practices exhibited by an organization's employees, management, and owners. It is the unique personality and essence of an organization, the collective fingerprint of the company that sets it apart from any other. Just as within a neighborhood, community, or nation, company culture is a blend of many factors and is always in a dynamic state of transition. It can incorporate tangible aspects, such as décor and physical workspace, to the more intangible elements, such as interpersonal communications, company mission statements, and approach to collaboration and input.

Company culture can be a secret weapon in the arsenal of success, but if not managed properly or not cultivated intentionally, it can be a contributing factor to problems, setbacks, and even company failures. Although everyone in the company has a contribution to the overall culture, the tone is typically set by the owners and managers of a business. Successful management of company culture can be a cornerstone of human resource development and employee retention.[30]

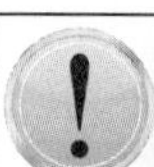

PITFALLS

Being Persistent versus Being a Pest

While it is important to be proactive when following up with an employer, there can be a fine line between being enthusiastic and being irritating. Recognize the boundaries and employ some patience. Regardless of the size of the company you are applying to, chances are that the person interviewing is a very busy one. It is all right to follow-up with a phone call a week to 10 days after your interview. But if you still aren't getting a response, it's okay to let go. Remember—rejection is protection, and there are plenty of other opportunities for someone with your talents and skills.

It used to be a business conundrum: Who comes first? The employees, customers, or shareholders? That's never been an issue to me. The employees come first. If they're happy, satisfied, dedicated, and energetic, they'll take real good care of the customers. When the customers are happy, they'll come back. And that makes shareholders happy.

—Herb Kelleher, former CEO, Southwest Airlines

Company culture is not dependent on size or number of employees: even if you have your own massage practice and are the only one in it, your business still has a company culture. Such a culture is usually tightly interwoven with your own personality and the experience you create for your clients. Later in the book you will learn techniques for helping to shape culture as an owner or manager. So why should you care about company culture as a job seeker? As an employee, company culture is something you will want to look at and consider closely in your job search, as it can have a serious impact on your professional experience. You will want to pay close attention to your comfort with the company culture and your fit within the organization.

Employee fit is the degree to which a person matches the position to be filled and the company culture in which he or she works. Employee fit is very important to employers, as they want to hire, train, and retain individuals who build their brand, boost their business, and benefit their bottom line. But fit is very important to you as well. Career experts agree that fit is an integral part of overall career success for any individual, as it affects performance, motivation, longevity, and income over time.[31] Ideally, you will want to work in a company whose culture is closely aligned with your own values. If you are someone who values interpersonal relationships, asking questions, and supportive environments, then you might feel more comfortable in an organization that stresses teamwork and a strong learning culture over an organization that is task oriented or number driven. Establishing a good fit between employee and employer is a win-win situation for everyone involved.

If you get a chance to do a formal or informational interview, there are many things you can do to assess fit. One of the most important things is to simply observe—how are employees interacting? How are customers or clients treated? How are *you* treated? How do you feel in the space? Simple observation can uncover a host of clues about a company's culture.

There are also many questions you can ask in an interview to determine company culture and gauge your fit within it.[32] You can expect that many of the questions interviewers will ask of you will be designed to determine the same information of you, as you learned earlier. Asking thoughtful, insightful questions about the company and its culture shows that you are interested in the position and the company, and concerned about more than just a paycheck. It can also show that you've done your homework. However, do not ask questions that are easily answered by the company's website, and do not dominate the interview time by grilling endlessly about what the company has to offer you.

EVERYTHING IS NEGOTIABLE

Because you have mastered the interview process, the job offers are pouring in. Before you say yes to any of them, take a moment to consider what they are offering you. Unless you were born to a wealthy family, happen to be an unparalleled investor, or are confident that the lottery jackpot is waiting for you and only you, your income is the one and only way to maximize your personal prosperity throughout your lifetime. Many professionals recognize this, and understand the important step of negotiating wages, salaries, and benefits before they accept a job. **Salary negotiation** is the process of discussing and arriving at a compensation package that is

PUT IT IN WRITING

Who's Interviewing Who?

It is important to remember that any interview is a two-way process—you are an invaluable asset to an employer and you should be evaluating the company just as much as it is evaluating you. The following is a list of some questions you might consider asking:

- What type of person is successful here?
- Are there any changes or improvements you would like to see made by the person who takes this position?
- Are there opportunities for further education and training within this company?
- What do you love about working here? What are some challenges for you?
- What is a typical work day like here?
- How is performance measured here?
- Apart from clients, who are some of the key people I would be working with?
- Can you tell me about the interactions of team members?
- In addition to massage, what other duties might I be required to perform?

What other questions can you think of that might help you gauge if a company is one you would like to work with? Write them down below.

____

____

____

____

____

mutually beneficial to you and your employer. Factors affecting a salary negotiation include experience and skills, geographic location, economic conditions, market competition, company guidelines, and industry standards.

Many massage therapists and holistic practitioners that go to work for someone else do not include salary negotiation in their career development. If they think of it at all, they mistakenly assume that salary negotiation is reserved for corporate suits and movie stars and has no role in their own holistic employment process and long-term career. But taking charge of financial well-being is important for any professional, regardless of industry (see Chapter 7 to learn more about personal finance). Even in a slack labor market and in a bad economy, don't assume you are without leverage in negotiating your compensation.

While it is true that there is less maneuverability in entry-level or highly competitive positions, everything, as they say, is negotiable in business. Nearly 80 percent of employees report negotiating salary, and 90 percent of human resources representatives say that salaries are negotiable.[33] The trick, say hiring and compensation experts, is to get a company to see your value and "fall in love with you" before you even think about discussing money.[34] A good company understands the value of its human capital and will want to invest in the right employees.

There are four basic tenets of salary negotiations: prepare, know your own needs, answer questions strategically, and look at the entire package. To prepare, you will want to do your research on what kind of money you can expect. Explore as much information as possible on industry standards, norms in your area, and the going rate for your skill set and market niche. What are industry standards? What are other companies paying massage therapists in your area? What is the salary range in this particular company? There are several ways you can find all of this information. The Bureau of Labor and Statistics offers salary data for massage therapists, as do professional trade associations such as AMTA and ABMP. Salary survey sites such as PayScale, Salary.com, and Vault can offer location-specific salary information based on what users have self-reported. Some of the detailed salary surveys can be costly, however, so you may want to weigh the merits of the information against the price tag.

You can also use online chat groups and listserves to inquire about salary standards for massage therapists or even for specific companies. Many massage therapists work for organizations that operate as nonprofits. If you are looking to work for a nonprofit organization, you can do a little sleuthing on the organization's financial information. By pulling up the company's 990 tax form (an annual return that all tax-exempt organizations are required to file with the IRS that is available to the public), you can get an idea of how much people are making within the company.[35] One of the best ways to find out company-specific earnings information is to go to your own network and ask people you know how much they are making at their own jobs.

You will also want to have a very solid handle on your own financial requirements. Sit down and analyze your own expenses and your financial goals, and the bare minimum you will need to make in order to take care of yourself. Some jobs may pay so poorly that you just should not take them, and it is okay to acknowledge that. Working hard for less money than you need will lead to burnout, resentment, and an unsustainable situation over time. You will save yourself and your employer time and money by recognizing that up front. During the interview process, you may be asked directly what your salary requirements are or what you made in your last job. You will want to answer all questions about compensation strategically. Do not give a specific number, but rather a ballpark spectrum. You will want to formulate a range that begins with your bare minimum and extends to your ideal. Engage common sense and ground your maximum number squarely in your research on industry norms—if an employer does not think they can afford you, you will take yourself out of consideration for the job. Providing a realistic range will allow you to look affordable enough to stay in the running while giving you some leeway to negotiate once the company sees how fantastic you are.

Finally, do not be strictly number-bound when negotiating your salary as a massage therapist. Look at all aspects of compensation that the company is offering you, such as health benefits, vacation time, wholesale prices on quality products, child care, discount on wellness services, and so forth. If an employer cannot afford to pay you an extra few dollars an hour, see if you can get an extra week of vacation time or an increased discount on products. When you add up all of the different perks, you may be making more than you originally thought.

However you ultimately do your research, preparation, and homework for your salary negotiations, make sure you do it. It will be a very important tool to help you advocate on your own behalf. Good research, preparation, and strategy are imperative in salary discussions, and a negotiation locked and loaded with hard facts will be difficult for any employer to dispute. And even if you are new to the massage profession, remember: the transferable skills that you bring from other areas of your life (marketing, sales, customer service, great network, management, administration, etc.) can be very strong points to leverage for the benefit to the bottom line of your new employer.

READ'EM THEIR RIGHTS

Any time you enter into a business relationship, you will be entitled to certain rights while assuming certain responsibilities and obligations to that employer. Through **labor law,** the federal and state governments set standards that regulate the rights of employees in both public and private employ. Employees across industries have many of the same basic rights: the right to not be harassed or discriminated against, the right to a safe workplace, the right to be paid a minimum wage, the right to be paid for overtime, and so forth.[36] (For more on your state or city-specific employee rights, speak with a labor attorney or visit the U.S. Department of Labor website at www.dol.gov.)

In the absence of a contract that states otherwise, most employment in the United States is *at-will.* **At-will employment** is an edict that outlines an employee-employer relationship with the understanding that either party can terminate employment at any time without legal liability. This means that you are able to give your notice to leave your job with your employer at any time, and they can break the relationship as well. However, employers cannot break the relationship for discriminatory reasons. An employer needs to have just cause, or a reasonable and impartial rationale for ending the relationship.[37] Employees typically have more latitude in labor law, and can leave a job without substantiating their decision with hard facts or documentation. However, if you sign a contract with an employer stating that you will work for them for two years and quit after three months, you are liable for breaching the employment contract.

Even if you don't have a contract, however, it is typically standard to give your employer two weeks' notice of termination. This gives the employer time to find a replacement to take over your position and ensure continuity of operations. Although emergencies often arise and life is not always predictable, it is very important that you give your notice professionally, respectfully, and in a sufficient time frame from your desired departure date. Anything less is highly unprofessional and can put your employer in a very bad position. No matter your feelings about your boss or your coworkers, leaving on bad terms can adversely impact your reputation as a professional (and it is a very small world when you have a bad reputation).

There are often city, state, and federal rules on your entitlements to breaks, work schedules, conditions, access to gratuities, and other provisions, which are particularly important for you as a massage therapist. Even if something is not covered by law, you have the right to inquire about certain labor conditions. You will want to know how much time you will be given between clients, and you should ask how or if you will be compensated for no-shows or last minute cancellations.

While working as an employee affords you a lot of rights, it also bears many responsibilities. You are being hired and compensated to represent the company and to help it build its brand. You do this through your customer service and delivery of excellent massage therapy sessions. In addition, there are many things that you are expected to do, such as be on time for your scheduled shift, wear the agreed-on attire, treat your coworkers respectfully, and contribute to a positive and productive work environment. You are required to be respectful of the materials provided for your work, as well as any physical property belonging to the company. Of course you are obligated to never harass, intimidate, or threaten anyone in the work environment. Some employers will provide an **employee manual,** a handbook outlining expectations, operating procedures, and guidelines that are unique to the company and to which all employees must adhere. It is also your obligation to have a clear understanding of your employers' expectations; if you are unclear or if an employee manual is not provided, you should always ask for clarification to avoid misunderstandings or problems.

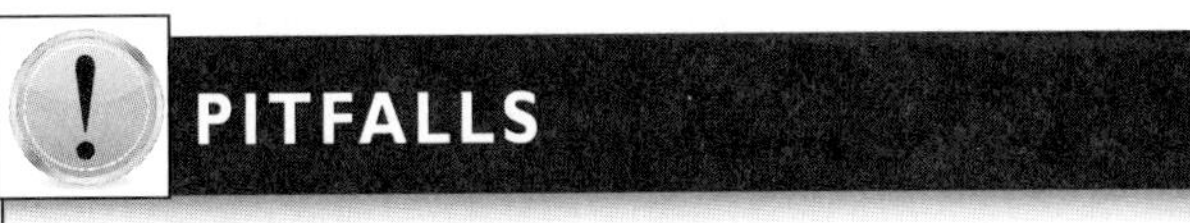

Illegal Interview Questions

To ensure that the hiring process is not discriminatory, several local, state, and federal laws regulate the questions that a potential employer can ask during an interview. Interview questions must relate to your ability to perform the job, and cannot pertain to factors such as your age, race, physical abilities, sexual orientation, gender, or socioeconomic status. An interviewer may ask you one of these prohibited questions due to ignorance (or in outright dismissal) of the employment laws. It is not the questions themselves that are illegal, but rather the end result that is the problem (i.e., refusing to hire you because of your age or sexual orientation). If you are asked one of these questions, you are free to answer or not answer, but keep in mind that there can be ramifications either way. One massage therapist got around this by jokingly asking, "Is that a trick question?" Making light of such questions can save you and help the interviewer save face.

Because many therapists run their own businesses *and* function as employees, many employers have begun to include noncompete agreements or clauses in their employment packets. A **noncompete clause** or agreement is part of a contractual relationship between an employer and an employee or independent contractor. In a noncompete clause, the employee/contractor agrees to not pursue a similar trade in competition with the employer. This is to dissuade therapists from "stealing" clients away. Remember, you are being paid to represent someone else's business, not to build your own. It is hardly professional (or ethical) to advertise your own business during a massage conducted at your employer's establishment.

MARKETING MATTERS

You are going to learn a great deal about marketing a massage business in Chapters 11 and 12. However, it is essential to understand the importance of marketing as an employee. Many therapists believe that once they go to work for someone else, they no longer need to worry about anything besides showing up, giving massages if they happen to be scheduled with clients, and going home. This may be true, but only if you have no investment in your career success at all. A true professional knows that whether you collect a paycheck or run a business, you are always marketing yourself. After all, you are the CEO of "ME, Incorporated," and everyone (including your boss) is a client in your business.[38] If you approach your professional career with indifference and laziness, then ME, Inc. may not be in business for long.

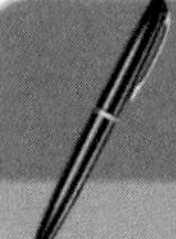

PUT IT IN WRITING

Employee Obligations

The following is a list of some other common obligations of the employee. Read through them, and see if you can't add a few more to the list.

- Be honest
- Report wrongdoing (by self, coworkers, clients, or managers)
- Communicate own scheduling needs and get cover when unable to work
- Safeguard confidential company information (trade secrets, financial data, etc.)
- Follow all safety guidelines
- Report any job-related illness or injury to employer

The list above isn't exhaustive—what else can you think of?

____

____

____

____

Later you will learn more about personal branding, which is a solid tie-in to this same concept. But for now just understand the importance of committing to marketing yourself even after you get the job as a cornerstone of career development. Every point of contact you have with a client, a potential client, a vendor, a competitor, or anyone else is an opportunity to market both yourself as an employee and the company you are representing. When you are networking and meet someone who is interested in massage, hand them a company card and tell them to come and see you. Do not confuse this with the ethical breach of stealing clients—you are promoting yourself as an agent of the company, and fortifying your own paycheck as you build your employer's business. Remember, it is hard to be successful in an unsuccessful company—the better your employer does, the more you will profit and flourish.

EVERLASTING LEARNING

Lifelong learning is the secret to successful individuals. No matter how much you already know, there will always be room to broaden your knowledge base. Just as you want to invest in your own marketing as an employee, you will want to make continuing education part of your professional repertoire. **Continuing education** is the ongoing participation in classes, workshops, apprenticeships, or anything else that deepens your knowledge and skill base as a professional practitioner. Continuing education can be offered by massage schools, association workshops or conferences, or through individual mentorship. Many states have continuing education (CE or CEU) included in their massage licensing requirements, and you will need to keep up with your CEs for membership in professional organizations like AMTA, ABMP, and NCBTMB. If you are doing a CE to satisfy a requirement, you will want to ensure that you are going through a provider that has been approved by the state or specific organization. As a professional, you are ultimately responsible for researching state and association requirements. You don't want to find out after you've spent your valuable time and money that you can't apply the experience to your CEs requisite.

But beyond fulfilling requirements, continuing your education is an incredibly important part of your professional development, your skill as a massage therapist, your personal brand, and your value as an employee. Even if you don't have to satisfy a checklist for licensure, you should still adopt an appreciation of lifetime learning for your own benefit. Successful professionals of every stripe and industry know the value of enriching their minds and the direct impact it has upon their achievements and income. And employers *love* to hire individuals who are committed to their own development and education. Not only are skilled practitioners more beneficial to the clients, a massage therapist who is forever honing his craft is far more productive, engaging, and passionate for the work that he does. And who wouldn't want to have that around the workplace?

Continuing education need not be limited to a class or a workshop. It is true that endless classes can be quite costly, and very few people can afford to fly to Bangkok for a month's class in Thai massage. However, you can keep yourself abreast of new modalities, industry standards, innovations, and new ideas in many ways beyond formal participation. Check out trade publications, business books, motivational CDs, instructional DVDs, or try a new style of bodywork as a client. You can even ask another practitioner to teach you a modality in which he or she specializes. In return, offer to teach her a technique you have polished to perfection. Continuing education is often more of a state of mind—a receptivity to lifelong learning—than a formal process.

This chapter has provided you with a lot of great tools to use in your professional development, both in a job search and throughout your career. As you have seen, a massage career offers so many wonderful options and directions. Research, preparation, self-promotion, and a commitment to continual expansion will take you to great heights in your career. Any company would be lucky to have you!

CHAPTER SUMMARY BY LEARNING OBJECTIVES

1. **Identify and explore options for massage careers** The world of massage offers the individual so many directions from which to choose. Because healing takes many forms and the industry continues to grow, there are as many different career paths in massage as there are massage therapists. Whether self-employed or working for someone else (or both), a career in massage has limitless options.
2. **Describe employment venues** There are many places to build a career as a massage therapist, and the setting you choose will depend upon your specialization and goals. From chiropractors to cruise ships, sporting events to hospices, the massage world really can be your oyster.
3. **Contrast status of employee, independent contractor, and room renter** An employee is someone who performs activities and services for an organization that controls what, when, and how those activities and services will be done. A room renter operates his or her own business out of an existing business, renting space from another company. An independent contractor provides services or performs activities for a company, but, like room renters, are not employees of that company. Independent contractors and room renters are self-employed, and responsible for their own taxes and insurance.
4. **Identify ways to find jobs** Many schools offer job boards or career fairs, and many employers place ads for open massage positions online. A great way to find jobs is to tap your network and to let people know that you are looking and what you are looking for. Other students may be able to provide great leads for you, particularly if they are working somewhere where you would like to interview.
5. **Create a captivating cover letter and winning résumé** Résumés and cover letters are your quintessential marketing package. A résumé is a document that demonstrates your abilities and provides a synopsis of your professional and academic credentials, as well as any relevant accomplishments and skills you may have. Cover letters provide an overview of the information in your résumé, and compel the employer to take the time to read the rest of your information.
6. **Explore interviewing and communications skills** An interview is a formal meeting that is designed to gauge the qualifications, skills, and fit of a potential employee by an employer, and vice versa. The goal of an interview is to take your two-dimensional résumé and cover letter to the next level, where you can expand on all of your great characteristics and skills, as well as the intrinsic value you will bring to any work situation. Interviews can be conducted either in person or over the phone. Both your verbal and nonverbal communication will be conveying information to an interviewer.
7. **Relate the concept of culture and the importance of "fit"** Company culture is the set of shared values, attitudes, and practices exhibited by an organization's employees, management, and owners. It is the unique personality and essence of an organization, the collective fingerprint of the company that sets it apart from any other. Employee fit is the degree to which a person matches the position to be filled and the company culture in which he or she works. Fit affects performance, motivation, longevity, and income over time. Ideally, you will want to work within a company whose culture is closely aligned with your own values.
8. **Evaluate the fine points of negotiation and examine your rights and obligations as an employee** Salary negotiation is the process of discussing and arriving at a compensation package that is mutually beneficial to you and your employer. Factors affecting a salary negotiation include experience and skills, company guidelines, and industry standards. Employees across industries have many of the same basic rights: the right to not be harassed or discriminated against, the right to a safe workplace, the right to be paid minimum wage, the right to be paid for overtime, and so forth. Your state may have massage therapy-specific labor laws. As an employee, you are obligated to be represent the company, be on time for your scheduled shift, wear the agreed-on attire, treat your coworkers respectfully, and contribute to a positive and productive work environment.
9. **Illustrate why marketing still matters as an employee** You are the CEO of "ME, Incorporated," and as such you will want to promote yourself as an agent of the company. This helps to fortify your income as you build your employer's business. Remember, it is hard to be successful in an unsuccessful company—the better your employer does the more you will profit and flourish.
10. **Explain the importance of continuing education and professional development** An ongoing commitment to continuing education is an incredibly important part of your professional development, your skill as a massage therapist, your personal brand, and your value as an employee. Even if you don't have to satisfy a checklist for licensure or professional membership, you should still adopt an appreciation of lifetime learning for your own benefit. Successful professionals of every stripe and industry know the value of enriching their minds and the direct impact this has on their achievements and income.

ACTIVITIES

Quiz: Professional Development Review

1. In order to help focus your interview stories into succinct narratives that illustrate your value to an employer, experts recommend you use the _____ method, which stands for _____.
   a. GOLD: Goals, Observations, Leadership, Drive
   b. STAR: Situation, Task, Action, Result
   c. LEED: Lie, Exaggerate, Embellish, Deceive
   d. RICE: Reveal, Inquire, Consult, Expose
2. A résumé that provides a summary of skills as well as a specific work history and time line is know as a _____ résumé.
   a. functional
   b. chronological
   c. combination
   d. targeted
3. Eye contact, posture, hand gestures, smiles, and other expressions of the body are powerful aspects of _____.
   a. nonverbal communication
   b. Vulcan mind melds
   c. verbal communication
   d. manipulating others
4. A _____ is an introduction and communication of intent that typically accompanies a résumé. It provides an overview of the information in your résumé, and compels the employer to take the time to read the rest of your information.
   a. thank-you letter
   b. candidate correspondence
   c. follow-up
   d. cover letter
5. The philosophy that past behavior is the best indicator of future behavior, and can be uncovered through the use of stories and narratives, is known as _____.
   a. cognitive behavioral counseling
   b. behavior-based interviewing
   c. negative conditioning
   d. a sound strategy for dating
6. An employer has the right to direct the result of the work of a/an _____, but not the means and methods of accomplishing that result. In other words, employers cannot dictate the schedule, dress code, or execution of strategies.
   a. employee
   b. job applicant
   c. independent contractor
   d. intern
7. True or False: An employer is responsible for paying all taxes for employees and independent contractors alike.
8. True or False: Working with clients in a hospice is the same as working with clients in a retirement home, and the clients' needs are the same.
9. True or False: Even though room renters and independent contractors are not technically employed by a company, they still reflect upon that company when they are doing services on the premises. Clients and customers often do not know the difference between employer, renter, or independent contractor when doing business with a company.
10. True or False: Employers are required to ask you your age, race, and sexual orientation.
11. True or False: In a tight labor market, there are more jobs than there are candidates to fill them. This is a great market for job hunters, but companies have to compete for quality talent.
12. True or False: Once digital dirt is "out there" on you, there's really nothing you can do to clean up your online image.
13. True or False: At-will employment means that as an employee, you can walk away from a job at any time, even if you have signed a contract.
14. True or False: At different times in their massage careers, many massage therapists will work as employees, business owners of their own practice, or both at the same time. These choices are equally valid in a massage career.
15. True or False: No one really pays much attention to a résumé, so it really doesn't matter how much effort you put into it or how much time you spend proofreading it. Your skills will speak for themselves.

Discussion Questions

1. What has your experience been with interviewing in the past? Do you consider yourself to be a strong interviewer? What are questions you can remember that might have tripped you up in interviews? How do you think interviewing for massage jobs will differ from jobs you have interviewed for in the past? In what ways do you think it will be the same?
2. Look at the different aspects of being an employee, a room renter, and an independent contractor. Discuss the pros and cons of the different business relationships, and evaluate which relationship might work the best for you. Why?

Case Study

Kahlil

Kahlil is graduating from massage school next month and will be leaving his current job as a wealth management specialist. He wants to work at an upscale spa, and has targeted several ones with whom he would like to interview. He is open to the idea of relocating if necessary, and so looks at Spa-jobs.com to see what other opportunities are available in luxury spas. Some of his classmates are planning to open their own practices, but Kahlil feels that he would rather work explicitly as an employee. Not only does he feel he needs to learn the industry, he doesn't want to assume the risk, manage the responsibility, or put forth the financial investment to own his own business.

Kahlil has spoken with his professors and many past graduates about the difficulties facing new graduates. The economy has been very bad in the last two years, and fewer and fewer people are spending money on massage. Kahlil does some research and discovers that some of the high-end spas he is targeting are actually doing better than some of the less expensive massage franchises. His willingness to relocate to communities with stronger economies is also helpful, but Kahlil knows that he has to work hard on his résumé to make it stand out. He enlists the help of his friend Brenda, who works in human resources at his current company, and together they craft a stellar résumé and cover letter.

Kahlil sends his résumé to his top two choices: Spa Tranquillité and Spa Mantra. The manager at Tranquillité receives his résumé first, and is very impressed with Kahlil on paper. When she searches for Kahlil's name on Google, however, she uncovers a news file about a white-collar criminal in Boston who has the same name. Unwilling to do anything to jeopardize the prestigious image of her spa, she discards Kahlil's résumé and moves on to the next one. Completely unaware of this other person with his same name, Kahlil wonders why he never heard from Spa Tranquillité.

Spa Mantra, on the other hand, is incredibly impressed with Kahlil's résumé and cover letter and do not uncover the article. The owner calls Kahlil in for an interview the following week. When he enters the spa for the interview, he is greeted very warmly by the receptionist and invited into the relaxation room while he awaits the owner. Here he is able to observe the employees interacting with guests and one another. He is impressed with the respectful way the employees all speak to one another, and very taken with the incredible customer service and emphasis on luxury and pampering. He is equally impressed with the sincere commitment to optimal and holistic wellness.

After a few minutes, Henry, the owner, approaches and invites Kahlil in to his office in the rear of the spa. Henry is very friendly and tells Kahlil that Spa Mantra is a family-run spa. He tells Kahlil that the spa has worked very hard to find the best therapists, and that the spa treats its employees very well. Looking over Kahlil's paperwork, Henry says "Kahlil is such a lovely and unique name. What nationality are you?" Kahlil tells him, and then Henry proceeds to the rest of his interview questions. Kahlil has practiced his responses, and has selected stories from his work as a wealth management specialist to highlight his fit in the company. He has also prepared some questions to ask Henry, and Henry is impressed with the quality of thought that Kahlil has put into his inquiries. At the end of the interview, the two men shake hands, and Kahlil asks if it will be okay to follow up with Henry in a week or so.

As soon as he gets home, Kahlil sends Henry a thank-you letter, reiterating his interest in the position, his strengths, and the value that he believes he will bring to Spa Mantra. Two days later, Henry calls and offers Kahlil the job, which he immediately accepts. He cannot believe his good luck to find his dream job so quickly, and he wants to get started immediately!

Case Study Questions

1. Do you think that Kahlil might have some transferable skills from his current job as a wealth management specialist that would be helpful in his new career as a massage therapist? If so, what are they? How can he communicate these competencies in an interview?
2. What kind of market conditions does Kahlil face? What does he do to overcome them? What might you do differently?
3. Why do you think Kahlil didn't get the job with Tranquillité? Do you think that this is fair? Do you think this could actually happen? What do you think Kahlil could have done differently? What would you do?
4. What do you think of Spa Mantra's company culture? Do you think you would fit in there?
5. Did you see anything problematic during the interview? How did Kahlil handle it? How would you?
6. Do you think Kahlil should have accepted the job offer immediately? What opportunity did he miss by saying yes right away? Is there anything you might have done differently?
7. How realistic do you think Kahlil's success is? Do you think most people get a job from their first interview? Have you ever done so? What characteristics can you identify that make people successful at interviewing, and how many of those characteristics does Kahlil have?

CHAPTER 3 Time Management 101

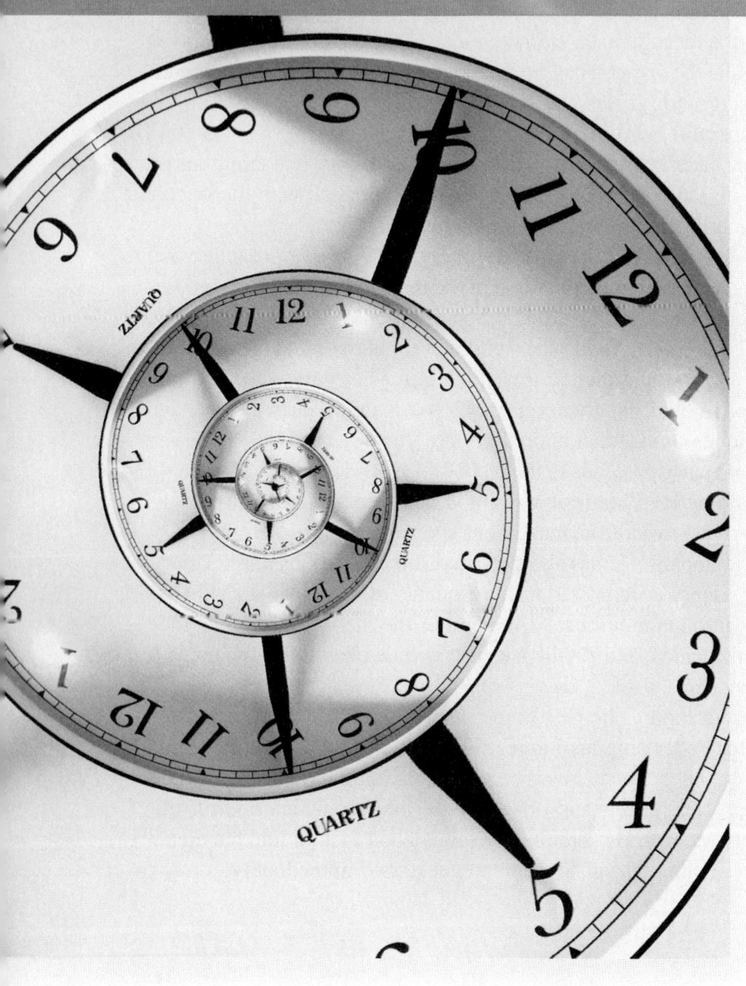

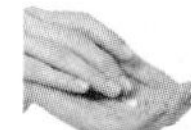

CHAPTER OUTLINE

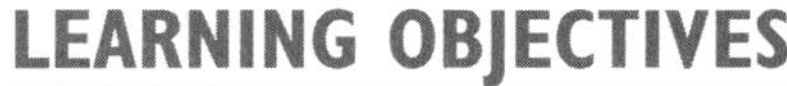

LEARNING OBJECTIVES

1. Define time management
2. Identify short-term and long-term time orientations
3. Evaluate the importance of prioritizing activities
4. Define the Pareto Principle and identify time wasters
5. Learn effective ways to overcome procrastination
6. Calculate what your time is worth
7. Explain what it means to work smart versus work hard
8. Discover and utilize tools to optimize time
9. Consider time management issues unique to massage therapists
10. Learn how to minimize interruptions
11. Explain the importance of organizing your workspace
12. Find balance in your schedule

KEY TERMS

action plan *51*
break time *53*
cancellation policy *53*
day planner *50*
long-term orientation *44*
no-show *53*
prioritizing *46*
Pareto Principle *46*
procrastination *48*
short-term orientation *44*
time log *51*
time management *44*
time orientation *44*
time wasters *47*
to-do list *51*
work-life balance *54*

Don't say you don't have enough time. You have exactly the same number of hours per day that were given to Helen Keller, Pasteur, Michelangelo, Mother Theresa, Leonardo da Vinci, Thomas Jefferson, and Albert Einstein.

—H. Jackson Brown

MANAGING YOUR TIME

One of the most important characteristics of a successful individual is his or her ability to manage time. **Time management** is the art of maximizing the hours in a day to be more efficient in achieving your goals. With the ever-increasing pace of the world, there are likely interminable demands on your schedule. You may find yourself feeling overwhelmed and overloaded, and often feel like you spin your wheels without actually accomplishing much. You may look around at all the obligations and aspects competing for your time in your life—work, family, friends, health, spirit, finances, education, travel—and wonder how anyone ever finds time to balance it all. But balance is rarely achieved by accident. Fitting everything in takes deliberation, calculation, and practice.

Time orientation is the relationship a person has to a timetable, but it also encompasses a broader world view. Time orientations can be quite different across cultures.[1] It is important to understand your own time orientation, which may help you interact professionally with people who regard time differently. Maybe you know some people who are late to everything, or others who get very angry when you make them wait. Or maybe you see things in a very black-and-white way and get frustrated when others are more ambiguous about time. These behaviors are rooted in a person's time orientation. Like anything else, people's connection to and orientation around time can vary from setting to setting for an individual. There are two different views on time; some people see time in the absolute and value reliability and promptness, while others have a more flexible regard for time, and schedules are approached in a more roundabout fashion.

In this fast-paced Western world, people tend to be fairly prompt and focus on the short term.[2] **Short-term orientation** is focused primarily on the present and immediate scope of a time line. This orientation often lends itself to the pursuit of instant gratification over the sacrifice for future gain, as the present mutes the importance of the past and future. **Long-term orientation** takes a more long-range view of a time line, and someone with this orientation is typically marked by patience, perseverance, and thrift.[3] Of course, all attributes and time associations are equally valid, but unexamined differences and beliefs among people can cause a lot of frustration and disharmony in a professional setting.

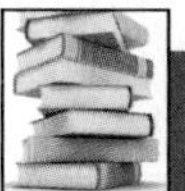

HELPFUL RESOURCES

As a business owner and a helping professional, cross-cultural differences can be very important to understand. Geert Hofstede has pioneered the field of intercultural business management. Check out his website to learn more: www.geert-hofstede.com.

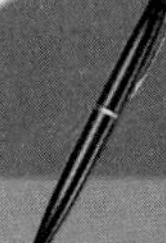

PUT IT IN WRITING

How Do I Manage Time?

1. Do I feel as though there are never enough hours in the day?
   1-not at all 2-rarely 3-sometimes 4-often 5-always
2. Am I good at time management?
   1-not at all 2-rarely 3-sometimes 4-often 5-always
3. Do I set aside time for planning and scheduling?
   1-not at all 2-rarely 3-sometimes 4-often 5-always
4. Do I worry about meeting deadlines?
   1-not at all 2-rarely 3-sometimes 4-often 5-always
5. Do I use a to-do list?
   1-not at all 2-rarely 3-sometimes 4-often 5-always
6. Do I prioritize my activities to ensure I accomplish important things?
   1-not at all 2-rarely 3-sometimes 4-often 5-always
7. Am I susceptible to distractions?
   1-not at all 2-rarely 3-sometimes 4-often 5-always
8. Do I find time to balance all the things that matter to me?
   1-not at all 2-rarely 3-sometimes 4-often 5-always

Now add up your scores:

32–40: Skip this chapter and write a time management book for others!

24–31: Time is on your side!

16–23: Pretty good time organization; with a little help you are on your way to success!

8–15: Although you have some time management skills, they could definitely use a polish.

0–7: Time is getting the best of you! You're ready to learn some skills!

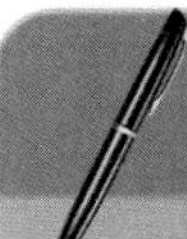

PUT IT IN WRITING

What Time Is It?

Before time can be managed effectively, it is important to understand your own relationship to it. Time orientation and the importance of the clock vary significantly from culture to culture and even from person to person. Before you set out to alter or control your schedule, it is important to understand your current and past association with time. Take this quiz to explore some of your attitudes.

1. When I make dinner plans with a friend for 7:00 pm,
   ____ a. I get to the restaurant half an hour ahead. Better early than late!
   ____ b. I get there whenever—it's no big deal. What's 45 minutes between friends?
   ____ c. I'm there at 7:00 sharp!
   ____ d. I try really hard to make it on time, but something usually distracts me and I arrive 15 or 20 minutes late.
2. When I start dating someone new,
   ____ a. I wonder what it will be like to grow old together.
   ____ b. I enjoy our time together with no future expectations.
   ____ c. I focus on getting to know them in the present, but pay attention to things that are important in my future.
   ____ d. I start picking out the china patterns.
3. I just won $20,000 in a local lottery. The first thing I'm doing is
   ____ a. spending it all on a shopping spree and vacation in Thailand.
   ____ b. putting it all into my retirement fund.
   ____ c. investing $2000 and spending the rest on a trip to Vegas with friends.
   ____ d. taking my husband out to dinner and using the rest for a down payment on that house we've wanted to buy.
4. I have a regular massage client who always shows up 20 minutes late. I respond to this by
   ____ a. rolling my eyes and resenting it—life is unpredictable, I guess.
   ____ b. telling her we cannot work together any more.
   ____ c. scheduling out a little time on the back end and working on my marketing materials while I wait. When she arrives, I explain the importance of arriving on time for her overall optimal benefit.
   ____ d. running an errand and then showing up late for her.
5. I just started working out with a trainer two weeks ago but haven't lost any weight yet. I
   ____ a. don't worry because I know it takes time to change my body. I'm prepared to work on this all year.
   ____ b. will give it a few more weeks, and then try something else.
   ____ c. QUIT! This is ridiculous!
   ____ d. figure it's because I spaced most of our appointments and never showed up. Oh well.
6. In my family of origin,
   ____ a. time was always very flexible—I don't think we owned a clock.
   ____ b. we were always the first ones at every party.
   ____ c. punctuality was a sign of respect. It was rude to not stick to schedules.
   ____ d. we were known for arriving fashionably late.
7. When someone arrives late to our meeting, I feel
   ____ a. indifferent... it's no big deal and I have a book to read.
   ____ b. very angry. How dare they waste what little time I have!
   ____ c. grateful—I arrived late myself and am relieved I'm not the only one.
   ____ d. a little frustrated, but glad to have the chance to catch up on my Blackberry.
8. The deadline for my project at work was yesterday, and I didn't finish or get anything turned in. I
   ____ a. will get it in today, but I didn't want to sacrifice quality over timeliness.
   ____ b. think I should probably get it done by tomorrow or next week. Hopefully.
   ____ c. had a deadline? Really?
   ____ d. am mortified that I didn't organize my time better. Submitting things late is very unprofessional!
9. An employee of mine habitually shows up late to work. I respond to this by
   ____ a. firing him. Tardiness is unacceptable in my company.
   ____ b. understanding that things come up and it's hard to always be on time.
   ____ c. developing an action plan together. While I understand that sometimes extenuating circumstances arise, I need him to be on time.
   ____ d. ignoring it. Who am I to complain about someone else being late?
10. When it comes to my retirement,
   ____ a. I just opened a 401k. I've just realized the importance of regular investing and I want to be prepared for my future as best I can.
   ____ b. Retirement?
   ____ c. I have been putting something away every month since I started my first job.
   ____ d. I try and save, but there never seems to be any money left.

Scoring guide:

Now that you've completed the quiz, go back and score it.

1) a = 4 b = 1 c = 3 d = 2 6) a = 1 b = 4 c = 3 d = 2
2) a = 3 b = 1 c = 3 d = 4 7) a = 2 b = 4 c = 1 d = 3
3) a = 1 b = 4 c = 2 d = 3 8) a = 3 b = 2 c = 1 d = 4
4) a = 2 b = 4 c = 3 d = 1 9) a = 4 b = 2 c = 1 d = 3
5) a = 4 b = 3 c = 2 d = 1 10) a = 3 b = 1 c = 4 d = 2

Now add up your scores:

33–40: The train conductor: tempest fugit tempest fugit! You have a very strong adherence to time, and you orchestrate your life around the clock. You often expect this same behavior of others and are easily frustrated when external forces throw off your

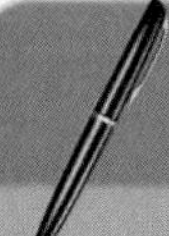

PUT IT IN WRITING

What Time Is It? (continued)

schedule. In business, it is good to be organized, but flexibility can be an important part of your success, as well as an enjoyable life.

24–32: Pleasantly punctual: you have a reverent relationship with time and show your respect for other people's schedules. You try to make the most of the situation, but like the train conductor, you have to be aware that others may not operate from this orientation. You may have to work to keep your boundaries while accepting others' relationship to the clock.

16–23: Stuff happens: I'll get there when I can. You try to keep your appointments, but distractions and interruptions easily deter your schedule. You don't think too much of showing up a little late for your appointments or turning work in late. It's good to be flexible, but be careful you don't develop a reputation for being unable to fulfill promises. This casual attitude could become a liability if not managed properly.

10–16: Hang loose, man: you are very much in the present moment, where time is fluid and things happen naturally. For you, strict adherence to the clock ruins the natural flow and circumvents creativity. Many people strive to reach this state of being, but it can make you seem unreliable or undependable. In business, it can deter people from wanting to build commitment-based relationships with you.

PRIORITIZING

Managing your time efficiently allows you to do more work in less time. It can increase your productivity and minimize your stress levels. It can free up time to spend with your family or the hobbies you never get around to doing. In any given day, there are always exactly 24 hours yet infinite ways to spend your time. No one can possibly fit everything in, and in order to manage your time effectively, it is essential to prioritize. **Prioritizing** is choosing the things that are the most important to you, and giving your energy and attention to those things first. Prioritizing ensures that the most essential things get done. When you prioritize, you allow the activities that you value less to stop zapping your time and energy. When you don't, low-priority activities can dominate your day (see Figure 3-1 ■).

The Pareto Principle is a well-known concept in the business world. Also known as the 80/20 rule, the **Pareto Principle** states that 80 percent of outcomes are generated from 20 percent of input; put another way, only 20 percent is vital while 80 percent is typically trivial. The concept is named for Italian economist Vilfredo Pareto, who developed a theory on the uneven distribution of wealth when he found that 20 percent of the people owned 80 percent of the wealth and resources in his native Italy.[4] Managers and businesspeople have long employed this theory to explain why 20 percent of the work consumes 80 percent of the resources while 80 percent of productivity come from only 20 percent of the workforce. Applicable to nearly every situation, the Pareto Principle can be a very useful concept to help you prioritize your activities and better manage your time. By using this concept, you can remember to spend 80 percent of your time on the 20 percent of effort that is ultimately important.

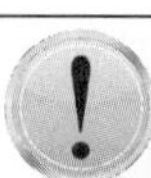

PITFALLS

Don't be fooled into thinking that being busy is the same as being productive. It is very easy to burden yourself with busywork without actually accomplishing anything. Concentrate on dedicating yourself to results-oriented activities, rather than on being busy.

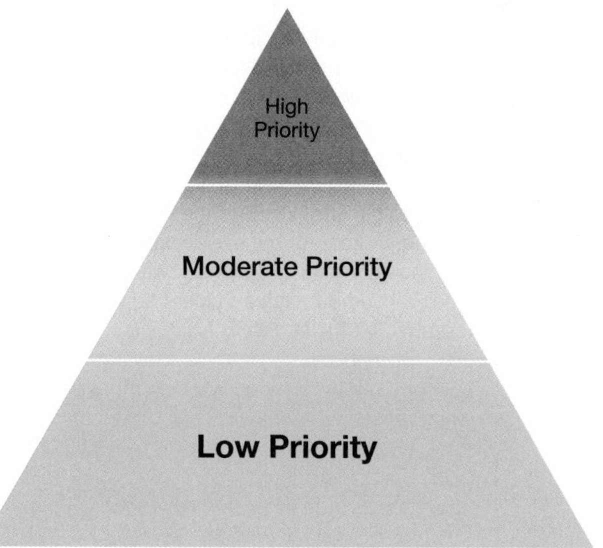

FIGURE 3-1

Without a plan, low-priority activities can absorb much of your time.

GETTING ORGANIZED

In order to grasp the importance of the Pareto Principle in your life, write down and take a look at the 10 things you did today. Don't worry about the order in which you did things, or even the meaning of any of it. Just write them down. When you finish, choose the one thing that is the most important to you for your day or your week. Here is an example to get you started:

What I did today:

1. Ate breakfast
2. Talked on the phone with Thalia
3. Spent one hour working on résumé
4. Caught up on e-mails
5. Went on job interview
6. Played around online
7. Watched the news
8. Packed lunches for the kids
9. Took kids to school
10. Went for a run

My #1 priority for today/this week: Get a new job

Percent of activities that directly support goal: 20%

Arguably, everything on that list could be construed as productive. But by prioritizing the most important thing for the day/week, only two things, #3 and #5, directly contributed to that goal. Again, the purpose here isn't to judge or even to eliminate the other 80 percent, but rather to be aware of how you spend your time. Now you try:

What I did today:

1. ______
2. ______
3. ______
4. ______
5. ______
6. ______
7. ______
8. ______
9. ______
10. ______

My #1 priority for today/this week: ______

Percentage of activities that directly support goal: ______

TIME WASTERS

When you chart out your day as you did in the exercise above, you will invariably find activities that are not only nonessential to your immediate goals, but altogether superfluous. These are known as **time wasters.** Something becomes a time waster only in relation to your goals and priorities, and can mean different things to different people. For example, someone could identify e-mail and reading magazines as unnecessary time wasters in their day; another person could spend hours e-mailing every day because they value networking or reading magazines to stay current with trends relative to his or her field. Wasting time is a subjective concept. However, some common examples of time wasters include:

- watching television
- sitting in traffic
- surfing the Internet
- talking on the phone
- playing videogames
- reading celebrity magazines
- waiting in line
- playing on MySpace or Facebook
- unexpected visitors
- meetings

Because time wasters can be caused by others, you may not be able to eliminate them altogether. The objective is to become aware of the limitations imposed when something divorced from your goals is eating your time.

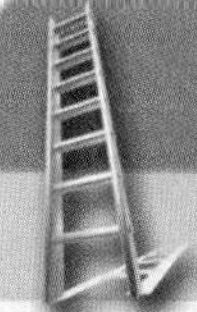

FIRST STEPS

If you want to get a good visual of the effect that time wasters have on your day, grab a pen, a piece of paper, and a pair of scissors. Start jotting down all the activities you do on a daily basis that are not task or goal oriented. This can be at your job or at home. Write randomly all over the page, rather than forming a linear list. When you finish, take your scissors and cut out the words of the things that are time wasters to you. When you finish, look at your piece of paper. What's left represents the time you allot to do the things that really matter to you.

PITFALLS

Naturally, it is important to take breaks and one cannot (and arguably should not) be productive all the time. But time wasters can overtake a day and prevent you from achieving your goals if you don't pay attention. There are invariably plenty of ways to relax and de-stress that are supportive of the things you value.

Never put off for tomorrow what you can do the day after tomorrow.

—Mark Twain

PROCRASTINATION

"What's one more day? I'll do it tomorrow." "Just one more episode and then I'll turn the television off." "The deadline isn't until Thursday. I'll just do it Wednesday night." Do any of those sound familiar? If so, you are already acquainted with the concept of procrastination. Merriam-Webster's dictionary defines **procrastination** as "the putting off intentionally and habitually of something that should be done."[5] Leaving the dishes until morning, postponing that important return phone call to a client or boss, waiting until the weather is better to go exercise . . . everyone finds themselves succumbing to procrastination from time to time. But just like time wasters, procrastination can begin to sabotage your success if left unexamined and misunderstood.

People procrastinate for many different reasons: feeling overwhelmed by a situation or by the abundance of options; feeling intimidated by the magnitude of what needs to be done; the easy distractions of busywork and time wasters; feeling overworked; or even resentment over externally imposed deadlines. Procrastination is not always intentional; it can be the result of unclear goals, conflicting objectives, or unrealistic expectations. Fear of failure can be a very strong driver of procrastination, as anxiety about moving forward into the unknown or unfamiliar can be immobilizing.

WHAT IS YOUR TIME WORTH?

One very strong deterrent to procrastination and time wasters is the hidden financial cost these can incur. If the old adage is correct and time really is money, how much is it costing you to watch that extra hour of television rather than work on your marketing plan or make those confirmation calls for tomorrow's appointments? Take a look at Table 3-1 ■, which is based on the typical eight-hour, five-day work week in a calendar year with two weeks of vacation. It does not include taxes or other intervening factors. It simply breaks down your income into daily, hourly, and minute units.

The most recent data show that the average massage therapist earns $40,330 annually for 15 hours of massage every week.[6] Though everyone knows that your wonderful massage

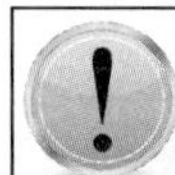

PITFALLS

Be gentle with yourself as you examine your behaviors and habits with time wasters and procrastination. As with so many of the exercises in this book, the goal is not to induce guilt or stimulate more anxiety over the way things *should* be done. It is human nature to avoid uncomfortable things, and have compassion for yourself as you go through the process.

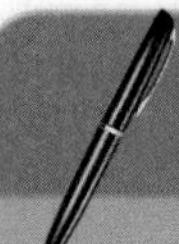

PUT IT IN WRITING

Procrastiwhat Now?

To help you pinpoint an instance of procrastination and examine some of the underlying issues, try this exercise. Think of the last time you put off doing something important to you. This could relate to your relationships, your professional career, your physical health, your household. Hang on to your answers—simple awareness of the things you avoid can be a great tool to help you get a handle on procrastination.

1. The last task I put off was ________________
2. When I think about not doing this task I feel ____________
3. The benefit to me of accomplishing this task is __________
4. The benefit to me of putting off this task is ____________
5. If I had to identify the sensation of procrastinating this task in one word, it would be ________________
6. If I had to identify the sensation of accomplishing this task in one word, it would be ________________

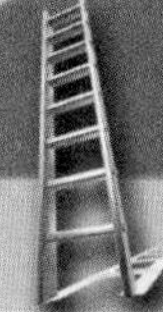

FIRST STEPS

Tips to Overcoming Procrastination

- Be clear about the outcome you are aiming for.
- Break tasks down into manageable components so as to not overwhelm yourself with unwieldy undertakings.
- Close your door (literally and figuratively) to outside distractions.
- Use the prioritizing work you did earlier to help clear your calendar of busywork that distracts you from getting the important stuff done.
- If possible, delegate lesser tasks to others so you can focus on what matters.
- Make a plan! Spend a little time each day outlining what you'd like to accomplish. Sometimes just having a schedule to look at deters procrastination.
- Build in breaks. Overworking yourself can set you up for procrastination and avoidance of important tasks if you feel too fatigued.
- Build in rewards. It can be really beneficial to bestow accolades and treats upon yourself when you accomplish things. Rewards can incentivize away procrastination.
- Phone a friend. Enlist the help of a friend or someone you trust to hold you accountable to your goals.
- Believe in yourself!

skills and incomparable business acumen render you far from average, let's use this number for purely illustrative purposes. Thus, every hour you elect to spend watching reality television or reading about the exploits of the latest celebutante ultimately costs you $20. Every day you spend wringing your hands for fear of failure rather than doing what needs to be done can carry a price tag of $160. To get a better understanding of the dollar value of your precious time, check out an online time value calculator (SmartMoney.com and MSN Money both offer these for free). When you understand the hidden costs of procrastination and time wasters, you become galvanized to rein them in.

TABLE 3-1 The Value of Your Time

If Your Yearly Salary is:	Every Day is Worth Approx:	Every Hour is Worth Approx:	Every Minute is Worth Approx:
$15,000	$60.00	$7.50	$.13
$20,000	$80.00	$10.00	$.17
$25,000	$100.00	$12.50	$.21
$30,000	$120.00	$15.00	$.25
$35,000	$140.00	$17.50	$.29
$40,000	$160.00	$20.00	$.33
$45,000	$180.00	$22.50	$.38
$50,000	$200.00	$25.00	$.42
$60,000	$240.00	$30.00	$.50
$75,000	$300.00	$38.00	$.63
$100,000	$400.00	$50.00	$.83

Adapted from Leadership-tools.com.

PITFALLS

Don't make the mistake of thinking that charging $60 for an hour of massage is the same thing as making $60 an hour. Doing so both gives you an inflated income estimation, an inaccurate time valuation, and fails to take into account the time you spend supporting and contributing to that one hour of massage (marketing, phone calls, administrative work, continuing education, etc.).

WORK SMART, NOT HARD . . . HUH?

It's true hard work never killed anybody, but I figure, why take the chance?

—Ronald Reagan

You have undoubtedly heard the expression "work smart, not hard." It is a sound motto indeed, but what exactly does that mean to you? In the professional world, the basic idea is to strategically and intelligently optimize your time so that you do not have to work as hard for a desired result. Like any adage, it can sound great in theory but fall short in practical application, especially if you aren't used to applying it. Rather than having to work hard at working smart so you don't have to work hard, cut out some of the guess work by looking at some simple suggestions for working smart.

- Learn from those who've come before; leverage the experience and resources of a mentor rather than recreate the wheel as a newbie.

- Use time-saving technologies, but use them wisely.
- Be ever-vigilant of the activities that contribute to and those that detract from your goals.
- Find people that can do the things that are not your strengths.
- Reevaluate the priority of the activities in which you invest your time and energy.

The truth is, there's nothing wrong with hard work, especially when you are starting a new career or launching a new business. Hard work is the cornerstone of much of the successes in this world, but does not guarantee success. In fact, it is often the case that working too hard can be counterproductive to success. Often people work hard because they have been taught that simply forging ahead will yield results, and that is not necessarily the truth. Working long and hard at low-energy activities can often be a substitute for a good plan and sharp focus. The good news is that you don't have to choose between smart *or* hard work, but elect for smart *and* hard work. Hard work is most valuable when it is an investment—in your career, your business, your relationships, your health, and so forth. And when hard work is coupled with smart work and efficiency, the sky really is the limit for you, your career, and your business!

TOOLS TO MANAGE TIME

Throughout the chapter you have been laying the foundation for successful time management. This short section will introduce a few tools to give you even more auxiliary support. You will find templates of all the tools available for you to use in Appendix B.

1. ***Day Planners and Successful Scheduling:*** Anyone serious about time management knows that a **day planner** is among the most important tools in an arsenal of success. Unless you are supernaturally adept at remembering every single detail, save yourself the brain cells by writing down your schedule. Planners can be electronic or tangible and paper-based depending on your preference (see Chapter 14 for more information on online scheduling). A sample planner is provided for you in Appendix B, though you should explore the scheduler that works best for you. Table 3-2 is a sample three-day planner.

   A few tips for effective and successful scheduling:

   - Be consistent. Spend time each morning reviewing your schedule for the day, and each night preparing your schedule for the following day.
   - Schedule high-priority tasks first. Use your to-do list.
   - Estimate the time you have available and contrast this with all you would like to do. Be realistic, and don't overwhelm yourself.
   - Schedule contingency cushion time for unexpected events (late clients, bad traffic). Part of effective time management is to not schedule so tightly that you induce anxiety if unanticipated things come up.
   - Schedule and take breaks. As helping professionals, it is so important to ensure you receive time to recharge and take care of yourself. Having it in the schedule helps!

   You will want to decide how you want to approach the management of your personal and professional schedule. If you have your own clients, you will likely maintain a schedule separate from the one where you schedule dates or dentist appointments. Depending on

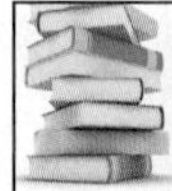

HELPFUL RESOURCES

A good read on working smart but not hard is *The 4-Hour Workweek* by Timothy Ferriss (2007, Crown Publishing). Another classic for professionals and entrepreneurs alike is *The Seven Habits of Highly Effective People* by Stephen R. Covey (2004, Free Press).

TABLE 3-2 Three-Day Planner

	Mon	Tues	Wed
6:00 am			
7:00 am	Wake up/shower	Wake up/shower	Wake up/shower
8:00 am	Breakfast/commute	Breakfast/commute	Breakfast
9:00 am	9:00 Jillian 90 min massage	9:00 Theresa 60 min massage	Gym
10:00 am	Finish/break	10:30- Stan 60 mins	Reiki class
11:00 am	11:00 Jan 90 mins	11:30 break	X
12:00 am	X	12:00 Marie 90 min prenatal	X
1:00 pm	1:00 Lena 60 mins	1:30 break	X
		1:45 Bill P. 90 mins	
2:00 pm	Break/confirm calls for Tues.	X	X
3:00 pm	3:00 Bill H. 60 mins	3:15 organize files	Coffee with Sharon.

the scale and scope of your practice, you may want to have a second schedule to organize your entire day. However, juggling two day planners can get complicated and you don't want to accidentally overbook or forget appointments by failing to duplicate your schedule consistently in both places. If you do have two planners, be very consistent in reconciling them.

2. *Time Logs:* Just as successful dieters have benefited from a food journal to monitor their intake of calories and comestibles, those looking to reform their relationship to time can benefit from a time log. A **Time log** helps you track and analyze the way you currently spend your time. Try and record your time as accurately as possible, accounting for the gaps between notable activities as well. Assign a level of importance (low, medium, or high) to each activity and its support of your goal. You may be surprised to learn where your time actually goes. Figure 3-2■ is a sample time log to help you get started. A blank log for you to work with is located in Appendix B.
3. *Action Plans and To-Do Lists:* Sometimes it can feel like there is so much to be done to accomplish a goal, and this can overwhelm you and distract and derail your time management. An **action plan** helps you clarify the goals you would like to accomplish and make the most of your time. Like a business plan or a marketing plan, an action plan is a tool to help you break your goals into actionable steps on a monthly, weekly, daily, or even hourly basis. Start by thinking of a goal you'd like to achieve in the near future. Once you've visualized the outcome of this goal (see Chapter 8 for more on creative visualization), write down all the actions you can think of that will help you achieve it. Prioritize this into a list of activities to be accomplished. This prioritized list becomes your to-do list. A **to-do list** is a catalog of the accomplishments that you would like to achieve. Having a to-do list helps you to encapsulate the activities that you need to do to accomplish a goal in one documented place. It allows you the gratification of checking off those activities as they are completed. Also like a business or marketing plan, an action plan is the most effective when it is reviewed and revised frequently. Figure 3-3■ is a sample action plan with an accompanying to-do list. See Appendix B for a blank form you can use.

Today's Date 9/18

Today's Goal see 3 massage clients and book a new one for tomorrow

Time	Activity	Time Spent	Importance Level to Today's Goal (low, med, high)
7:00	Went for a run	40 mins	Med
7:40	Showered	20 mins	Low
8:00	Breakfast	60 mins	Med
9:00	Commuted to work	45 mins	Med
9:45	Prepared for first appointment	15 mins	Med
10:00	Mike M: massage	75 mins	High
11:30	Jenny P: massage	75 mins	High
12:45	Read magazine	60 mins	Low
1:45	Confirm calls	15 mins	Med
2:00	Follow-up on client referral	5 mins	High
2:05	Call friend	25 mins	Low
2:30	Sukiko: massage	75 mins	High
3:45	Commute home	45 mins	Med
4:30	Play on Internet	90 mins	Low
6:00	Work on website	45 mins	High
6:45	Dinner	60 mins	Med
7:45	Watched movie	120 mins	Low

FIGURE 3-2

A log can help you track your time and maximize your day.

Action Plan

Today's Date 3/25

Statement of Goals Generate two new clients by Friday, April 3.

Implementation:

What needs to be done?	By when?	Priority?
1) Register for search engine opt. class at community center	Thurs 4/2	5
2) Follow-up with woman from Whole Foods who was interested	Today	1
3) Start client referral program	Sun 3/29	4
4) Sign up for chair massage at race this Sat.	Thurs 3/26	2
5) Tell book club members about Newcomer special at meeting Tues.	Tues 3/31	3

Assessment:

How will I know when the task is complete?

1) Will have attended class and learned tools
2) Will have called woman
3) Will have informed all clients in database of referral program via email
4) Will have called organizer and signed up
5) Will have made an announcement and handed out cards at book club Tues.

To-Do List

Activity	Priority (1–5)
Follow up with woman from Whole Foods	1
Sign up for chair massage at race Saturday	2
Tell book club members about special	3
Start client referral program	4
Attend search engine optimization class	5

FIGURE 3-3

An action plan and to-do list can help you set, prioritize, and accomplish your goals for the day.

MINIMIZE INTERRUPTIONS

With so many things competing for your attention in any given moment, it may seem impossible to accomplish everything on your to-do list. Emergencies will arise, friends will drop by, children will need attention, and clients (hopefully) will call. With all of its conveniences, technology has made communications available across the world and around the clock. The perpetual use of cell phones, e-mail, and Blackberries can make a person feel obligated to be constantly available to the world, and all the distractions can deter anyone from getting the important things done. There are, however, many ways to minimize interruptions and keep you on track.

> *By prevailing over all obstacles and distractions, one may unfailingly arrive at his [or her] chosen goal or destination.*
>
> —Christopher Columbus

If you are in an office or workspace with a lot of traffic from others, there are a few tricks to minimize distractions. If you are using a computer, center it on your desk so that people can see when you are working and will be less inclined to interrupt. Don't leave too many chairs in your office, as they invite people to come in and chat. Often

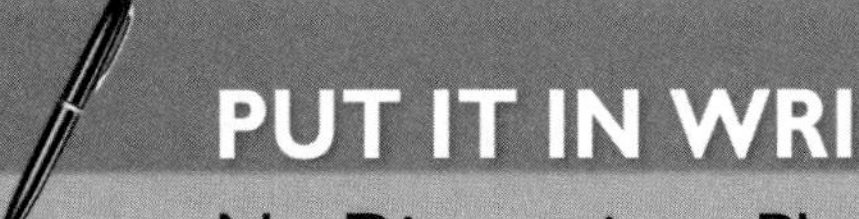

PUT IT IN WRITING

No Distractions Please!

Distractions are a normal part of life, but they do not have to prevent you from achieving your goals if you manage them properly. Think of your experiences with trying to do a project but having to postpone it or cancel it altogether due to distractions. Whether extenuating or commonplace, write down five distractions that you recall.

1. ______
2. ______
3. ______
4. ______
5. ______

For each distraction, see if you can find a creative way you could have forestalled that interruption to get your work done.

1. ______
2. ______
3. ______
4. ______
5. ______

Take a look at your five ideas for preventing those distractions. The next time you start a project, try to employ those ideas and see if you don't get more done!

you will simply want to close your door to all distractions, both literally and figuratively. Turn off all radio and television programs (unless you are one of those people who are genuinely helped to focus by white noise—even then, keep the volume on low). Close your e-mail, silence your cell phone or Blackberry, and put a "do not disturb" sign on your door.

MAXIMIZING THE MASSAGE THERAPIST'S TIME

While most of the suggestions in this chapter can be applied to most people, there are a few challenges and tools that are unique to massage therapists. Whether you are an employee, a contractor, or a business owner, chances are pretty good that your income will be proportionate to the number of clients serviced. In most instances, no clients equals no money. Things like last-minute cancellations and no-shows can affect your bottom line and waste your precious time.

A **no-show** is a client who cancels or fails to show up for an appointment without giving notification. No-shows and late cancellations can be a problem in the massage industry, and can easily cut into your profits as it is difficult to recover the lost income. However, there are many ways that you can reduce their frequency and boost your business. Most holistic businesses have a **cancellation policy,** a written statement of procedures and responsibilities for no-shows or cancellations made within a specific time period before an appointment. Terms on cancellations policies vary, but they typically include the imposition of a partial or complete payment requirement. It is a good idea to include your cancellation policy on client intake forms, and to remind clients of it when making appointments. Just having a cancellation policy will not necessarily eliminate no-shows, however. A few more tips for reducing no-shows and maximizing your schedule:

- Set an appointment time that is convenient for your clients' schedules. Give them a few different options so that they are able to choose the best time.
- If the client is coming for the first time, take the time to make him or her feel welcome and comfortable. Provide as much information as possible, and offer to answer any questions he or she has before the appointment.
- Create and use a welcome letter or a welcome kit, explaining all the information a new client might like to know and what the client can expect from working with you.
- Include an FAQ page on your website that addresses all of the common questions clients have about massage in general and your practice in particular.
- Confirm appointments a day or two in advance, either by phone or by e-mail notification. Many online schedulers will provide this service for you automatically.
- Engage clients in the ongoing treatment process. This can be done by giving clients assignments between appointments, such as various stretches or exercises.

Another important time management tool for massage therapists is the use of adequate break time. **Break time** is the scheduled period between sessions when massage therapists are able to change sheets, transition clients, or attend to physiological or personal needs. Break time is a very important concept for massage therapists, as insufficient space between appointments can lead to poor customer service and a burned-out therapist. Over the long

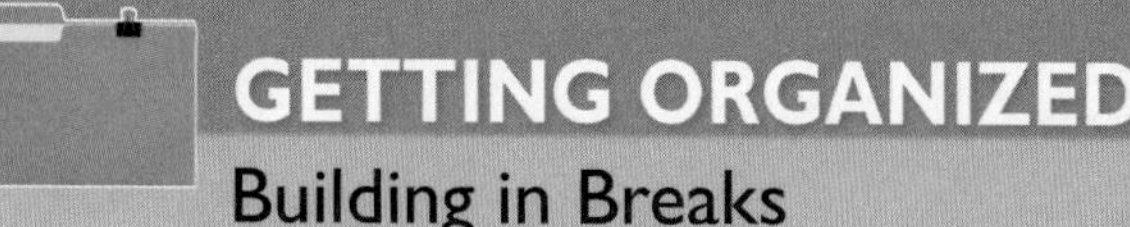

GETTING ORGANIZED
Building in Breaks

Whether you are working as an employee, a contractor, managing others, or running your own business, scheduling and respecting break time will definitely be your business. Make it a habit to build in breaks between massage sessions early. Whether you are using an electronic or paper schedule, create one now that includes fixed breaks, and keep a copy of it to help you remember this crucial ingredient to career success.

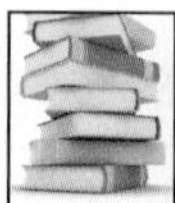

HELPFUL RESOURCES

Looking for more information on organizing and designing your workspace? Check out the *Zen of Organizing* by Regina Leeds (2002, Alpha Books) or *The Inspired Workspace: Designs for Productivity and Creativity* by Marilyn Zelinksy (2002, Rockport Publishers).

term, this can result in lost customers, illness, and therapist burnout. Preserving just a few moments between sessions can actually end up saving you a lot of time in the long run.

ORGANIZE YOUR WORKSPACE

As hard as you are working to minimize distractions from the outside, make sure you deal with one of the biggest distractions of all—a messy workspace. Whether you are an employee, a business owner, or both, you will still want to take control of your work area as best as you can. It may sound trivial or trite, but having a well-organized workspace can make a huge difference in your effectiveness and your time management. Creating order and harmony in your workspace brings more of a flow into your work and helps you to be more efficient. Think how difficult it is to get anything done when your desk is piled with papers and massage sheets clutter the floor. Obviously, if your primary workspace is the room where you have direct client contact and perform your massages, having a well-organized, attractive workspace is essential. Your clients are coming to see you for restoration and healing; you don't want them to see a cluttered, disheveled room.

If you are going to have your own business, you will explore more of the basics for designing and creating your ideal massage space in Chapter 9. But for now just consider the relationship between organizing your space and managing your time, as well as a few simple tips.[7] Always put things back in the same place, and keep all your supplies organized. You might consider buying organizing containers for your linens, your oils and lotions, or any other tools you use in massage. A storage cabinet is useful to house both your tools and your client files. To save time and trouble in the long run, establish early on an efficient system for filing and recordkeeping, ensuring current client files are easily accessible. Label all your files clearly and arrange them alphabetically for quick retrieval. Some therapists find color coding their files by client category and frequency is a helpful technique. Try not to let mail stack up, but rather open it as it arrives and sort it by priority.[8] Even if you work for someone who handles these things, offer to help organize the work environment if you don't think your boss is keeping things coordinated.

If you are also managing your massage business from a traditional-style office, consider the following suggestions for optimal design. Clear your desk of all papers and materials that are not relevant to your immediate task at hand. Have trays to organize work by priority. Have a calendar and your day planner visible, so you always remember your appointments and can track your time efficiently. When you are finished working in your space, always tidy it up before you leave for the day, taking note of what you need to work on tomorrow.

FINDING BALANCE IN THE SCHEDULE

When you are getting started with a new business or starting a new career, it is easy to lose sight of balance. Innumerable things will need to be done, and as the entrepreneur or professional of record, you are ultimately the one to do them. But trying to fit it all in can lead to increased stress, overwork, and eventual burnout. **Work-life balance** is the equilibrium achieved when one is able to strike an accord between professional and personal obligations. Most professionals and entrepreneurs will tell you that they have to work hard to maintain the boundaries to ensure their work-life balance. And those same professionals and entrepreneurs will also tell you that that work-life balance is integral to their productivity and ultimately to their overall success.

You will explore this concept in more detail in relation to self-care in Chapter 5, but for now just keep in mind the importance of work-life balance when developing your time management program. Remember the ultimate goal of time management is to augment your efficiency so you can devote more time to other aspects of your person and have a smooth ride on your Wheel of Life.

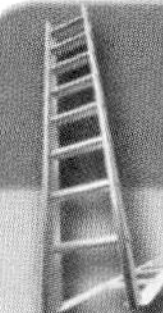

FIRST STEPS

As you get started with all the tools you have learned for time management, keep in mind the following tips to help you maintain your work-life balance.[9]

- *Master one word—NO.* You really don't have to do it all, and with all the work you have done to prioritize the things that are important, you have every right to say "no" to the things that are not on that list. Ultimately, saying "no" to the things that you don't want to do is the best thing for everyone involved.
- *Don't cram your schedule.* Many people treat their schedules like a clown car, wedging every imaginable thing in. Allow for the unexpected and give yourself some wiggle room by planning breaks and keeping things simple. You are not trying to win a productivity contest—you are trying to stay balanced.
- *If you can't participate, delegate!* As difficult as it may seem to give up control, it's okay to hand over tasks to others. Friends, family members, and coworkers may not do it the same way, but entrusting them with details can help you devote your time elsewhere.
- *Be realistic.* Don't set yourself up for failure by loading your to-do list or giving yourself unobtainable goals. This will only discourage you and undermine your work-life balance.
- *Write down personal commitments.* Schedule your personal commitments—to your health, your loved ones, your spirit, to anything other than your business—into your personal planner. If it helps you stay accountable to your commitments, you can even make mini-contracts to those other areas of your life.
- *Keep evaluating what matters.* Continue to reassess your activities and their contribution to your goals. It's easy to slip back into patterns and to reintroduce time wasters, but ongoing evaluation of what matters will help you stay focused.
- *Accept help.* If someone offers to watch your kids or another therapist offers to take care of your clients so you can go on vacation, let them. Gracious acceptance of help from others is often very difficult to do, but it is key to maintaining balance.
- *Use technology when it is appropriate.* Technology can be an invaluable part of time management, but managing your use of it is a fundamental key to maintaining balance. Find technologies that save you time without letting them suck your time.
- *Ease up on perfectionism.* Time management is not a science; it is an art and an ongoing process. Do not obsess about maximizing every second in your day and be compassionate with yourself if you fall short of your goals. Enjoy the process!

CHAPTER SUMMARY BY LEARNING OBJECTIVES

1. **Define time management** Time management is the art of maximizing the hours in a day in order to be more efficient in achieving your goals. Time management is about optimizing effectiveness and focus while minimizing distractions and derailments to accomplish goals. Time management is an important component of running any successful business.
2. **Explore short-term and long-term time orientations** With a monochronistic orientation, time is very focal and regarded as fixed, and things tend to get done in a linear fashion. When a person is monochronistic, punctuality is very important. Short-term orientation is focused primarily upon the present scope of a timeline. This orientation often lends itself to the pursuit of instant gratification over sacrifice for future gain, as the present mutes the importance of the past and future. With a polychronistic orientation there is a flexible regard for time, and schedules are approached in a more circuitous fashion. Past and future supersede the present. Long-term orientation takes a more long-range view of a timeline, and someone with this orientation is typically marked by patience, perseverance, and thrift.
3. **Evaluate the importance of prioritizing activities** Prioritizing activities helps arrange in order the things that are the most important and directs energy towards those activities. Prioritizing ensures that the most essential things get done first, so that time or energy is not wasted on nonessential activities.
4. **Define the Pareto Principle and identify time wasters** The Pareto Principle states that 80 percent of outcomes are generated from 20 percent of input; time wasters are activities that are nonessential to immediate goals, and often superfluous altogether. Examples of time wasters include surfing the Internet aimlessly, extensive talking on the phone, watching television, or playing video games.

5. **Learn effective ways to overcome procrastination** Procrastination is the behavior of deferring important activities until a later time. When done habitually, procrastination can become a saboteur of success and goal achievement. Procrastination can be the result of unclear goals, conflicting objectives, or unrealistic expectations. Clarifying desired outcomes, breaking tasks into manageable components, minimizing distractions, prioritizing work, planning, and scheduling breaks are some of the many ways to avoid procrastinating.
6. **Calculate what your time is worth** One very strong deterrent to procrastination and time wasters is the hidden financial cost they can incur. By breaking income down into daily, hourly, and even one-minute increments, one can put a dollar amount on the value of the time that is being spent in ways that do not support goals.
7. **Explain what it means to work smart versus work hard** Hard work alone is not the secret to success, and people can spin their wheels working hard if they are not also working smart. Examples of working smart include leveraging the experiences of others, using time-saving technologies, regarding time as an investment, and being strategic about all choices.
8. **Discover and utilize tools to optimize time** Day planners help organize a schedule and can be electronic or manual. Time logs help track and analyze the way time is currently being spent. Action plans help clarify the goals one would like to accomplish and help make the most of one's time. Like a business plan or a marketing plan, an action plan is a tool to help you break your goals into actionable steps on a monthly, weekly, daily, or even hourly basis. A to-do list is a catalog of the accomplishments and activities needed to be done to accomplish a goal.
9. **Consider time management issues unique to massage therapists** Having a cancellation policy and taking supportive measures can help to minimize cancellations and no-shows, thereby maximizing therapists' time. Scheduling sufficient breaks between clients is another important time management tool, as it can help to improve client retention and decrease therapist burnout.
10. **Learn how to minimize interruptions** Many things compete for your attention when you are trying to get things done—emergencies may arise, people will drop by, and the phone will ring. Technology often makes people feel that they need to be available 24/7. Interruptions can be minimized strategically to help accomplish goals and stay on track. Techniques for minimizing interruptions include arranging your workspace to discourage disturbances; turning off cell phones, pagers, and Blackberries; and putting a "do not disturb" sign on your door.
11. **Learn the importance of organizing your workspace** Having a well-organized workspace can make a huge difference in your effectiveness and your time management. Establishing efficient filing and recordkeeping systems will save you time, and a clean space can cut down on stress. Obviously, if your primary workspace is the room where you have direct contact with clients and perform your massages, having a well-organized, attractive workspace is essential.
12. **Find balance in your schedule** Work-life balance is the equilibrium achieved when one is able to strike an accord between professional and personal obligations. Work-life balance is a tenuous pursuit for many professionals and entrepreneurs, but it can be integral to their productivity and the overall success of their careers and businesses.

ACTIVITIES

Beyond the Classroom

1. Are you familiar with all the technology available to help you save time? Explore some of the gadgets, software, and tools available out there and see if any of them might help you manage your time better. Consider enrolling in a class that will help teach you how to use relevant technologies to optimize your time even more.
2. Can you identify areas of strength in the organization system you already have? How about areas of weakness? Are there any changes you would like to make? How will reorganizing your workspace help you to be more efficient?
3. Look around your group of friends and coworkers and identify someone who seems to always get things done. Does this individual have a work-life balance that you admire? Ask the person what techniques, tools, and tricks he or she uses to manage time.
4. You have heard the expression "you can have it all." But the truth is, no one can be everywhere and do

everything. What things are you able to sacrifice to get control of your time? What things are you unwilling to give up in order to gain a few more minutes in your day?

5. One of the tricks of time management, particularly as it relates to prioritizing and maintaining a good work-life balance, is the ability to say "no." But many people struggle with this ability. Take an inventory of yourself in the past—is saying "no" something that has been comfortable or uncomfortable for you? Why do you think that is? What messages have you learned about setting strong boundaries with your time?

Case Study

Gail

Gail has been a massage therapist for four years, and has created a very successful massage practice with a thriving clientele. Seeing the growth of her business, Gail has decided that she wants to hire other practitioners and open a wellness center in her area. She knows that she has a lot of work to do to get her new center open: find a location, write a business plan, explore the reorganization of her legal structure, interview potential staff, do budgeting, meet with a business coach, and so many other things she hasn't even thought of yet.

Things are going great in her personal life, too. Together with her partner, Shontell, Gail has a 4-year-old son named Charlie. Gail is a very devoted mother and loves to spend as much time with her son as she can. Shontell works in finance and works very long hours, so Gail picks him up and drops him off from day care every day. She is very grateful to have her family in town, as well as Shontell's mother and sister. They have a very full social calendar filled with friends and regular events at their church.

Gail tends to be fairly organized with her time. She is very good at identifying and preempting distractions to the task at hand. She keeps her massage office and her filing system very well organized, with everything in its place. She always shows up for meetings on time, and in all four years only made one late cancellation with a client, when Charlie had the flu. She usually uses a day planner to track her schedule, but often relies on memory to keep appointments. She never uses to-do lists because she feels uptight trying to stick to a list. She and Shontell talk a lot about their future together, and both women have established retirement accounts and educational funds for their son. She would like to exercise more, but can never seem to find the time.

Table 3-3 ■ shows what her time log looked like when her business planner asked her to track her time for a day.

TABLE 3-3 Time Log

Time	Activity	Time Spent	Importance Level to Today's Goal (low, med, high)
6:00	Got on the computer and surfed the net, did e-mail	90 mins	
7:30	Shower	20 mins	
8:00	Fed Charlie, ate breakfast	60 mins	
9:00	Took Charlie to school	45 mins	
9:45	Drove to work	15 mins	
10:00	Prepared for first massage	30 mins	
11:30	Tim R. massage	60 mins	
12:30	Break	15 mins	
12:45	Malia T. massage	60 mins	
1:45	Break	15 mins	
2:00	Peter J. massage	60 mins	
3:00	Break	15 mins	
3:15	Massage cancellation—talked on phone to friends instead	60 mins	
4:15	Got online to research LLCs, S-Corps, and C-Corps for wellness center organization	30 mins	
4:45	Drove to get Charlie	15 mins	
5:00	Drove home	45 mins	

TABLE 3-3 Time Log (continued)

Time	Activity	Time Spent	Importance Level to Today's Goal (low, med, high)
5:45	Cooked dinner	20 mins	
6:05	Dinner	45 mins	
6:50	Called business consultant to set up meeting	10 mins	
7:00	Watched tv while Charlie and Shontell went to park	60 mins	
8:00	Get Charlie ready for bed—storytime	30 mins	
8:30	Read a chapter of book on interviewing	30 mins	
9:00	Read *People* magazine	45 mins	
9:45	Got ready for bed	15 mins	
10:00	Bedtime		

Case Study Questions

1. What do you think Gail's main goal is right now?
2. Identify some of the activities that Gail might do to support that goal.
3. Prioritize those things. Go back to her time log and prioritize her activities as low, medium, or high priority. Are there activities that she should be doing but isn't? Write a list of those high-priority things she could be doing to achieve her goal.
4. Could Gail delegate some of those activities?
5. If she did delegate, who could she enlist to help?
6. Identify some of Gail's time wasters.
7. Identify some of Gail's proactive time management skills already in place.
8. How would you describe Gail's time orientation?
9. Be Gail's new business coach. How would you help her manage her time as she grows her business?
10. In your first meeting with Gail, you are going to put together an action plan and encourage her to use a to-do list. What will it look like? Fill in the blanks in Figure 3-4■.

Action Plan

Today's Date ________

Statement of Goals/Objectives ______________________________
____
____
____

Implementation:

What needs to be done?	By when?	Priority?
1) ______________	______	______
2) ______________	______	______
3) ______________	______	______
4) ______________	______	______
5) ______________	______	______

Assessment:

How will I know when the task is complete?

1) ______________________________
2) ______________________________
3) ______________________________
4) ______________________________
5) ______________________________

To-Do List

Activity	Priority (1–5)

FIGURE 3-4

Action plan and to-do list.

CHAPTER

4 Professional Issues

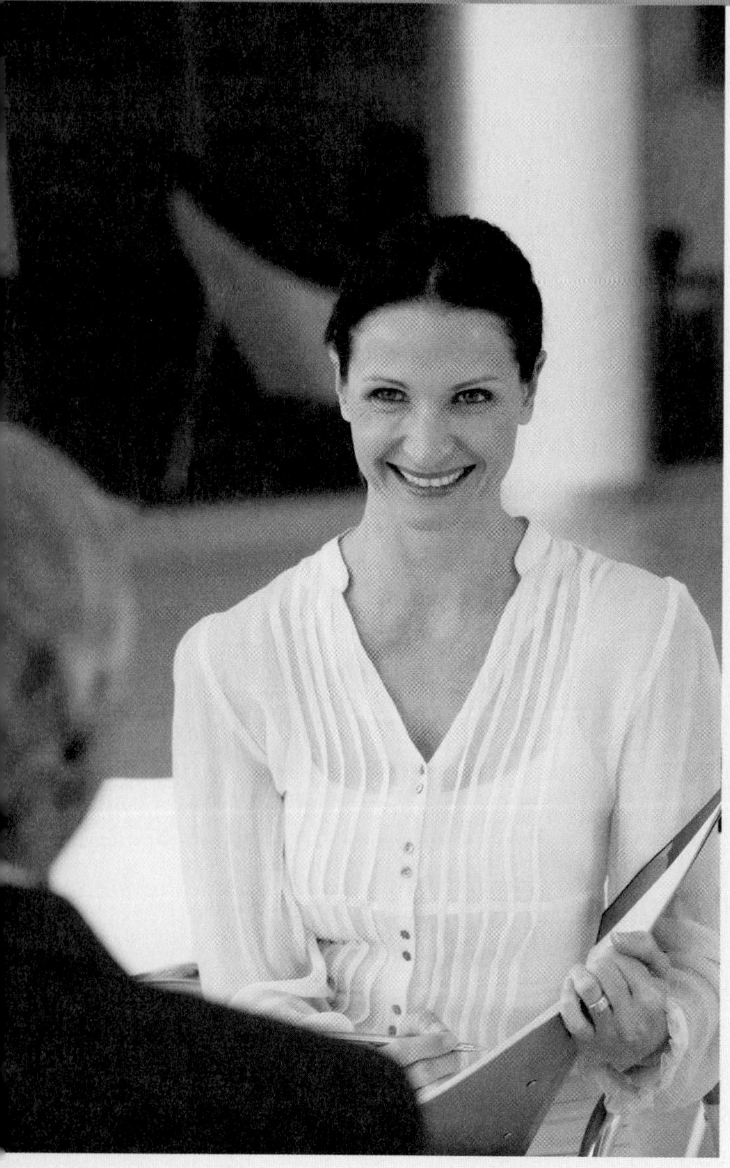

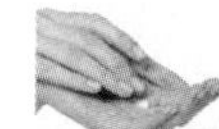

CHAPTER OUTLINE

Learning Objectives
Key Terms
Ethics and Professionalism in Massage Therapy
Get It in Writing: Documents and Recordkeeping
The Therapeutic Relationship: What You Need to Know
Define Different Boundaries
Haunted by the Specter of the "*Other* Kind of Massage": Identifying and Preventing Sexual Misconduct
It's a Woman's World: Unique Challenges for Male Therapists
The Land of Opportunity: Good Prospects for Male Therapists
License to Heal: Licensure, Exams, and Certifications
Members Only: Professional Associations and Publications for Massage Therapists
Chapter Summary by Learning Objectives
Activities

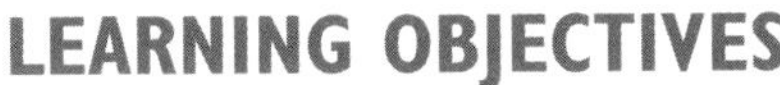

LEARNING OBJECTIVES

1. Define and explore ethics and professionalism for the massage therapist
2. Distinguish important documentation and the importance of keeping records
3. Explore the complexity of relationships between massage therapist and client
4. Define different boundaries for the massage therapist
5. Characterize sexual misconduct and identify preventative courses of action
6. Analyze gender and the massage therapist
7. Evaluate opportunities for the male therapist
8. Identify requirements for licensing, certifications, and national exams
9. Explore relevant professional associations and trade publications

KEY TERMS

boundaries *66*
boundary crossing *67*
boundary violation *67*
concentration certification *70*
confidentiality *63*
countertransference *65*
credentials *70*
documentation *64*
dual relationship *66*
ethics *62*
financial boundaries *67*
gender discrimination *69*
HIPAA *63*
hippocratic oath *62*
informed consent *63*
legal boundaries *67*
national certification *70*
personal boundaries *67*
power differential *65*
professional association *71*
professional boundaries *66*
professional license *70*
recordkeeping *64*
right of refusal *63*
right to privacy *62*
right to safety *63*
right to self-determination *63*
sexual misconduct *68*
SOAP notes *64*
therapeutic relationship *65*
trade publications *71*
transference *65*

ETHICS AND PROFESSIONALISM IN MASSAGE THERAPY

> *The meaning of good and bad, of better and worse, or right and wrong, is simply helping or hurting.*
>
> —Ralph Waldo Emerson

As a massage therapist, a great deal of your success will relate to the development and sophistication of your professionalism. Beyond the realm of practical skill and business applications, you will be exposed to many levels of professional issues, both in theory and in practice. Professional issues can range from the very structured and straightforward, such as licensure requirements or trade member associations, to more complex matters, such as ethics and relationship boundaries. Whether clear-cut or complicated, addressing professional issues will be a very important part of your career as a massage therapist.

One very important aspect of professionalism is the subject of ethics. **Ethics** is an area of philosophy which addresses questions of morality, specifically the issues and definitions of right and wrong. Ethics typically translate into codes of behavior and guidelines for daily life, and many of the collective ethics evolve into laws.[1] Ethics have been a source of debate and deliberation for millennia, and it can be very difficult to encapsulate the broad range of debate into a succinct definition. One thing that most scholars agree on: ethics in the absolute can be difficult to pin down.[2]

Although ethics in general can be complex and relative, in a professional context you are often provided with guidelines for appropriate ethical behavior. Fortunately for you, many professional organizations have worked for years to clarify and standardize professional ethical codes (see Appendix B for the codes of ethics for the National Certification Board for Therapeutic Massage and Bodywork, American Massage Therapy Association, and the Associated Bodywork and Massage Professionals). This cataloging of professional ethics has helped to standardize behavior, clear up ambiguities, and establish increased credibility in the industry. Like so many other medical and healing professions, the ethics that govern massage therapy are based in the Hippocratic Oath. The **Hippocratic Oath** is a pledge in which new physicians promise to treat all people fairly and with the best intentions, to preserve all life, and to maintain patient confidentiality. The oath is named after the ancient Greek physician Hippocrates, who, in the fourth century BCE, practiced and believed adamantly in holistic approaches to healing the body. Hippocrates was a big supporter of massage therapy in curing ailments and supporting optimal health.[3] Although the famous words "First, do no harm" are not technically in the Hippocratic Oath (in such an order), they reflect the protective primacy of its spirit and the essence of ethics in massage therapy.[4] At the core of massage ethics is the health, safety, and well-being of the client. See Appendix B for full texts of both the modern and classical versions of the Hippocratic Oath.

A large part of personal and professional ethics relates to clients' rights, including right to privacy, right to safety, and right to self-determination (see Figure 4-1 ■).[6] **Right to**

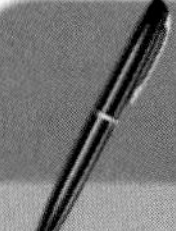

PUT IT IN WRITING
Ethics Exploration

Take a moment to ponder the following questions, evaluating some of your beliefs, motivations, and the ways you might react in certain scenarios.[5] This information is for you only. Do not judge your responses at this point, only observe and record them.

1. Do you think it is appropriate to see a client socially or outside of a therapeutic context?
2. Do you think it is appropriate to supplement income with certain products, such as oils, CDs, or liniments? If so, do you think it is appropriate to recommend them to clients?
3. Are there certain topics that you feel should be left out of conversation during a massage? What are they?
4. Do you think it is appropriate to give and receive gifts from clients?
5. Do you think it is ethical to offer discounts or pay clients for referrals? How about paying other practitioners?
6. Do you think it is appropriate to date a client?
7. What needs does being a massage therapist fulfill for you?
8. How much responsibility does the massage therapist have for the well-being of a client?
9. How much responsibility does the client have for his or her own health and well-being?
10. Do you think it is appropriate to flirt with a client, or have a client flirt with you?
11. When you listen to clients' problems, how much do they affect you?
12. When you recognize that a client's needs are beyond your scope of practice, how do you proceed?
13. How would you handle sexual feelings for a client?
14. Do you think there are different rules of comportment for male and female therapists? If so, why? And what are they?
15. How close can you get to a client without crossing any of your personal or professional boundaries? Where is the limit?

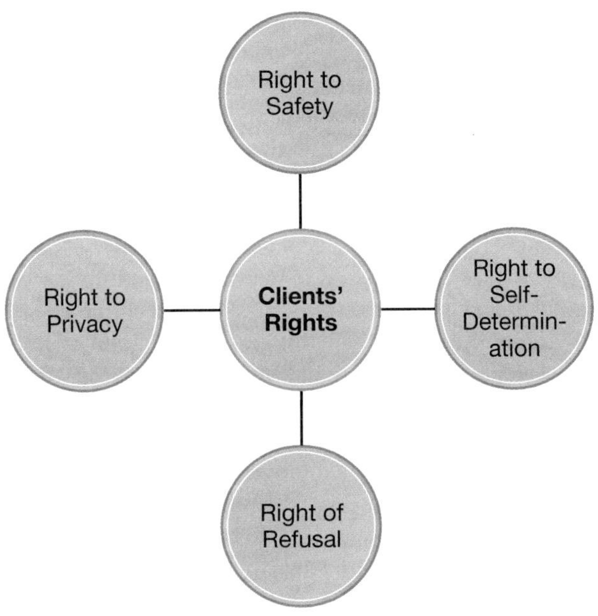

FIGURE 4-1

Four of the basic rights of clients.

privacy is the entitlement to protect personal or sensitive information and to reveal that information selectively. This has become particularly important in the digital age where information is so fungible (convertible) and accessible. In Chapters 10 and 15, you will learn about protecting yourself and your clients' security online, but for now consider privacy a fundamental aspect of your professional massage career. In a client session, allowing the client to disrobe and dress in private, as well as observing steadfast draping techniques, are all important elements of privacy.

Privacy also involves your commitment to therapist-client confidentiality. **Confidentiality** is an assurance that any information communicated between therapist and client is privileged and protected. Confidential information must not be shared with any other party without express consent. Confidential information can be communicated in many ways, including what a client tells you verbally or writes on an intake form, or even what you observe about their physical state during a massage session. In order to protect client privacy and ensure medical confidentiality, the United States Congress passed the **Health Insurance Portability and Accountability Act (HIPAA)** in 1996.[7] HIPAA requires that all medical providers inform clients about their privacy rights, explain why any information is collected, and make clear how information will be used and safeguarded. It also obliges healthcare providers to get written permission to communicate any information to third parties, such as insurance carriers or other medical providers.[8]

Clients' **right to safety** is the entitlement to be treated in a manner that safeguards health, welfare, and well-being. As part of this right, practitioners should always operate with the best intention for the client, and should never practice beyond his or her scope of expertise. All equipment should be in good working order, and all tools and resources included in the massage should be as safe as possible for the client. The cleanliness and sanitation of the environment also relates to the right of safety; clients have the right to expect disinfected linens, and therapists should always observe good personal hygiene to minimize the spread of disease and the exposure to any infections.

The **right to self-determination** establishes that clients have ultimate responsibility and control over their own health.[9] They should expect to be provided with all of the relevant information in order to make educated decisions about their own course of treatment. **Informed consent** is a process by which a client is informed of all aspects of treatment, as well as his or her rights therein. From this information, a client voluntarily confirms willingness to participate in the treatment method. The type of information provided by the practitioner typically includes information such as the goals of therapy, potential benefits and potential risks, proposed duration of treatment, and the financial requirements and terms of therapy.[10] As part of the informed consent, clients should understand that they have the right of refusal. The **right of refusal** affirms that clients can reject, decline, or terminate treatment at any time and for any reason. They should understand that they are under no obligation to continue treatment with you if they do not want to. Incidentally, therapists maintain this right as well, and are not required to work with any client that threatens any of their own rights.[11] A word of caution, however—this does not mean that you can refuse to work with clients for discriminatory

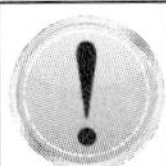

PITFALLS

While confidentiality is a crucial part of your practice, clients should be made aware that their records can, in fact, be subpoenaed by a court of law. They should also know that you are required to breach confidentiality if you believe there is a threat to the safety of the individual or others, or if you suspect abuse. Don't forget to give this information to clients as part of the informed consent.

GETTING ORGANIZED

If you are accepting insurance or will be working in a scope of practice affected by HIPAA, you should have all the information and requirements easily accessible. You can go to www.hipaa.org to read all the frequently asked questions and requirements, as well as to download checklists and forms. Keep these on file so you will have them on hand when needed.

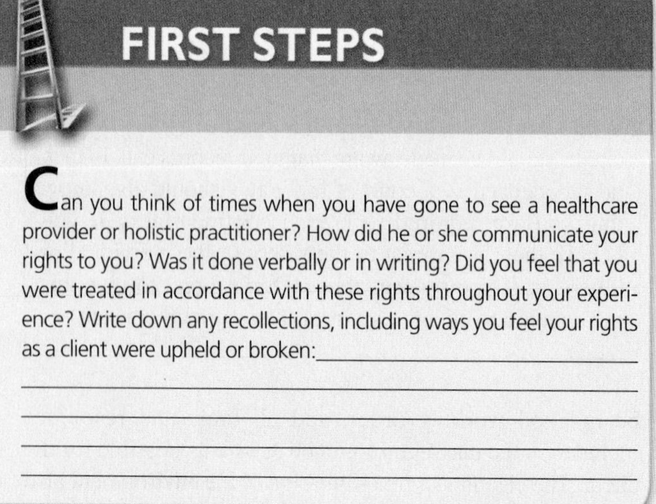

FIRST STEPS

Can you think of times when you have gone to see a healthcare provider or holistic practitioner? How did he or she communicate your rights to you? Was it done verbally or in writing? Did you feel that you were treated in accordance with these rights throughout your experience? Write down any recollections, including ways you feel your rights as a client were upheld or broken:____________________

reasons. Doing so can open you up to discrimination claims by rejected clients. If you decide to refuse a client or terminate a therapeutic relationship, you would be wise to properly document the situation and your reasons for doing so in order to protect yourself from potential claims.

GET IT IN WRITING: DOCUMENTS AND RECORDKEEPING

An important element of professionalism as a massage therapist is the fastidious keeping of good documentation and records. **Documentation** is the written record of anything that happens within your practice, from tracking finances to keeping detailed notes of client sessions.

Recordkeeping is the process of organizing, filing, and storing of that information for future use. Good documentation and recordkeeping can serve four major purposes: first, these will help you better serve your clients by providing a more systematic and efficient treatment plan. These will also relieve your brain of unnecessary taxation. Even with the best memory, it can be hard to remember everything that was done or said in every session with every client. Keeping session notes gives you a reminder of treatment goals, specific client information, techniques employed, and outcomes from previous sessions.

Good records are also very important if you are working with other healthcare practitioners, such as a chiropractor or a physician. Keeping detailed notes will help you track the client's progress collectively and create a comprehensive treatment plan for him or her (only with the client's permission to share confidential information, of course!). It also increases professional credibility with other healthcare providers if you not only speak their lingo, but have it documented as they do. Third of all, detailed recordkeeping is essential if you are accepting insurance or are subject to the HIPAA rules discussed earlier in the chapter. And finally, having consistent documentation and systematic recordkeeping will protect you in the event that you are ever in a lawsuit or audited by the IRS. In the legal world, good documentation can be invaluable. Always remember the importance of confidentiality in your documentation and in the use of recorded information.

For the massage therapist, the better part of documentation will be done through SOAP notes. An acronym for *Subjective, Objective, Assessment, and Plan,* **SOAP notes** are standard methods of documentation among healthcare providers. Soap notes provide a format for tracking therapist action and client progress. If you are working in a clinical setting, you will likely be required to work with SOAP notes frequently. Even if you don't, it is still a good idea to get in the habit of using SOAP notes for all of your client sessions (particularly if you have a lot of repeat business). The "Getting Organized" box gives a snapshot of the anatomy of a SOAP note.

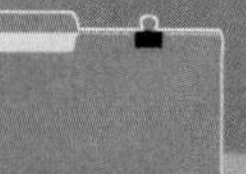

GETTING ORGANIZED

SOAP Notes

As you get used to documenting your sessions through SOAP notes, this is a good little "cheat sheet" to keep on hand in your *Business of Massage Therapy* notebook.

S: *Subjective:* Any information about the client that is provided in his or her own words. This information might include information such as motivation for therapy, recent physical strain, current ailments, medical history, or specific concerns.

O: *Objective:* Any information about the client that is observed by the therapist. This might include information such as postural and gait analysis, muscle tonicity, range of motion, or anything else detected by the therapist. This is also the place to document what occurred during the session and what techniques were used.

A: *Assessment:* A record of the immediate results of the bodywork session. Examples might include diminished hypertonicity, a reduction of adhesions, or hyperemia in the tissue. Of course, it is not a diagnosis, as that is beyond the scope of practice for massage therapists.

P: *Plan:* Here is where you record goals for subsequent sessions or the next course of action. Exercises, follow-up appointments, specific care instructions, or future requests of the client are recorded here.

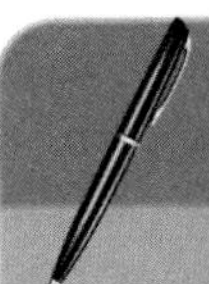

PUT IT IN WRITING

SOAP It Up!

Read the following account by Lynne, a massage therapist, and then help her write her SOAP notes. Lynne doesn't have a P (plan) for her notes: make one for her!

> The other day Ravia came to get a massage from me. It was her third visit, and when we spoke before the session began, she mentioned that she was feeling an increased pain in her right calf. She said that she had been running increased distances in preparation for her upcoming race. She was also sleeping less and feeling very stressed at work, and complained of headaches. During the session, I noticed that there was pronounced hypertonia and spasticity in the gastrocnemius and fibularis longus, much more hypertonic than the last session. I also noticed that there was mild hypertonicity in the neck muscles, particularly the scalenes and SCM. I performed petrissage and percussion in the legs, and used some focused NMT on trigger points between shoulder blades and along occipital ridge. I noticed that the distal muscles of the leg relaxed within a few minutes. The neck muscles were more problematic, and only released slightly. I didn't get to properly address it, but Ravia's rhomboids were laden with adhesions and she had excessive shortening in her pectoralis major and minor. After the session, Ravia reported feeling much more relaxed, and reported that though her legs were tender, her headache was gone. She said she felt a little light-headed and very tired. I wonder what exercises I might recommend, or what the next course of action in her treatment plan might be.

S: ____

O: ____

A: ____

P: ____

THE THERAPEUTIC RELATIONSHIP: WHAT YOU NEED TO KNOW

Relationship dynamics can be very interesting anywhere in life, and the world of massage therapy is no exception. As bodyworkers, the question of how to build a therapeutic relationship and successfully care for clients while maintaining boundaries in the relationship is an ongoing challenge. When a client comes to you as a helping or healthcare professional with the intention of engaging holistic services and effecting change in their physical or mental health and well-being, the two of you enter into a **therapeutic relationship**. Therapeutic relationships are quite different from other types of relationships, as they serve a unique function. Often times the relationship between a therapist and a client is a key component of the healing process itself.[12] Although therapeutic relationships exist between a client and any holistic, medical, or mental health provider, massage therapists need to be aware of the unique challenges to the relationship that are often inherently part of their profession. The prolonged physical contact and time spent alone in massage lends a level of intimacy that is lacking in most other therapeutic professions, and this can sometimes complicate relationship issues quite quickly.

One common occurrence in the therapeutic relationship is transference. **Transference** is the shifting of emotions or feelings that are based in a past relationship and transferring them onto a present relationship. Transferred feelings can be positive or negative, and occur on both conscious and unconscious levels for clients in regard to their therapists. Transference is quite common in a therapeutic relationship, and can happen for a number of reasons. Often transference is based on mental associations. An example of transference might be a client that distrusts you because you remind him or her of a heartbreaking ex-girlfriend or an abusive teacher they once had. A client might also assign positive feelings to the therapist based on past relationships, and become overly attached or reverent.[13] It is important for therapists to be aware of this occurrence, as both negative and positive transference can impact the effectiveness of treatment and cause unintended consequences.

On the other hand, it is not only clients that are vulnerable to bringing past associations and transferred feelings into the relationship; therapists can do it, too. **Countertransference** happens when a therapist begins to transfer his or her own feelings onto the client. Just as with transference, this can result in an adverse reaction or an excessive affection. It can also lead to a need to over-deliver to clients, or to feel that you are a powerful and sure-fire healer for someone else.[14] This, too, can result in a troubled and ineffective therapeutic relationship. As a therapist, you will want to be constantly vigilant of the possibility or presence of transference and countertransference with clients (see Figure 4-2 ■).

It is also very important to understand and respect the power differential between clients and therapists.[15] A **power differential** occurs when the therapist is regarded as a specialist endowed with knowledge and skill that the client does not possess; this takes place to varying degrees in nearly all therapeutic relationships. In most cultures, society grants a certain degree of power to professionals and experts, particularly in the medical and therapeutic fields. When clients come to you to solve a problem, they are typically doing so because they regard you as a professional with the skill and expertise to solve their problems. These assumptions automatically place you in a position of power, whether or not it is sought or even consciously acknowledged. In addition, the

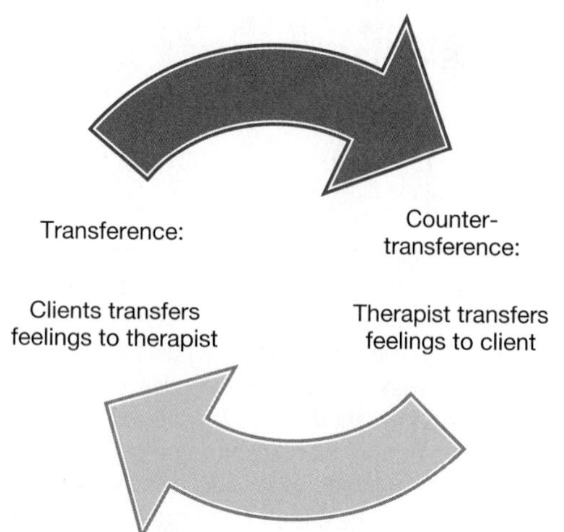

FIGURE 4-2

Transference and countertransference are common occurrences in the therapeutic relationship. It is important for therapists to always be aware of this.

mere fact that clients are placing their physical bodies, often partially or fully disrobed, into your care indicates a power differential.[16] When engaging with clients and administering therapy, it is important to be aware and respectful of this power differential.

Another frequently encountered interpersonal challenge for practitioners is the commonality of dual relationships. A **dual relationship** exists when a therapist has interactions or associations with a client beyond the therapeutic context. Having a client that is also a friend, a colleague, a teammate, a parishioner, or a family member can place you in a position of playing multiple roles in addition to that of massage therapist.[17] Doing this can dilute the importance and effectiveness of your therapeutic role, limit or jeopardize the treatment process, and can become interpersonally damaging to the therapist and the client. Understand the possible consequences or relationship losses that can come about as a result of dual relationships.

DEFINE DIFFERENT BOUNDARIES

In order to protect the integrity and clarity of the therapeutic relationship, it is essential that the therapist define and maintain strong boundaries. As you recall from Chapter 1, **boundaries** are the limits that define and clarify personal and professional space and maintain areas of comfort while upholding integrity between individuals. They can be communicated verbally, energetically, physically, or in writing. However, not everyone is able to readily identify their own boundaries, nor communicate them to other people. Boundaries exist on many levels, including professional, personal, financial, and legal (see Figure 4-3 ■).[18]

Professional boundaries are limits that protect the nature of the therapeutic relationship, define the roles of therapist and client, and preserve the integrity of each party. Although professional boundaries serve both therapist and client, it is the therapist's responsibility to rigidly maintain them. According to massage ethics experts, there are five subcategories or secondary boundaries within professional boundaries. These include intellectual, physical, emotional, sexual, and energetic boundaries (see Figure 4-4 ■).[19] Many of these boundaries are dictated and defined by law or by a professional code of ethics.

PITFALLS

Although massage therapists may not always be as culturally revered or as financially compensated as other medical professionals, they must bear in mind that they are still held to very high ethical and professional standards. Because many therapists find themselves in a position of trying to stay afloat financially, and because the work is so highly personal, many therapists tend to scrimp in the therapeutic relationship and boundary departments, often blurring the lines. Although it may be tempting to do this, keep a long-range vision and remember that a short-term payout does much less for your career than a long-term professional reputation and ethical career.

PUT IT IN WRITING

Multiple Roles

If you are already seeing clients, take a moment to do this exercise. You may have never considered it before, but it is possible that you are playing more roles than just that of massage therapist. Is a client also your friend, neighbor, personal trainer, or mother? Write down all the clients you are seeing currently, and flesh out as many possible roles as you may be playing. Evaluate if you experience or foresee any conflicts because of this.

Client's Name:	Other Relationships:
______	______
______	______
______	______
______	______

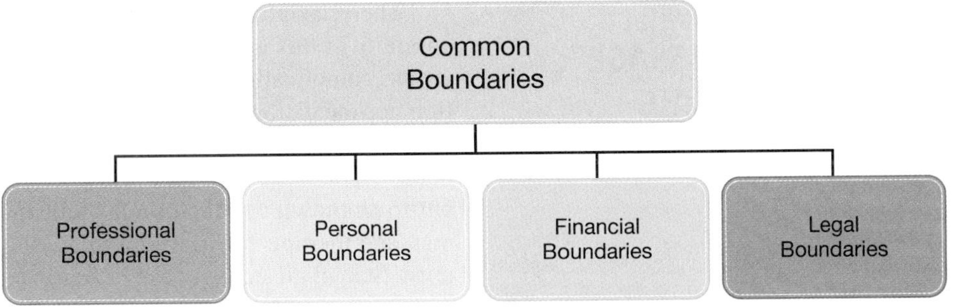

FIGURE 4-3

Some of the common boundaries to keep between therapists and clients.

Personal boundaries are established by an individual in order to protect his or her own comfort and safety in any capacity (mentally, physically, emotionally, sexually, and so forth). Unlike professional boundaries, personal boundaries are much more subjective and specific to an individual. **Financial boundaries** are limits that exist between individuals to protect their economic integrity. This is an important one for many therapists, and often one that goes unnoticed or unmentioned. You will explore more about the internal and external dynamics of finances for the massage therapist in Chapters 7 and 13, but in the meantime just understand that many massage therapists sacrifice their own financial well-being by not being clear on their boundaries.[20] Examples of this include undervaluing services, setting a cancellation penalty but never enforcing it, or repeatedly discounting for certain clients even when you cannot afford to do so. On the other hand, massage therapists can take advantage of their power differential and exploit a heightened sense of trust by recommending unnecessary products they are selling, scheduling needless or excessive sessions beyond a client's need, or trying to engage clients in additional and non-therapy-related financial relationships.[21]

Beyond the boundaries mentioned above, massage therapists are obviously bound to follow the legal parameters under which they operate. **Legal boundaries** are the limits that are imposed by each city, state, or country in order to preserve the legal rights of an individual and the security of a community. Legal boundaries can be explicit laws or implicit understandings within those laws. For example, in some cities it is a violation of a legal boundary to perform massage within your home or the home of a client, or to do massage in locations not expressly authorized by legal authorities.

Many therapists have maintained that crossing the line on any boundary can often happen slowly and subtly, whether on their behalf or that of their clients. A client could come for years before revealing romantic feelings for a therapist, and a therapist could have weekly sessions with a client that evolve into a close social contact. Because "boundary creep" can be quite common in this profession, it is so important to stay aware and to stay centered in your overarching and primary mission as a massage therapist.

When any of the various boundaries are breached, it is either a boundary crossing or a boundary violation. According to massage ethics authors Sohnen-Moe and Benjamin, the difference between the two is the intent of harm or the likelihood of harm.[22] A **boundary crossing** is an overstepping of a limit that may or may not be harmful to an individual, while a **boundary violation** is a transgression that induces harm. An example of a boundary crossing might be a therapist who talks constantly about him or herself (one of the top complaints of massage clients, by the way).[23] Such behavior pushes the limits on professional and personal boundaries, and may irritate a client to the point where he or she may not return to the chatty therapist's table. However, it is unlikely that the client feels harmed or violated by the behavior. An example of a boundary *violation* might be disclosing confidential information without permission, or inappropriately touching a client's private areas. Sexual misconduct of any kind is a violation of the boundaries and ethics of massage therapy. Speaking of which . . .

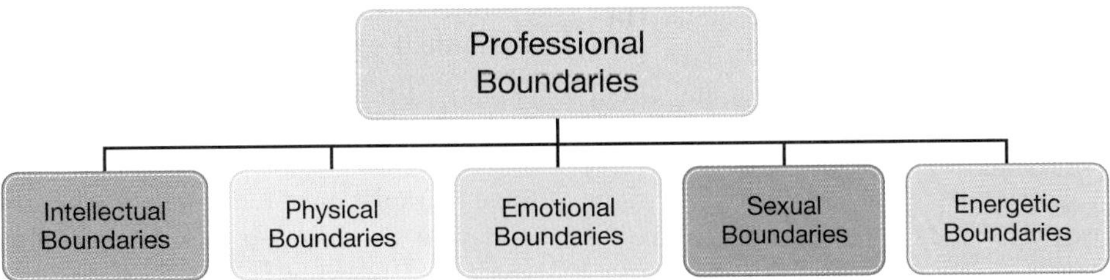

FIGURE 4-4

Professional boundaries are limits that protect the nature of the therapeutic relationship, define the roles of therapist and client, and preserve the integrity of each party.

HAUNTED BY THE SPECTER OF THE "*OTHER* KIND OF MASSAGE": IDENTIFYING AND PREVENTING SEXUAL MISCONDUCT

The price one pays for pursuing any profession or calling is an intimate knowledge of its ugly side.

—James Baldwin

While massage has innumerable upsides, it can also be a frustrating career. Even after decades (and some might argue millennia) of establishing therapeutic legitimacy and proof as a scientifically proven health modality, it is a simple fact that there are still people out there who simply cannot extricate massage from sex. Although this issue has waned significantly in recent years and instances of solicitation for sexual favors have dramatically decreased, recent events such as the "Craigslist Killer" and the prominence of back-page classified ads for "massage" serve as a reminder that the industry still faces this challenge. As skilled as you are, and as innocent as your intentions surely are, you may wish this "other massage" issue would just go away. However, public ignorance and sexual misconduct are challenges that must be looked squarely in the face and addressed by all in the profession.

Sexual misconduct is any behavior or activity that aims to sexualize the relationship between a client and a therapist. Sexual misconduct can be initiated and perpetuated by either party, and exists along a continuum of severity from minor to serious. Of all the boundaries listed above, crossing a sexual boundary is perhaps the most treacherous. A client that crosses this boundary can leave a therapist feeling violated, disrespected, and fearful. A therapist crossing this boundary is exploiting the power dynamic and is completely breaching professional (and usually legal) boundaries and standards. Sexual activity with a client is strictly prohibited by nearly every professional organization, professional code, governing body, and licensure law.

Although there is nothing inherently wrong with sex, it invariably has no place in a therapeutic relationship. The occurrence of sexual overlap in massage and the professional challenge that this presents is not a new phenomenon of the modern era. Earlier in the chapter you read about Hippocrates, who established the oath that is still adhered to even today. Sexual boundaries between practitioner and client were of enough concern in Hippocrates' day, that he actually included them into his oath:

> In every house where I come I will enter only for the good of my patients, keeping myself far from all intentional ill-doing and all seduction, and especially from the pleasures of love with women or men, be they free or slaves.[24]

The reason that it is important to acknowledge the antiquity of this issue is that it reflects an important truth: sexual complications are neither a contemporary aberration nor the distorted reality of select deviants in the contemporary post-puritanical age. All humans are sexual beings, and the key point here is not to disparage or judge, but to acknowledge the crucial schism between sex and massage therapy.[25] Clarity on this issue with clients is a must. Sexual misconduct can be devastating to your career and professional life. In addition to the professional and legal ethics mentioned above, sexual misconduct could result in a damaged reputation, loss of licenses, and even a malpractice lawsuit.[26]

So how do you as a therapist navigate the waters? The best advice is to do your best to steer clear of boundary issues altogether. Open communication is fundamental in preventing misunderstandings or uncomfortable situations. Establish clear cut boundaries at every point of contact. If you have your own practice, you will want to stress the therapeutic nature of your service in all of your marketing collateral and on your website. During face-to-face interactions with clients, be aware of your body language and your tone. While many therapists are spirited extroverts, you don't want your behavior to be construed as flirting or as a come on. During the session, of course, maintain clear physical boundaries through draping and appropriate touch.

With all of these measures, it is typically rare for unwarranted advances to take place during a session. However, it not beyond the realm of possibility and it is important to have a protocol for response. If you suspect a client is making sexual advances at any point, stop the session immediately. When he or she is off the table and dressed, tell the client your interpretation of what has been said or done, and give them the opportunity to explain or clarify. You have the right to terminate the therapeutic relationship if you feel that a boundary has been violated; if your feelings of violation are severe enough, you may want to contact local authorities.

According to massage industry specialist Patricia J. Benjamin, there are a few conditions in which sexual relationships with a client might be permissible. If a person with whom you already have a sexual relationship (such as a romantic companion, a partner, or a spouse) becomes a client, this is a different scenario from that described above. Of course, bringing such an individual on as a client presents the challenge of dual relationships discussed earlier.[27] If you truly have irrepressible feelings for a client and want to enter into a sexual relationship, the NCBTMB stipulates that a massage therapist must terminate the therapeutic relationship and wait a minimum of 6 months before beginning a sexual relationship.[28] Waiting helps minimize the potential dangers by separating the roles and giving both parties time to evaluate the sexual relationship with some good perspective.[29]

IT'S A WOMAN'S WORLD: UNIQUE CHALLENGES FOR MALE THERAPISTS

> *A successful man is one who can lay a firm foundation with the bricks others have thrown at him.*
>
> —David Brinkley

In an ideal world, therapy would be gender blind. Unfortunately, that is not always the case, and male therapists face unique challenges within the profession. Many male therapists report that they are the recipients of gender discrimination at various points along their career path. **Gender discrimination** is a separation, restriction, or exclusion based upon culturally developed gender norms which keep an individual from benefiting from full human rights. There is currently a disproportionate ratio of male to female therapists working in North America. According to a study by the U.S. Department of Labor in 2006, 84 percent of all massage therapists are female.[30] The study also found that female massage therapists have much better job prospects than men, as many clients (both male and female) felt more comfortable being physically touched by female therapists.

In spite of these statistics, there are countless male massage therapists who have found great success in their profession, and who have become leaders at every level of the industry. Many maintain that if male therapists expect to have problems finding jobs or anticipate a struggle to grow a practice, they will likely find such challenges. If they refuse to surrender to limitations and expect a thriving career, they will have one.[31] Regardless of where you fall on the positive thought continuum, it does help both male and female therapits to be aware of the role gender can play for a massage therapist, as well as the unique opportunities and experiences within the massage profession.

The sociocultural reasons that males encounter more resistance within the profession are beyond the scope of this book, but a few common themes emerge. First of all, some female clients have experienced abuse or violation by a male figure, and are very uncomfortable entrusting their physical safety to a man. Homophobia can play a part in resistance on behalf of male clients, who may not want to be touched by other men. Body image can also be an issue for individuals who are uncomfortable with men seeing their bodies.[32] Some people have just been conditioned to identify women as more nurturing figures, and are unable to see men in this role. However divorced any of this might be from reality, fairness, or from the actual character and skill of the male massage therapist is irrelevant. Clients' comfort and safety is always the most essential part of the equation.

At the same time, much can be done by those within the profession (both male and female) to educate clients about the benefits of working with male therapists. One major complaint among men working in a spa or group practice environment is the receptionist who asks a client "would you prefer a male or female therapist?" The argument is that the existing stigma automatically swings the clients' vote to the female therapist. However, a receptionist can level the playing field with an informed option such as "Ed, who specializes in sports massage, and Kate, who specializes in reflexology, are both available at 1 pm. Which would you prefer?" As one male therapist states, "If asked to choose between a male and female therapist, 9 times out of 10 a client will ask for the woman. Without all the information, human nature is to go with the most familiar option, and in this industry, it is female therapists. People might be more familiar with hamburgers than Kobe beef, but when given all the information, a lot of people go for the Kobe. At least they can make an informed choice!"

Men make fabulous massage therapists! Due to their inherent physical strength, male therapists are the preferred choice for many clients. Male energy is also an integral part of human energy and the therapeutic process, and working with men in a safe, nurturing environment can be very healing for both men and women.

THE LAND OF OPPORTUNITY: GOOD PROSPECTS FOR MALE THERAPISTS

In spite of all the data and reported stigma in the massage industry, men have wonderful opportunities within the profession—many of which are not available to women. Many clients prefer a male therapist over a female therapist. For example, many men, both heterosexual and homosexual, are not comfortable with women, and feel safer working with a man. Some deeply religious men, such as Catholic priests or Orthodox Jewish men, abide by moral precepts of not commingling the sexes in many contexts, particularly in such an intimate one as massage.[33] Many athletes prefer the natural strength of male therapists, who they believe to be more capable of deep work than women. And of course, there are always gender-blind clients, who genuinely have no preference either

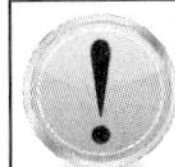

PITFALLS

Many female therapists assume that they are not adversely impacted by the gender bias in massage therapy; in fact many enjoy the benefit of the bias—more clients—without thinking of it all. But discrimination in any form can have negative effects for everyone involved. All of the "isms" (racism, ageism, classism, homophobia, sexism, religious intolerance, etc.) affect everyone and need to be addressed by everyone (especially those in privileged positions). For more on this issue, grab a copy of *The Social Psychology of Interpersonal Discrimination* by Bernice Lott and Diane Maluso (1995, Guilford Press).

way but are simply interested in the skill and capability of the therapist. There are plenty of those clients out there.

If you are working with male and female therapists in a spa, clinic, chiropractor's office, or any environment where another person has control over your appointment schedule, take the time to educate the person scheduling the appointments (as well as management) on your unique skills. You might even offer a free session so they can experience your work and give you a recommendation. Explain the problem with the standard "would you prefer a male or female" question, and provide alternatives.

There are a few recommendations for new male therapists just starting their own practices. If possible, starting in a group practice or in a wellness center with other holistic practitioners is helpful. Not only does this increase your credibility, it also provides a layer of psychological safety for clients to have other individuals around. It is also a great idea to select and develop a targeted area of expertise, rather than being a generalist therapist.[34] Being an expert in one thing and having a clarified vision of your target market will help you grow your business more quickly (see Chapters 11 and 12 for more information on target markets). Chair massage is a great way to grow a practice for a male therapist, as people tend to be less gender particular when they are fully clothed. Once they experience your touch through a chair massage, they will be more likely to become regular clients.

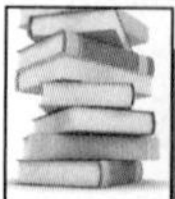

HELPFUL RESOURCES

Requirements for massage therapists are always subject to change, so make sure you stay abreast of modifications to applicable laws in your area. Check with your local governing or licensing agency. For an up-to-date guide of state requirements, go to www.massagetherapy.com or www.massageregister.com.

LICENSE TO HEAL: LICENSURE, EXAMS, AND CERTIFICATIONS

In most professions, an individual's skill is often measured not only in technical application but in the credentials she or he possesses. **Credentials** are qualifications that demonstrate an individual's competency and experience in a particular area. Credentials can be granted by schools, governments, or trade organizations, and include such things as diplomas, local and national certifications, professional affiliations, specialized certifications, licenses, advanced education, and so forth. These credentials provide a standardized way for the public, educators, employers, and other professionals to gauge an individual's background and experience. While many credentials can be optional (Reiki Master or a position on a national massage trade board), some of the credentials, such as diplomas, licenses, and continuing education, are the minimum standard for practicing. At present, only eight U.S. states allow massage therapists to practice without any kind of state regulation, and every state has its own regulations and requirements for massage therapists.[35] As if that didn't sound complicated enough for a nomadic therapist, some states even allow individual cities to devise their own additional regulations for practicing therapists.

As massage therapy has continued to flourish, more and more government agencies are getting involved in the development and enforcement of regulation and professional licensure of massage therapy. You will learn about different kinds of business licensure in Chapter 10, but first you may need to obtain a professional license. A **professional license** is an authorization granted to trained and qualified individuals to perform their occupation in a designated jurisdiction. This is done for multiple reasons, such as to provide a professional standard for both therapists and consumers. Many authorities maintain it helps to keep the "other kind" of massage out of the community. Of course, with the ever-increasing volume of practicing massage therapists, the amount of revenue that is generated by regulating and granting professional licenses is certainly a consideration for many cities and states.

In addition to graduation from an accredited school and an hours prerequisite (500–1000 hours for example), many states require a national certification for licensure. **National certification** is the confirmation of professional characteristics, values, and expertise as assessed through external examination by a certifying organization. While there are various organizations that certify for different modalities, two predominant organizations provide licensing exams to certify massage therapists and bodyworkers at the national level.

The National Certification Board for Therapeutic Massage and Bodywork (NCBTMB) was established in 1992, and administers the National Certification Exam (NCE). For many years, the NCBTMB was the only national certification authority in the United States. In 2007, however, the Federation of State Massage Therapy Boards (FSMTB) was organized and presented an alternative exam, the Massage & Bodywork Licensing Examination (MBLEx). Many states that require national certification for licensure recognize both of these organizations. While more states currently accept the NCE, recognition of FSMTB and adoption of the MBLEx are happening quickly. Because of the professional credibility associated with these nonprofit organizations and their examination process, many therapists that operate in states without the requirement still elect to take an exam and become nationally certified (for a list of the major massage therapy organizations, see Appendix B).

In addition to local and national certifications, many therapists pursue certifications in specific concentrations. **Concentration certification** is the confirmation that an individual has trained and acquired some level of mastery in a specific modality or bodywork system. Depending on the source, there are between 80 and 200 registered bodywork modalities.[36] Therapists can get certified in anything from deep tissue to prenatal massage, or from Anma to Watsu. Because there are so many different concentrations and so many people and groups organizing certification standards, the value, quality, and importance of these certifications can vary significantly.[37]

Staying current with techniques and keeping up with your continuing education requirements is important, but many therapists attend classes and collect certifications in different modalities as though they were on an Easter egg hunt. While it is wonderful to have a voracious mind and to be passionate about pursuing new techniques and knowledge, you must be grounded in your motivation for doing this. If you are chasing these certifications because you think it will bring you more clients, be forewarned that the vast majority of massage clients are familiar with only the most basic modalities (Swedish, deep tissue, sports massage, etc.). The more bodywork beads you string on your necklace, the more you will have to educate your clients.

In addition, the financial investments may be much greater than the actual return. Keep the perceived value of the client in mind—some clients will simply not care about the expert bodywork systems you have mastered, but only whether or not you can solve their immediate problems. Some therapists also find that mastering one or two techniques and focusing on a certain market is much more beneficial for their practice than dabbling in every modality out there. If you decide to obtain additional concentration certifications as part of the continuing educations requirement for licensure or association membership, make sure that the classes are accredited by the governing bodies before laying out any money. Of course, if you have a genuine interest and passion in learning something new and expanding your bag of tricks, by all means do it! Just be sure you are doing it for the right reasons.

MEMBERS ONLY: PROFESSIONAL ASSOCIATIONS AND PUBLICATIONS FOR MASSAGE THERAPISTS

I won't belong to any organization that would have me as a member.

—Groucho Marx

Nearly every industry has a group that organizes, provides services, sets standards, and advocates on behalf of the professional, and massage therapy is no different. A **professional association** is an organization that seeks to advance a profession and its members. Almost always nonprofit, professional associations provide services to their members and represent publicly their best interests. They often offer continuing education opportunities for professionals, and advocate for the profession in government policy. In the United States, there are hundreds of different professional groups for massage therapists (see Appendix B for a partial list of popular associations). The three main groups are American Massage Therapy Association (AMTA), Associated Bodywork and Massage Professionals (ABMP), and International Massage Association (IMA).

As a massage therapist, there are several benefits to being a member of a professional association. You can get listed in bodywork directories, where potential clients might find you, and some groups offer professional liability insurance. In addition, many associations provide job boards where massage therapists can find great positions. Many offer business development resources and marketing tools, such as websites.

Getting involved with local and national trade associations is a great way to network with other massage professionals as well. Some associations have over 50,000 members throughout the United States and in countries around the world. You can publish articles for association publications, which enhances your credibility and positions you as an expert in your field. If you love talking to groups about your specialty or industry-specific issues, being a part of professional organizations may lead to some great speaking opportunities as well.[38]

One of the best ways to polish your professionalism is to stay current with news and trends within the industry. A great way to do this is through trade publications. **Trade publications** are magazines, journals, newspapers, or books that intend to provide a target audience with industry-specific information and reports. Trade publications are offered online or offline (i.e., a glossy magazine or newspaper), and can provide you with invaluable industry data and trends to help you identify challenges and opportunities within your career or business. Many associations offer both online and offline

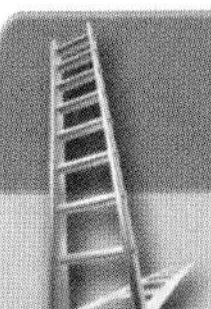

FIRST STEPS

Learning about all the various associations and certification groups might leave you with some questions about which ones to choose (if you live in a place that allows you to choose, of course). If that is the case, visit the websites of the associations listed in this chapter or in Appendix B. Make a comparison table or spreadsheet of all the things that they do and do not offer, and include the criteria that is most important to you (such as insurance coverage, trade publications, directory listings, etc.). From there, you can evaluate the associations and certification groups that best fit your needs.

publications that include up-to-date information relevant to the industry; most of the best-known and award-winning massage magazines are published by professional associations. AMTA puts out *Massage Therapy Journal,* and ABMP issues *Massage and Bodywork.* Some therapists prefer to subscribe to publications that are not affiliated with any group but serve solely to inform members of the industry. *Massage Magazine* and the online *Massage Today* are both unaffiliated publications.

Great job! In this chapter you've tested your ethical mettle and learned a great deal about the professional issues faced by massage therapists. Remember that ethics, professional development, and recordkeeping are not things that you learn once and are done with, but rather represent an ongoing commitment to upholding professional standards. With strong professional development skills, a knack for documentation, unflappable professional ethics, and solid boundaries, there is no stopping you in your new career!

CHAPTER SUMMARY BY LEARNING OBJECTIVES

1. **Define and explore ethics and professionalism for the massage therapist** Ethics addresses questions of morality, specifically the issues and definitions of right and wrong. Many of the professional ethics of massage therapists have been universally agreed upon and codified by professional massage organizations. Like so many other medical and healing professions, the ethics that govern massage therapy are based in the Hippocratic Oath, which promises to treat all people fairly and with the best intentions, to preserve all life, and to maintain patient confidentiality. Good ethics and professionalism are essential ingredients for a successful massage career.
2. **Distinguish important documentation and the importance of keeping records** Documentation is the written record of anything that happens within your practice, from tracking finances to keeping detailed notes of client sessions. Recordkeeping is the process of organizing, filing, and storing that information for future use. Good documentation and recordkeeping help you to better serve clients, establish goals, and track progress, work with other healthcare practitioners, work with insurance providers, and can protect you in a legal situation. SOAP notes are one of the most important documents for massage therapists.
3. **Explore the complexity of relationships between massage therapist and client** As bodyworkers, the question of how to build a therapeutic relationship and successfully care for clients while maintaining boundaries in the relationship is an ongoing challenge. Therapists need to be aware of common issues such as power differentials, dual relationships, transference, and countertransference.
4. **Define different boundaries for the massage therapist** In order to protect the integrity and clarity of the therapeutic relationship, it is essential that the therapist define and maintain strong boundaries. These can be communicated verbally, energetically, physically, or in writing. Boundaries exist on many levels, including professional, personal, financial, and legal.
5. **Characterize sexual misconduct and identify preventative courses of action** Sexual misconduct is any behavior or activity that aims to sexualize the relationship between a client and a therapist. Sexual misconduct can be initiated and perpetuated by either party, and exists along a continuum of severity from minor to serious. There are things that therapists can do to prevent misconduct by either party, such as clear communication, clear boundaries, and vigilant interpersonal awareness.
6. **Analyze gender and the massage therapist** According to a study by the U.S. Department of Labor in 2006, 84 percent of all massage therapists are female, leaving male therapists to face unique challenges within the profession. Many male therapists report that they are the recipients of gender discrimination at various points along their career path. Both male and female therapists can work together to respectfully educate clients and equalize the profession.
7. **Evaluate opportunities for the male therapist** Many clients prefer a male therapist over a female therapist for myriad reasons, such as comfort levels, religious convictions, and physical strength. Many clients are simply gender-blind and are happy working with a talented therapist, regardless of gender.
8. **Identify requirements for licensing, certifications, and national exams** A professional license is an authorization granted to trained and qualified individuals to perform their occupation in a designated jurisdiction. National certification is the confirmation of professional characteristics, values, and expertise as assessed through external examination by a certifying organization. Two predominant organizations provide licensing exams to therapists and bodyworkers at the national level: NCBTMB and FSMTB. However, licensing regulations vary and are determined by local and state authorities.
9. **Explore relevant professional associations and trade publications** In the United States, there are hundreds of different professional groups for massage therapists (see Appendix B for a partial list of popular associations). The three main groups are American Massage Therapy Association (AMTA), Associated Bodywork and Massage Professionals (ABMP), and International Massage Association (IMA).

ACTIVITIES

Quiz: Identifying Professional Issues: Words and Concepts

1. A boundary crossing is _____.
   a. an overstepping of a boundary that may or may not be harmful to an individual
   b. an overstepping of a boundary that is definitely harmful to an individual
   c. a place on the highway where cars stop to let boundaries cross
   d. a targeted attack on a client
2. Right to _____ is the entitlement to protect personal or sensitive information and to reveal that information selectively.
   a. safety
   b. informed consent
   c. party
   d. privacy
3. The five subcategories of professional boundaries are:
   a. logical, environmental, sensual, financial, and feelings
   b. intellectual, physical, emotional, sexual, and energetic
   c. physiological, safety, belonging, esteem, and self-actualization
   d. personal, professional, financial, legal, and emotional
4. A massage therapist that repeatedly undervalues his service or does not enforce his own cancellation policy is not respecting his own _____ boundary.
   a. legal
   b. financial
   c. client
   d. emotional
5. The Hippocratic Oath is _____.
   a. a vow exchanged between massage educator and student
   b. a promise made by clients to follow treatment
   c. a pledge taken by holistic and traditional medical providers
   d. a promise made between hippopotami
6. SOAP notes are used by health professionals and include information that is:
   a. Subjective, Objective, Assessment, and Plan
   b. Personal, Impartial, Evaluative, and Map
   c. Succinct, Optional, Accurate, and Proper
   d. Indifferent, Subjective, Diagnostic, and Improvised
7. The two main organizations that standardize and administer national licensing exams include the _____ and the _____.
   a. American Massage Therapy Association (AMTA), Association of Bodywork and Massage Professionals (ABMP)
   b. International Massage Association (IMA), American Association of Alternative Healing (AAAH)
   c. National Certification Board for Therapeutic Massage & Bodywork (NCBTMB), Federation of State Massage Therapy Boards (FSMTB)
   d. Day Spa Association, Esalen Massage and Bodywork Association
8. _____ is an assurance that any information communicated between therapist and client is privileged and protected.
   a. Secrecy
   b. An open-door policy
   c. Indiscretion
   d. Confidentiality
9. If a massage therapist treats a client who is also a friend or family member, a/n _____ occurs.
   a. bad situation
   b. ruined friendship
   c. optimal relationship
   d. dual relationship
10. True or False: Once you obtain a business license, you do not need to worry about getting a professional or occupational license.
11. True or False: Even though it is taboo to have a sexual relationship with a client, it doesn't result in any major repercussions.
12. True or False: The ratio of male to female therapists is very disproportionate and male therapists often experience gender discrimination from clients and other professionals.
13. True or False: HIPAA requires that all medical providers inform clients about their privacy rights, explain why any information is collected, and make clear how information will be used and safeguarded.
14. True or False: Massage trade publications can be an invaluable resource for massage therapists who want to keep current with trends in the industry.
15. True or False: Only clients are susceptible to transferring feelings, aversions, or attachments onto a therapist.

Discussion Questions

What would you do: Get together with a partner, and choose two of the scenarios below. Discuss how you each might handle the situations. Try to look at all of the circumstances, and give the matter thorough consideration.

1. You are a male student in massage school, and during class you have been spending a lot of time with Jerusha, your classmate. You often sit together and pair up when practicing new techniques. You realize that you find Jerusha very attractive, but are not sure if pursuing a relationship with a classmate would jeopardize professional ethics. After class one day, Jerusha asks you on a date. What do you do?
2. Chris and Kwame are close friends who both come to see you for regular massage. Chris has recently been diagnosed with cancer, and has disclosed this information to you. During a session, Kwame begins to press you for information about Chris's recent withdrawal, and to ask how his massage treatments have been going. You know that Chris and Kwame are very close, and assume Kwame already knows about the cancer. What do you do?
3. John is one of your close friends from school. He is incredibly friendly and personable, and people seem to gravitate to him constantly. At lunch, John tells you that he hangs out with many of his clients and that he is planning to go on a fishing trip with one of his clients next week. What do you think of this? Do you say anything to John, and if so, what?
4. You are a female therapist. Mitch, a young professional about your age, has been referred to you by another client. You recognize an immediate attraction to Mitch, and become almost agitated during his session. You do your best to ignore your feelings and act professionally. However, Mitch schedules several more appointments, and each time you recognize the same attraction. What do you do?
5. Elise is a client who started coming to you for relief from her chronic headaches. She is quiet and withdrawn, and stays silent during her massages. During your first session, you notice bruises on her arm, which she explains as a result of a fall. After a few more sessions, more mysterious bruises appear which Elise quickly explains away. You begin to suspect an abusive situation, although Elise does not disclose anything to you. What do you do?
6. You are a female massage therapist who is having routine backaches. A colleague recommends that you go to see another therapist, George, who specializes in low back pain and offers great prices. You quickly book an appointment, and get in the next day. You chose not to mention that you are a therapist. Although the session begins well, George begins to employ techniques (such as crossing private areas with forearms to work acceptable areas with hands) and work in areas that make you incredibly uncomfortable. In the immediate situation, what do you do? And when the session finishes, what do you do?

Case Study

Delena

Delena has been practicing massage for six years, and prides herself on her professionalism and love for her career. She specializes in sports massage, athletic performance enhancement, and injury recovery. She operates a small but successful practice, and has a clientele comprised evenly of male and female clients. An amateur athlete herself, she loves helping her clients maintain active lifestyles and achieve optimal performance.

One of Delena's clients is Rob, a good-humored and intelligent man who comes to see her once a week. He has been coming to see her just over two years with the goal of maintaining and supporting very rigorous athletic training. Although Delena is about 20 years younger than Rob, they have always had a very natural rapport and have easy conversations during his sessions. About a year and a half into their therapeutic relationship, Rob invited Delena and her boyfriend to join him and his wife, Kate, for a museum exhibition. Although Delena didn't usually socialize with her clients outside of work, she really wanted to see the exhibit and accepted the free tickets. The four of them had a great time during the evening, and another invitation to a ski weekend ensued. Soon the two couples were hanging out more frequently; Rob and his wife had a great deal of money, and were happy to treat the young couple to dinners, concerts, and cultural events. Although Delena wasn't sure about developing a dual relationship, she really admired Rob and Kate's relationship and was captivated by the lifestyle and resources of the older couple.

As their relationship evolved, Rob began to open up more to Delena during massage sessions. He began to disclose problems he was having with Kate, initially sharing things as regular marriage challenges. In time, however, he shared stories of Kate's drug and alcohol abuse, revealing more and more of an unhappy and dysfunctional picture than Delena ever imagined. Several months went by, and as she listened to Rob during his sessions, she remembered issues in her own parents' marriage. In time, Rob began asking Delena out for lunch to "talk through his emotions." Delena was so compelled to help and to be there for Rob as a friend that she began meeting him for lunch. However, she couldn't help but notice that both of their demeanors were changing during their lunches, and that their behavior was bordering more and more on flirtation. They began communicating frequently throughout the day. Delena waved concerns away, telling herself that they were just friends. Besides, she was being honest with her own boyfriend about the relationship and that nothing physical ever occurred between them.

Rob then started bringing Delena gifts, some from his travels and some "just because." When her car broke down, Rob even lent her his own. Delena basked in the glow of this attention and friendship, ensuring herself that she hadn't crossed any "real" boundaries. However, the bond between them was growing more and more emotionally intimate, and she had to admit to herself that she was thinking of Rob romantically. *Still,* she justified to herself, *nothing physical has happened. I haven't violated any boundaries. We're just good friends. I can't help the way I feel.*

One day, just before leaving for a trip, Rob insisted that he had to see her and invited her to lunch. At lunch he told her that he had fallen in love with Delena—who truly understood him as no one had in years—and was leaving his wife. Though no sexual or romantically physical contact whatsoever had passed between them, he was saying he loved her and talking about leaving his wife for her. Delena was at once delighted and mortified. What had she done? And what would she do next?

Case Study Questions

You are Delena's close friend and she has come to you with this story. She is seeking your advice, but before you can give it, answer the following questions.

1. Do you think the situation between Rob and Delena is realistic? Do you think it is possible for a therapist not to notice or acknowledge when boundaries slide gradually?
2. At what point do you think Delena first crossed a line in her therapeutic relationship with Rob?
3. What role, if any, do you think transference and countertransference played in this situation?
4. Do you think the fact that there was no physical contact or sexual intimacy changes the situation at all?
5. What do you think Delena should do in this situation?
6. Do you identify with either Rob or Delena at all? Have you ever been in a similar situation? If not, can you imagine yourself being in one? What did you do or would you have done differently?

CHAPTER 5

Self-Care

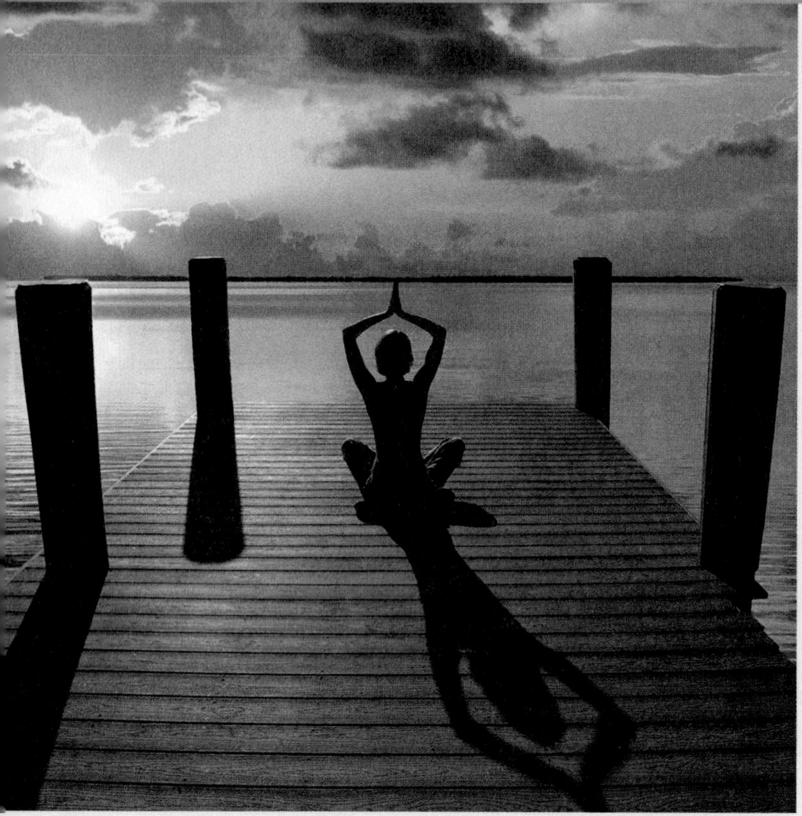

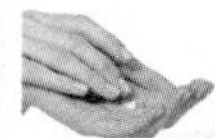

CHAPTER OUTLINE

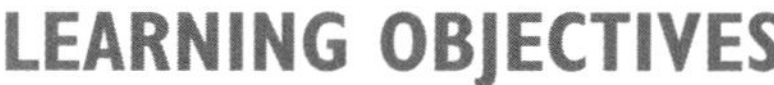

LEARNING OBJECTIVES

1. Illustrate the importance of taking care of the caretaker
2. Explain the concept of "healthy selfish"
3. Identify foreseeable stressors for massage therapists
4. Examine techniques to manage stress
5. Define and create a self-care mission statement
6. Craft a self-care plan
7. Develop a good support system
8. Examine internal versus external nurturing
9. Review the importance of boundaries

KEY TERMS

accountability partner *84*
business stressors *80*
career stressors *81*
compassion fatigue *80*
healthy selfishness *79*
self-care *78*
self-care mission statement *82*
self-care plan *82*
stress *81*
stressor *80*
support system *84*

SELF-CARE

While you probably became a massage therapist so that you could help other people, if you are going to have any sustainable longevity in your career, it is imperative that you put yourself at the top of your priority list. Longtime healers know that taking care of the caregiver is one of the most important secrets of success. **Self-care** is the practice of putting your own needs first and nourishing your own spiritual, emotional, mental, and physical health before another's. At first blush, it may seem like a chapter on self-care doesn't necessarily belong in a book about business, or at most could be a paragraph in the chapter on professional development. However, far too many therapists fail to make self-care a priority, and failure to do so can be incredibly detrimental to you, your clients, your career, your business, and your life. It can be a major factor of burnout, illness, injury, job dissatisfaction, and career departure.

One of the primary reasons to practice self-care is to set a good example for your clients, who will often be looking to you for self-care guidance. Although you will likely coach your clients on ways to care for themselves, reduce stress, and find balance, often holistic practioners do not practice what they preach and pay little attention to their own ongoing self-care. As one therapist observed, "It's hard to sell what you won't buy." This can result in subsequent mental, physical, and emotional burnout, which is a prime catalyst for leaving the profession.[1] Jillian Guthrie, founder of Healers in Balance, says that many holistic professionals suffer from a malady known as "forget thyself," in which the practitioner puts all emphasis on helping others and fails to recognize that he is deteriorating mentally, physically, emotionally, financially, or spiritually.[2] And how beneficial to others or successful in your own career can you be when that happens?

Conventional typecasting holds that self-care is a much more difficult concept for women, who are traditionally taught to be the caregivers of society. However, interviews with many male therapists have revealed that they, too, struggle with the concept and implementation of self-care often just as much as

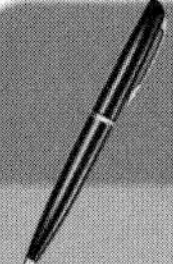

PUT IT IN WRITING
Self-Care Quiz

It can be challenging to fit in everything that needs to be done in a day, let alone ensure your own self-care. How good are you at nourishing yourself and finding balance in your life?

1. I have a circle of friends to whom I can go and talk when I need to process things in my life.
   1-not at all 2-rarely 3-sometimes 4-often 5-always
2. I make it a habit to exercise several times a week.
   1-not at all 2-rarely 3-sometimes 4-often 5-always
3. I enjoy many hobbies that bring me joy and diversion.
   1-not at all 2-rarely 3-sometimes 4-often 5-always
4. I am connected with my body and know how to respond positively when it communicates signals such as stress, pain, hunger, or fatigue.
   1-not at all 2-rarely 3-sometimes 4-often 5-always
5. I participate in my own regular spiritual discipline, which fortifies me.
   1-not at all 2-rarely 3-sometimes 4-often 5-always
6. My diet supports my optimal health, and I incorporate fruits, vegetables, and whole foods into my meals.
   1-not at all 2-rarely 3-sometimes 4-often 5-always
7. I surround myself with positive people who encourage and support my goals.
   1-not at all 2-rarely 3-sometimes 4-often 5-always
8. I take frequent breaks and can recognize when I need one to regenerate.
   1-not at all 2-rarely 3-sometimes 4-often 5-always
9. When I leave work, I really leave work. I am able to draw a line between my personal and professional time.
   1-not at all 2-rarely 3-sometimes 4-often 5-always
10. When it is necessary to preserve my health and sanity, I can say "no" without feeling guilty.
   1-not at all 2-rarely 3-sometimes 4-often 5-always

Use the score key below to tally up your results.

46–50: There is nothing standing in the way of you and your commitment to taking care of yourself, and you serve as an example to your clients. You are in a great position to thrive in your holistic career. Great job! This chapter can help reinforce the positive habits you already have implemented.

37–45: On the whole you are very dedicated to taking care of yourself and are therefore in a better position to care for your clients. A few things may divert your attention from self-care mastery, but this chapter aims to help you get there.

28–36: You have some pretty good self-care techniques in place, but you would like to learn some ways to stay committed and to stave off foreseeable stressors so your self-care goals aren't thrown off track so easily. Keep reading!

19–27: You try to take care of yourself, but you are easily distracted from regularly nourishing yourself and often pulled by the whims of others. This chapter will help you make self-care a more focal priority in your practice.

10–18: You tend to put everyone else's needs ahead of your own and find that when it's your turn there is little left. But do not despair. This chapter will teach you great tools to make a change.

their female colleagues. In fact, many men said that the concept of self-nurturing was particularly difficult, as they are not always provided the tools, techniques, or external permission to do so. Thus, self-care is an area that both male and female therapists need to be committed to developing if they are serious about a thriving career in massage therapy.

HEALTHY SELFISH

For many people, putting oneself at the top of the list and taking care of "me first" feels counterintuitive. After all, isn't putting yourself above everyone else selfish, and not the trait of a good healer? In short, absolutely not. One of the best expressions to come out of self-help and psychotherapy in recent years is the term *healthy selfish*. **Healthy selfishness** is the practice of systematically ensuring one's own needs are cared for before attending to the needs of another. The paradox of this concept is that it is imperative to be selfish before you can be any good to anyone else or even think about being an effective contributor to anyone's healing process. If you are stressed out, injured, financially burdened, or ill, you have little to give to your clients, your family, your friends, or anyone else.

If you've ever flown on an airplane and are one of the rare few who actually listen to the flight attendants' safety demonstration, you know that when those little masks fall from the overhead compartment, it is crucial that you secure your own oxygen mask before helping another. After all, what good are you to anyone else if you yourself cannot breathe? The flight attendants themselves know to always preserve their own well-being first in the event of an emergency, and are told throughout their training "you are the most important person on that plane." In your massage therapy career, YOU are the most important person. No matter what your vocational calling, not taking care of your own needs first will put you on the fast track to burnout.

If you are like most other therapists who are attracted to this profession, you pursued this path because you want to help others. You will likely be advising clients on ways to optimize their own health, to cut back on stressors, and to take better care of themselves. But how successful can you be if you do not commit to a self-care plan yourself? Your effectiveness as a massage therapist, an employee, and even a business owner will increase dramatically if you make self-care a cornerstone of your practice. Thus healthy selfishness needs to become a tenet of your career and a driving factor in the choices you make.

> *The perfect man of old looked after himself before looking to help others.*
>
> —Chuang Tze

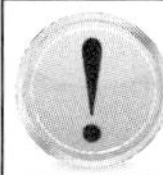

PITFALLS

Even when you are clear on the need for self-care, it is not uncommon to get some external pushback from those around you when you first begin to put yourself first. Selfishness is a dirty word for many people, and it can feel threatening to others to hear "no" from you when it isn't a word you use much. But remember, there is a very big distinction between narcissistic selfishness (which validates your needs at the *expense* of others) and healthy selfishness (which honors your needs for mutual benefit). Being able to articulate this concept to others not only helps them give you the space to self-nourish, it can help them understand the importance of it in their own life.

So where to begin? Do you have to start greedily hoarding or throwing elbows to be healthy selfish? Of course not. Healthy selfishness may be something as simple as getting more fruits and vegetables in your diet. It may be going to a yoga class, going for Mexican food with a friend, reading a book, watching a movie, taking refuge in nature, saying no to the PTA president, or painting your toenails. Everyone has their own ways to self-nourish, and you need to discover your own (see the "First Steps" exercise that follows). One suggestion that is highly recommended and one you likely have had drilled into your head during massage school: get lots of bodywork yourself. Not only will it help you maintain your body throughout all the physical demands of your career, it will help you to be a better therapist by experiencing different techniques.

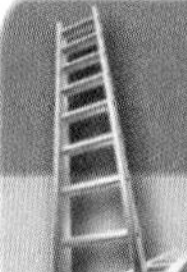

FIRST STEPS

When it comes to defining optimal self-care, there are a lot of "shoulds" out there. Rather than getting bogged down in the mire of someone else's lists of what is good for your self-care, take some time to really examine the things that energize and nourish YOU. Close your eyes and visualize things that you love to do, things that really bring you alive. See yourself doing or receiving these things, and engage as many senses as you can in your image. When you have a good image, write it down here, including as many details as possible:______________________________

____

____

This is your first step to a sustainable self-care plan: having self-defined activities to nourish yourself that are not prescribed by anyone else. Before you implement a laundry list of "shoulds" into your plan, take time to ensure the things you include are things you really love and will stick with.

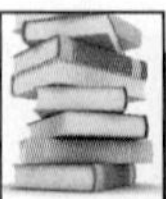

HELPFUL RESOURCES

Sometimes it can be helpful to read about ways that others have made self-care a priority in their lives. It can be easier to parlay tips from others into sustainable habits of your own. Check out *Healthy Selfishness: Getting the Life You Deserve without the Guilt* by Drs. Rachael and Richard Heller (2005, Meredith Books) or *Self-Nurture: Learning to Care for Yourself as Effectively as You Care for Everyone Else* by Alice Domar and Henry Dreher (2001, Penguin Books).

Many people who are not accustomed to putting themselves first can get very frustrated at the beginning of implementing a self-care regimen and give up before they really begin. It can be challenging to interrupt external caregiving patterns and grant yourself permission to be "healthy selfish," especially if you have never done if before. Be patient in the beginning, and understand that self-care is an ongoing investment in your career and to your overall well-being.

IDENTIFY STRESSORS

Any career can come with a lot of demands, challenges, and stressors, and massage therapy is no different. Later in this chapter you will learn more about the effects of stress, but surely you already have a fairly good grasp on what it is and what it does. One of the best ways for handling and countering anxiety and pressure is to anticipate their sources. This enables you to be prepared with proactive responses and preemptive planning that will support your self-care. A **stressor** is any event, person, situation, or change that provokes a stress reaction in the body and mind. Stressors can be anything that an individual perceives as a threat, irritation, or obstacle in achieving a desired goal. They can be environmental (overcrowding), relational (divorce), or even mundane (lost keys). Take a moment to consider the potential stressors that often take a toll on massage therapists (see Figure 5-1 ■).

Massage can be a very *physically* demanding job, and over time it can have a substantial impact on the body. There is a massive output of energy in every massage you administer, and you may be on your feet for hours and hours at a time. In addition, you may be rushing between appointments to change the sheets, talk with clients, and attend to administrative duties and biological needs. Even with incredibly sound body mechanics, the physical requirements of this career require a great deal of balancing self-care.

> *When health is absent . . . Wisdom cannot reveal itself. Art cannot become manifest. Strength cannot be exerted. Wealth is useless and reason is powerless.*
>
> —Heraphilies

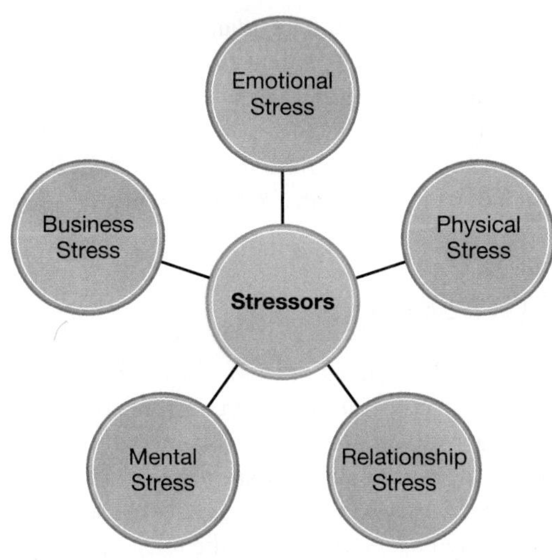

FIGURE 5-1

Stressors can come in many forms; some of the most common ones are emotional, physical, financial, business, relationship, and mental stress.

Massage can also be very difficult on you *mentally*. You are constantly assessing the optima treatments for clients' ever-shifting physiological conditions. You are constantly engaging your intellect and assessing your knowledge of the anatomy, physiology, pathology, and kinesiology you learned in school and beyond in order to service your clients in an effective and therapeutic manner. You will also need to be very aware of updates and new technologies in your area of specialization. And your commitment to continuing education will ensure that your learning curve often slopes up (see Chapter 2 for more on continuing education).

Even the most seasoned and professional massage therapists will admit that there are *emotional* challenges present in their business. Because massage is such a personal service, it is not uncommon to be effected by the suffering of your clients, especially if you are dealing with clients with chronic pain or disease. Caregivers and holistic healers of all kinds can be susceptible to what psychologists call **compassion fatigue**, in which one's constant exposure to the pain and affliction of others in the absence of balancing measures results in a decreased ability to care effectively for oneself. This term is used interchangeably with secondary post-traumatic stress disorder, and is a common affliction of those in healing professions.[3]

And of course, managing a career or owning your own practice can bring a whole other realm of professional pressures and over time that stress can have a very detrimental effect on your body, mind, relationships, and career. There are many kinds of stressors associated with being both an employer and an employee.[4] **Business stressors** are the situations, events, and circumstances relating to running a business that put special demands on a business owner. These include the pressure to market and attract clients, manage other individuals, pay all the bills, pay taxes, and so forth.

A bad economy affects everyone, but when you own the business, financial responsibilities and stress can seem much more acute. After all you are assuming more risk and responsibility when you own a business than when you work for someone else. This is especially true with massage, which is often described as a feast-or-famine industry.

But you don't have to be the boss to have work-related stress. **Career stressors** often have an adverse effect on employees, and can include job insecurity, insufficient income, an overwhelming and unrealistic workload, or unpleasant working conditions.[5] If you are working with other people, you will invariably have to deal with the ups and downs of interpersonal dynamics. The working relationship with a manager or boss can be a source of real stress for many employees if there is a personality difference or conflict. Feeling undervalued, underrespected, or underpaid for the hard work you are doing can also be a major career stressor. If left unchecked, job stressors can be a significant contributing factor to burnout and exodus for massage therapists.

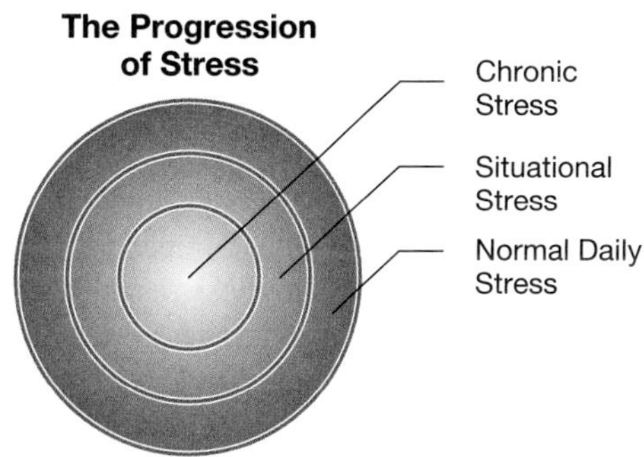

FIGURE 5-2

If not managed, regular daily stresses can progress into chronic stress.

GETTING A HANDLE ON STRESS

As you saw in the last section, stress is an inevitable part of life. **Stress** is a mental or physical reaction to the people and situations in life, and the perceived pressure that these things can bring to an individual. Events that present obstacles to the achievement of one's goals, environmental changes, life transitions, and myriad other factors can trigger a stress response.[6] Not only is stress unavoidable, it is a normal part of life and can be a catalyst for a lot of positive things in life. It has certainly helped the human race survive throughout its existence, saving our ancestors from saber tooth tigers, natural disasters, and starvation. Stress can motivate you to move forward and give you the incentive to make changes in a situation. Intense and prolonged stress, however, can present a very serious problem (see Figure 5-2 ■.)

A stress response is triggered in the body when an individual perceives any kind of danger or demand. Powerful neurochemicals and hormones are released in the body and prepare it for immediate action—this is the "fight or flight" response. The sympathetic nervous system is kicked into high gear: heart rate increases, pupils dilate, skeletal muscles increase strength, mental activity soars, and the body perspires.[7] This is certainly helpful when your life is in danger, but the body often cannot tell the difference between real and perceived threats. You may not have a tiger chasing you, but your body may offer up the same reaction to more trivial menaces. A looming deadline, a job interview, a bad economy, a screaming child, a traffic jam, a bounced check—anything can trigger the physiological stress response in the body. Prolonged, unmanaged stress can be incredibly detrimental to health and can debilitate

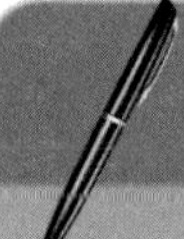

PUT IT IN WRITING
Challenges and Stressors

There are many other challenges and stressors in massage therapy that were not mentioned in the preceding paragraphs. Take a moment and see if you can anticipate some of the challenges that you might face in your career or in your business. Come up with three things for each of the categories below

Physical tolls: ________ ________ ________

Mental tolls: ________ ________ ________

Emotional tolls: ________ ________ ________

Spiritual tolls: ________ ________ ________

Business stressors: ________ ________ ________

Career stressors: ________ ________ ________

Now is the chance for you to preempt the challenges you face by coming up with creative ways to counter them. For each of the additional stressors you came up with above, write down a solution or a counter for each one below.

Physical tolls: ________ ________ ________

Mental tolls: ________ ________ ________

Emotional tolls: ________ ________ ________

Spiritual tolls: ________ ________ ________

Business stressors: ________ ________ ________

Career stressors: ________ ________ ________

you. It can lead to psychological disorders such as post-traumatic stress disorder or acute stress reaction.[8] It is very hard to be a successful healer or massage professional when you are coping with chronic stress.

Many people deal with stress through drugs, alcohol, nicotine, food, or other self-medications. Ironically, these coping mechanisms usually exacerbate stress responses,[9] and the addictions that follow add fuel to the stress fire. In fact, many people are actually addicted to the stress itself. Studies have found that the adrenaline rush that accompanies stress can be habit forming.[10] If you are an individual who has had chronic stress in your life, you may need to do some work to handle that dependence before you can focus on nourishing yourself. Although many people think that these are the same things (nourishing yourself = reducing stress), some people need to deal with underlying stress addiction issues before they can settle into a self-nourishing routine.[11] Below are a few techniques for handling acute and chronic stress:

- Seek medical attention
- Psychotherapy
- Hypnotherapy
- Avoid alcohol, drugs, caffeine, and nicotine
- Meditation
- Yoga
- Energy work
- Massage

> *Take care of your body with steadfast fidelity.*
>
> —Goethe

A MISSION OF SELF

In other sections in the book, you will learn the importance of mission statements and their role in business plans, marketing plans, and nearly any kind of plan. Here you will be exploring the value of creating your own self-care mission statement. A **self-care mission statement** is a written declaration of the purpose of self-care in your career. Often the cornerstone of a self-care plan (see the next section), this mission statement can help you connect to the underlying principle of nurturing yourself, define what it means for you, and keep grounded in your commitment to putting yourself first. It's like a mini-contract with yourself to be healthy selfish so that you can paradoxically be of better service to others.

Although your self-care mission statement will be your own and will be worded however you like, you will want to include three key elements: the purpose of self-care, the application of self-care, and the values behind self-care. The purpose explains why it is important to nurture yourself; the application will give an overview of how you will apply self-support, and the values reflect the beliefs you hold that are aligned with the concept of self-care. Below is an example of a massage therapist's self-care mission statement:

> In the spirit of the healer, and with the goal of being a positive change agent in the lives of my massage clients, I commit to nurturing my own body, mind, and spirit in an ongoing and sustainable manner. I understand that the better I am to myself, the better I can be for others. Through healthy boundaries, creative play, and awareness of my limitations, I make a continuing commitment to evaluate and improve upon my self-care plan.

A SELF-CARE PLAN

If you struggle to include self-care in your everyday routine, or if you would like to improve your commitment to taking care of yourself, you might consider a self-care plan. A **self-care plan** is a blueprint of your self-care goals, the reasons you want to achieve them, and how you are going to go about implementing actionable steps to achieve those goals. This plan is driven by your self-care mission statement.

By now you understand that self-care is far more than a fluffy concept or New Age rhetoric; it is rather a mindset that can really make or break a successful career, a sustainable business, and a fulfilling life. As such, you may decide for yourself that something so important warrants some intentional planning on its behalf. Crafting an official plan and making it part of your career strategy will not only help you organize and schedule time to take care of yourself, but will cement your ongoing commitment to healthy selfishness. This section will give you a few ideas on how to craft your own self-care plan.

It's best to keep your plan simple—not only will this make it easier to follow, it will make it easier to create in the first place. Many therapists find that a simple one-sheet checklist makes a great self-care plan; this is something they are able to implement into everyday life, and it is easy to modify. Be specific in the things that nourish you, and include information about the resources or tools you will need to accomplish each thing. For example, rather than write "hike" on your plan, write "a two-mile hike in Mt. Falcon park with hiking shoes, walking hat, sunscreen, and iPod." The more specific you are, the easier it will be to put your plan into practice. And remember, self-care strategies can be anything that nourishes you, not just following generic self-care guidelines.

It may help to think of the ways to nourish the different parts of your life. Refer back to the Wheel of Life exercise in Chapter 1 to refresh your memory of the things you value most. This will help you brainstorm ways to nourish and support the many facets of who you are as a complex person, and help you to achieve more balance in your life. The template in the "Getting Organized" box has sections devoted to mental, physical, spiritual, and social self-care. Keep it interesting for you, and vary the plan frequently. Remember, you do not have to spend a fortune to feed your body, mind and spirit. If you're looking for some ideas that won't break the bank, check out Appendix B for a list of self-care activities on a budget.

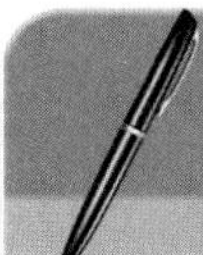

PUT IT IN WRITING

Self-Care Plan

The following is a list of ideas generated from the self-care plans of several massage therapists. Read through them, and then brainstorm more of your own ideas in the space provided.

- Schedule sufficient breaks between appointments
- Leave the car at home two days a week and walk instead
- Get a massage every other week
- Floss teeth
- Eat five fruits and/or vegetables a day
- Sleep 8 hours
- See my grandparents every weekend
- Meditate/pray
- 30 minutes of exercise every day
- Turn off TV three nights a week and read a book instead
- Write in my journal before bed each night

Now what would you like to include in your plan? Write out some ideas here:____

____

____

____

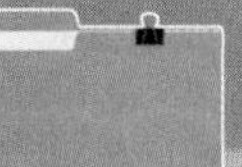

GETTING ORGANIZED

Self-Care Plan Template

The first lines of a sample self-care plan template have been filled out by Marta, a massage therapist, but the rest is for you to fill out. This provides a guide to craft your own self-care plan. Make any changes you like to reflect areas of importance to you, but be sure to include as many specifics as possible to ensure that you put your plan into action. Revamp your self-care plan frequently to keep it fresh, relevant, and useful to you, and store it in your *Business of Massage Therapy* notebook for easy reference. (You can also find a self-care plan template in Appendix B.)

A. Mental (continuing education, read a book, take a class, write an article, learn something new, etc.)

	Pursuit	When	What I need	Completed
1.	Read new book on lymphatic drainage	every night before bed	book, glasses	✓
2.				
3.				
4.				
5.				

B. Physical (exercise, diet/nutrition, sleep, massage, health care, etc.)

	Pursuit	When	What I need	Completed
1.	Yoga class	every Tues. at 7 pm	strap, mat, loose clothes, punch card	✓
2.				
3.				
4.				
5.				

C. Social (time with spouse/partner, family occasions, book club, dinner with friends, networking events, etc.)

	Pursuit	When	What I need	Completed
1.	Date night with husband	every Mon. night	cocktail dress, pearls, strappy shoes	✓
2.				
3.				
4.				
5.				

D. Spiritual (prayer, meditation, religious groups, retreat, pilgrimage, etc.)

	Pursuit	When	What I need	Completed
1.	Semana Santa in Antigua, Guatemala	April 2012	airline tickets, passport, suitcase, camera, etc.	
2.				
3.				
4.				
5.				

You have to stay in shape. My grandmother, she started walking five miles a day when she was 60. She's 97 today and we don't know where the hell she is.

—Ellen Degeneres

DEVELOP A GOOD SUPPORT SYSTEM

No matter how solid your self-care plan, how involved your checklists, or how committed you are to watering every single seedling inside of you, it is easy to get derailed and distracted from self-care initiatives. There will always be clothes to be washed, children to be fed, pets to be watered, bills to be paid, e-mails to return, and all the other cogs that need attention in order to make that Wheel of Life go round. Throw in the unforeseen circumstances, emergencies, special events, and surprising opportunities and it can be incredibly difficult to stay focused on your commitment to self-care. After all, no one can do it all.

A great strategy for staying on track with your plan is to leverage your support team. If you don't already have a support system in place, you may want to develop one. A **support system** is a network of resources and people who offer mutual assistance to one another, and help sustain one another through the highs and lows of life. A support system can be comprised of family members, friends, colleagues, professional groups, religious figures, or anyone that you trust to be there for you when you need them. You can work with household members to make the distribution of housework more equitable, or explain to your children that you aren't to be disturbed when you're writing in your bedroom. Communicate your support needs to those in your immediate circle.

Many people also enlist accountability partners from their pool of support to stay true to their plan. An **accountability partner** is a trusted friend, family member, or colleague who helps you stay responsible to the self-nurturing goals that you have set for yourself. Similar to coaches and mentors, accountability partners check in with one another often to ensure that they are fulfilling all of the tasks and goals to which each person has committed. For example, if you would like to make exercise a regular part of your routine, ask a friend to be a workout partner and meet you at the gym three times a week. A 2008 Gallup poll showed that nearly 70 percent of people who have successfully lost

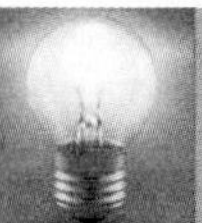

BRIGHT IDEAS
Mapping Your Support

It can be very helpful to have a visual of the satellites of good people orbiting around you and creating your support network. Figure 5-3 ■ is an example of a great support map. Take a look at it, and then create your own.

Now fill out your own (Figure 5-4 ■). Include people you already have in your network, as well as individuals or relationships you would like to develop. Add additional circles if you need to.

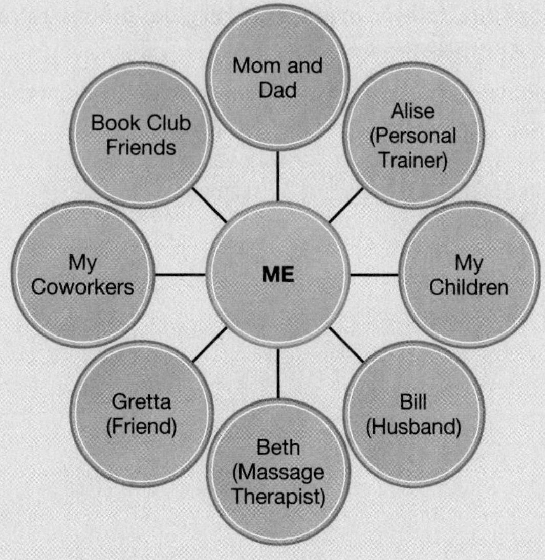

FIGURE 5-3

An example of a massage therapist's support map.

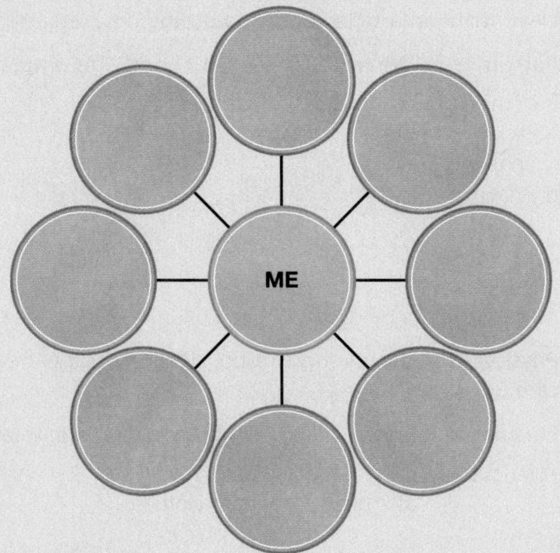

FIGURE 5-4

Blank support map.

weight had direct support from friends and family, and 57 percent had accountability partners.[12] Having another person to whom you are accountable can make a huge difference in your success. Accountability partners are a great idea for any goals you set for yourself personally and professionally (or any kind of goal, for that matter).

Your support system can also include professionals who offer reliable services that make your life easier and more manageable. Babysitters, mechanics, doctors, massage therapists, hairstylists, and accountants can all be a part of a solid support system. And your resources in your support network don't necessarily even have to be people. Guidebooks, libraries, the Internet, and even your own journal can help support your endeavors, enhance your efforts, and free up the time you need to devote to your own self-care. When you have a web of good resources and reliable support, the solution to any problem is at hand and your self-care fulfillment becomes easier.

INTERNAL AND EXTERNAL NURTURING

As wonderful as it can be to be surrounded by supportive friends, loving family, and nourishing accountability partners, it is important to not become overly reliant on others for your own self-care. One reason for this is that not everyone has the aforementioned network. You may not have family, or may be geographically removed from the people you love the most, unable to reach out to them for a cup of coffee or a date at the gym. Perhaps you are not a very social person, and find that you need only a few people to provide the support you need. You also might not always have the time to engage other people in your self-care routine. Your day may be so crammed full of obligations and to-dos that you don't have a spare moment to talk but still need outlets for taking care of yourself. All of these may be true, but the most important reason is that you must always be grounded in your ability to give yourself what you need first and foremost, without overly relying on external energies to see you through. Self-reliance is the backbone of self-care.

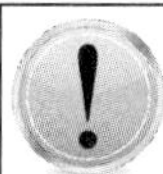

PITFALLS

Many massage therapists will complain that they just do not have the budget for self-care. They would love to go to the spa, get a pedicure, take a trip to Hawaii, or spend hours in therapy. But they just can't afford it. However, nurturing yourself doesn't have to be expensive. Just as with insufficient time, insufficient funds can be little more than an excuse to not take care of you first. See Appendix B for low-cost and no-cost self-care tips.

Some people find their internal strength through their religion or spirituality. Others find it through introspection. Meditating, journaling, listening to music, and working in the garden are all ways that professionals find to develop inner peace. In what ways do you go within to tap into your strength, soothe your wrinkles, and find your everyday sanctuary?

REVIEW THE IMPORTANCE OF BOUNDARIES

In Chapter 4 you learned all about boundaries within the therapeutic relationship, and in Chapter 3 you explored the concept of time wasters and minimizing distractions. This same concepts actually applies to self-care as well. If you are serious about incorporating self-care into your life for the long term, you are going to have to polish your ability to set boundaries. Boundaries are the emotional, mental, and physical space that is placed between oneself and others. Just as you always want to respect the boundaries of your clients, so too will you want to honor your own. Setting clear boundaries can help you avoid injuries and burnout as a massage therapist, and it can help to protect the space required for optimal self-care.

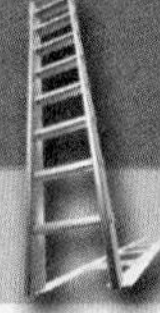

FIRST STEPS

The Sanctuary Jar

This exercise will help you step away from the buzz of the world and retreat into your personal haven. Find a large jar, several pieces of paper, scissors, and some colorful markers. Tear the paper into little scraps, and use the markers to write out all of the things you love to do (draw from other exercises and examples in the chapter if you are having a hard time brainstorming). Write down only things that you can do alone, and keep it simple. Many of the activities could be things that can be done around the house, such as soak in the tub, read a book, bake cookies, paint your toenails, or sing in the garden. Or they could be things that bring you out of doors, like a long walk, a concert, a bike ride, or a hike in the mountains. Try and choose activities that are practical, accessible, and not too difficult to engage in. Fold up all the scraps of paper and place them in your jar. Every day (or several times a week) pull a scrap out of your jar. This grab jar makes your self-care rituals into a game—you never know what you're going to get. And if you don't like what you pull out one day, grab again!

You can only take a client as far as you are willing to go.
—Julie Onofrio, LMT

So what are the ways that you can create boundaries around your self-care plan? Start with creating psychological space for yourself throughout the day. Designate a certain time each day to be "technology free." In a Twitter/Facebook/Blackberry-jammed world, it can often feel like you are perpetually available to everyone else. For one hour a day, give yourself permission to turn of your cell phone, turn off the computer, and shut down any of the media through which the endless noise filters in. It is quite likely that just about anything or anyone can wait for an hour. This will free you up to be more present in the moment, and less beholden to every wave that passes.

You can also give yourself permission to carve out little pockets of "you" time throughout the day. No matter how busy the workday, you can always close your office door and take a few deep breaths. In addition, you need to let go of the desire to be all things to all people. No matter how foreign it feels or how much it hurts, you must learn to say "no."

This chapter has provided you with a lot of tools and techniques to help you cultivate a solid self-care routine. However, all the tools in the world won't help you if you do not take the time to engage them. Doing this will help you be a better massage therapist, a better professional, and an all-around happier person. Even a few minutes a day of healthy selfishness can make all the difference in the world. As you will hear again and again throughout this book, your success will be a composite of many factors, but the most important one is always you.

CHAPTER SUMMARY BY LEARNING OBJECTIVES

1. **Illustrate the importance of taking care of the caretaker** Longtime healers know that taking care of the caregiver is one of the most important secrets of success. Self-care is the practice of putting your own needs first and nourishing your own spiritual, emotional, mental, and physical health before another's.
2. **Explain the concept of "healthy selfish"** Healthy selfishness is the practice of systematically ensuring one's own needs are cared for before attending to the needs of another. The paradox of this concept is that it is imperative to be selfish before you can be an effective contributor to healing.
3. **Identify foreseeable stressors for massage therapists** A stressor is any event, person, situation, or change that provokes a stress reaction in the body and mind. Stressors can be anything that an individual perceives as a threat, irritation, or obstacle in achieving a desired goal. Massage therapists can be affected by career and business stressors that are associated with work conditions. They can also be susceptible to physical, mental, and emotional stress due to the nature of the work.
4. **Examine techniques to manage stress** Stress is a mental or physical reaction to the people and situations in life, and the perceived pressure that these things can bring to an individual. While a normal part of life, excessive stress can be debilitating to the body, mind, and spirit. Although many self-care strategies work to minimize stress, people with prolonged and chronic stress may need to deal with their stress issues first before beginning a self-care plan.
5. **Define and create a self-care mission statement** A self-care mission statement is a written declaration of the purpose of self-care in your career. Often the cornerstone of a self-care plan, a self-care mission statement can help you connect to the underlying principle of self-care, define what it means for you, and stay grounded in your commitment to putting yourself first.
6. **Craft a self-care plan** A self-care plan is a blueprint of your self-care goals, the reasons you want to achieve them, and how you are going to go about implementing actionable steps to achieve those goals. A self-care plan is driven by your self-care mission statement.
7. **Develop a good support system** A support system is a network of resources and people who offer mutual assistance to one another, and help sustain one another through the highs and lows of life. A support system can be comprised of family members, friends, colleagues, professional groups, religious figures, or anyone that you trust to be there for you when you need them. It can also include service professionals, books, or online resources.
8. **Examine internal versus external nurturing** A good support system is very beneficial to achieve self-care goals, and accountability partners can help you stay connected and committed to your plan. However, it is equally important to be able to have an internal source of strength and self-nourishment.
9. **Review the importance of boundaries** Boundaries are the emotional, mental, and physical space that is placed between yourself and others. Just as you always want to respect the boundaries of your clients, so too will you want to honor your own. Setting clear boundaries can help you avoid injuries and burnout as a massage therapist, and it can help to protect the space required for optimal self-care.

ACTIVITIES

Discussion Questions

1. Do you regard yourself as a good self-care taker? What sorts of things do you already do to ensure that your mind, body, and spirit are all cared for?
2. Name three people who are masters at self-care and seem to find ways to strike a balance in many areas of their life. These could be friends, family members, or colleagues. What do these people do to create boundaries and ensure that their self-care is not derailed?
3. What do you think of the term "healthy selfish"? Do you think it is a good way to describe putting yourself first, or can you think of a better way to say it?
4. Take a moment to consider your current or previous job (before you began working as a massage therapist). What was the attitude about self-care in that environment? How did that attitude affect you?
5. When you were growing up, did your parents or caregivers carve out time for themselves? Do you remember your mother going on vacations with friends, or perhaps your father closing the bathroom door for a soak in the tub once a week? What patterns of self-care did you have modeled for you in your young life?
6. What role do you think gender plays in successful self-care plans? Do you think it is easier for men or women to be healthy selfish? Explain your answer.
7. Look at other professionals in other industries. These could be doctors, mechanics, researchers, lawyers, actors, analysts—whatever. Do you think some professions encourage more healthy selfishness? If so, which are they?

Beyond the Classroom

1. Look through massage trade magazines such as *Massage Magazine* or *Massage Therapy Journal*. Seek out any articles about self-care for the massage therapists. (If you do not receive these magazines, many of the articles can also be found online.) How common a theme is this topic in massage media? Do you think it gets enough attention? Too much? How helpful do you find the articles?
2. Interview a massage therapist who has been in the business for at least five years (whether as an employee, business owner, or both). Ask him what his self-care routine has been over the years, and what challenges he has faced in keeping with it. If he does not have a routine or does not incorporate any self-care techniques, ask him how he thinks this has affected his massage career.

CHAPTER

6 Networking

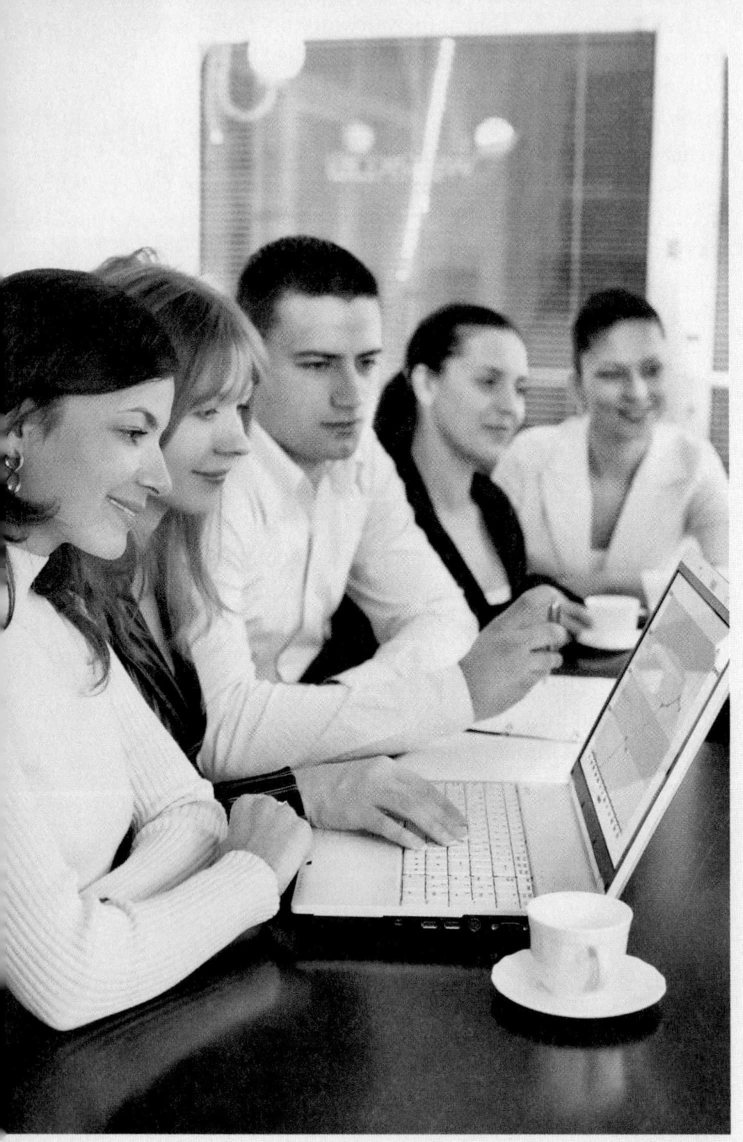

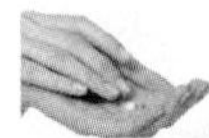

CHAPTER OUTLINE

LEARNING OBJECTIVES

1. Define networking
2. Name the three key ingredients in networking success
3. Explain the importance of networking for your career and the importance of networking authentically
4. Define personal brand and the function of brand loyalty
5. Identify ways to build your own personal brand
6. Demonstrate some of the "dos and don'ts" of networking
7. Illustrate ways to connect with other healing professionals to promote one another collaboratively
8. Explore the usefulness of the Internet, online forums, and social networking for your career
9. Illustrate the value of mentor relationships
10. Discover how to protect yourself professionally

KEY TERMS

brand loyalty *93*
connector *93*
E-networking *96*
exposure *90*
extrovert *91*
image *90*
introvert *91*
mentee *97*
mentor *97*
netiquette *97*
network *90*
networking *90*
online forums *96*
personal brand *91*
scam *99*
skills *90*
social networking *96*
strategic partners *90*

THE IMPORTANCE OF NETWORKING

> *We do not accomplish anything in this world alone . . . and whatever happens is the result of the whole tapestry of one's life and all the weavings of individual threads from one to another that creates something.*
>
> —Sandra Day O'Connor

It may seem like overkill to have an entire chapter devoted to networking. But if you are serious about succeeding in your career, networking is one of the most crucial skills you will need to develop. It is often one of the more underdeveloped skills in the massage community. **Networking** is the art of connecting with other people and building strategic alliances that benefit you, your career, and your business. The beauty of networking is that the benefits can exponentially spread to everyone with whom you network as well. Your **network** is a collection of all the people you know, and consists of personal, professional, educational, and community contacts. In your career, networking is an ongoing process that helps to ensure a constant flow of customers, partners, and opportunities. Networking is important for any profession, though arguably more so in a field like massage therapy, where the service offering is more intimate and the ebb and flow of clientele can be dramatic.

KEY INGREDIENTS OF NETWORKING SUCCESS

Success in personal and professional life is a blend of so many factors; however, many experts will tell you that success is often a seasoned recipe of three primary elements: Skills, image, and exposure. **Skills** are the unique talents that you have that generate value for your clients, employers, or others. For example, if you are accomplished at giving prenatal massages to alleviate the physical discomfort of pregnant women, that is your skill. **Image** is the combination of aspects about yourself that you project to others and that becomes instrumental in the perception others have of you. Many factors work in concert when developing an image: personal appearance, body language, voice, demeanor, clothing, confidence, and behavior are only some of the things that contribute to your overall image. In networking, **exposure** refers to the frequency of contact you have with others. Exposure can be either direct (face to face) or indirect (when someone reads an article you have written or hears about you through word of mouth). Figure 6-1 ■ illustrates the interrelated components of the three keys to success.

When considering the relationship between skill, image, and exposure and assessing their role in your career success, it is important to keep in mind that they are quite interdependent. If you have met someone at several different functions but your image is not compatible with what they value, you may find little success. All the skill in the world doesn't matter if people never hear about you. And even if you have the most polished and pleasing of personal images, if you don't have substantive skills that will solve a problem for others, they will figure out the deficit quickly and seek services elsewhere.

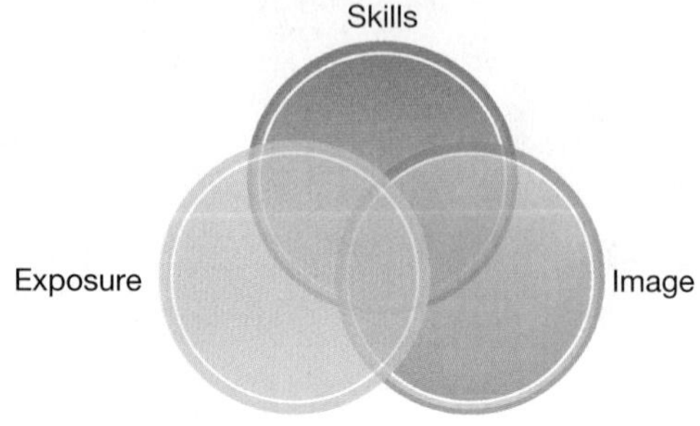

FIGURE 6-1
The three keys of success: Exposure, image, and skills.

WHY NETWORKING MATTERS TO YOU

Many massage therapists that go to work for someone else often make the mistake of believing that they don't need to do anything to promote themselves or their skills; after all, the business isn't their own, and the employer is doing all the marketing and business development. Spending all that energy building someone else's business is a waste of time for an employee. Right?

Wrong. As you saw in Chapter 2, whether you are working for yourself or for an employer, networking is an equally important part of your career development. Networking is a part of self-promotion and marketing. It is important in any profession, and in one as interpersonal and individualized as massage therapy, it is crucial. You should never put your professional development or career potential in the hands of someone else. Employers will want to ensure that clients are coming into the business, but you will want to do whatever you can to make sure they come to see *you.* Later you will learn more about the importance of word of mouth in marketing your skills, earning you referrals and ensuring you business (as both an employee and a business owner). But how will you ever get referrals if people don't even know about you?

Networking can also help you to connect with **strategic partners**, individuals or businesses with which you can ally to enhance each other's success. Perhaps you will encounter clients who need a service you cannot provide, such as nutrition counseling, chiropractic, prenatal care, and so forth. As you network, you begin to meet other service professionals who can add value for your clients, and these individuals can become strategic partners. Strategic partners fortify your toolbox and augment the value you can bring to your clients and your company. Networking now can also result in leads, job offers, new clients, useful resources, or collaborative partnerships later. Networking is one of the most important tools in your promotional and professional arsenal.

For some people, networking comes naturally and can be a very enjoyable process. Some personality types just lend themselves to the act of networking. **Extroverts** are individuals who are energized or nourished by contact with other individuals. The word comes from *extra,* the Latin word for "outside of," and *vertere,* the Latin word for "to turn."[1] Extroverts often look outside of themselves for fun, conversation, and enjoyment, and seem to fade when they are alone too much. They tend to think while they speak, and are quick to engage others, even complete strangers, in conversations.[2] Being drawn to and animated by others can be very advantageous in networking.

Of course not everyone is a natural at networking. If you are uncomfortable in social events, dislike small talk, and feel drained around others, you may be an introvert. **Introverts** are people who are sapped being around other people yet feel energized by being alone. Being an introvert is not necessarily synonymous with being shy or socially inept; introverts can have great social skills and enjoy conversation, but still become drained in social situations. This can make networking more challenging. But if you are an introvert, do not despair or give up on networking altogether. Doing so could thwart your overall career success. Check out the "Helpful Resources" box for books designed to help introverts use innate strengths and characteristics to their advantage.

AUTHENTICITY IN NETWORKING

The rest of this chapter is devoted to exploring and developing networking tools, but before you can engage these, you need to grasp a very important concept. Whether introverts or extroverts, many massage therapists and holistic healers resist the networking process because they feel that it equates with being insincere or having self-serving motives. However, this misses the true intent of networking, which is to build a community. Constructing a professional network and selling your personal brand to potential employers, clients, and strategic partners can absolutely be aligned with living an authentic life.

If you think about networking as a stuffy event where artificiality reigns and business cards clog the air, you may want to reconsider the art in the context of holistic business. Businesses, like communities, are interdependent ecosystems, and they rely on one another. The fact is, you, your career, and even your business will need a network to survive, and you as an individual are the cornerstone of your networking campaign. Other people and businesses need you, too. Everything is interconnected, and when you look at networking from this perspective, you can't help but be authentic in your efforts to make contacts. In business as in life, no one is an island and everyone depends on everyone else to not just survive, but thrive. If you approach this world of networking with the idea that business is abundant and there is enough work for everyone, your rewards will be exponential.

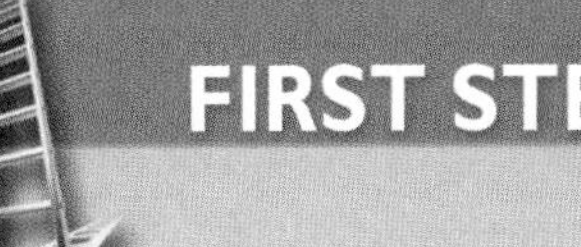

FIRST STEPS

To keep you grounded in authenticity while orienting you toward building a network to support your massage career or holistic business, try this exercise. Identify a networking event in your area that will put you in contact with people you would like to include in your professional ecosystem. Perhaps potential employers or clients might be there, or maybe you would like to find people to barter services with. Before you go to the event, establish your goal as making an authentic connection (whatever that means to you) and exchanging information with just one person there. Making one authentic connection can make all the difference for you and your business—imagine what more will do.

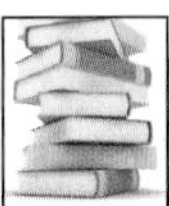

HELPFUL RESOURCES

There are many books designed to help introverts leverage their inherent strengths in networking situations. Check out *Confessions of an Introvert: The Shy Girl's Guide to Career, Networking, and Getting the Most Out of Life* by Meghan Wier (2009, Sphinx Publishing), *Introvert Power: Why Your Inner Life is Your Hidden Strength* by Laurie A. Helgoe (2008, Sourcebooks), and *The Introvert Advantage: How to Thrive in an Extrovert World* by Marti Olsen Laney (2002, Workman).

BUILDING A PERSONAL BRAND

As you will explore in Chapters 11 and 12, developing and maintaining a successful brand is a large part of good marketing and is the cornerstone of a successful company. Experts say that the average person in North America can be exposed to over 16,000 advertisements every day.[3] Companies rely heavily upon advertising to brand their products and services in the minds of their target market—and so can you. Success through branding can also hold true for successful professionals. When you are networking, you are in essence building a personal brand. A **personal brand** is the unique combination of the components that make up who you are and what you have to offer others. A brand consists of all the factors that make you stand out as the unique and incomparable person that you are—your personality, your appearance, your skills, your humor, your individual style.

> *You are the storyteller of your own life and you can create your own legend or not.*
>
> —Isabel Allende

The fact is, you have already been building your brand over the years, perhaps without even realizing it. The associations to which you belong, the company you have kept, the way people react to you, the stories you tell, the way you

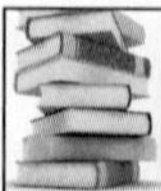

HELPFUL RESOURCES

There are many books on the market devoted to networking. Check out *Never Eat Alone* by Kevin Ferrazi and Tahl Raz (2005, Random House) or *The Brand That Is You* by Peter Montoya and Tim Vandehey (2008, McGraw-Hill).

make others feel, the things for which you are remembered—these are all related to the personal brand you have built. Your brand is your reputation in the community, the image you put forth, and the perceived value to others that you will bring to a situation. It can even be the way you dress, your body language, and the confidence you do or do not exude.[4]

When considering the ongoing crafting of your image and brand as a massage therapist, keep in mind the kind of clients you want to attract. The more you want to appeal to the general public, the more you may want to steer your image into the neutral zone. While there is nothing wrong with religious symbols, tattoos, piercings, dreadlocks, or any other forms of self-expression, keep in mind that some presentations are not acceptable (and can even be offensive) to some clients. Don't ever feel you have to conform into something you are not, but remember that you are there to serve the client, and should consider softening in areas where others might not feel welcome or comfortable.

It is said in business that it is much cheaper to retain existing customers than it is to attract new ones.[5] This conviction holds that once a customer develops allegiance to a brand, they will continue to support it. What is it about certain

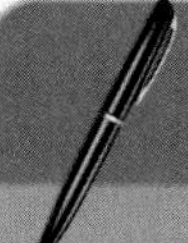

PUT IT IN WRITING

The Brand That Is You

Take some time to explore your own personal brand. Think about the brand you have built for yourself, as well as the brand you would like to build in the future.

1. I think about how my behavior and appearance reflect on me in professional settings.
   a) all the time b) some of the time c) rarely d) never
2. I think about how my behavior and appearance reflect on me in private settings.
   a) all the time b) some of the time c) rarely d) never
3. I can identify five unique components of my personal brand.
   a) all the time b) some of the time c) rarely d) never
4. If asked to, I could write a personal position statement.
   a) all the time b) some of the time c) rarely d) never
5. I am consistent in my behavior and image when I am around others.
   a) all the time b) some of the time c) rarely d) never
6. The way I present myself is consistent with my values and goals.
   a) all the time b) some of the time c) rarely d) never
7. I can readily identify the ways in which my personal characteristics are different from those of coworkers, collaborators, and competitors.
   a) all the time b) some of the time c) rarely d) never
8. I frequently receive accolades, rave reviews, and praise for my performance.
   a) all the time b) some of the time c) rarely d) never
9. Whether at work, school, or in my personal relationships, people respond to me in a similar fashion.
   a) all the time b) some of the time c) rarely d) never
10. Those in my network are able to recognize and express my value.
    a) all the time b) some of the time c) rarely d) never

Scoring Guide

For each a) answer, give yourself a 1.
For each b) answer, give yourself a 2.
For each c) answer, give yourself a 3.
For each d) answer, give yourself a 4.

Sum up your answers, and see where you are with your personal brand.

10–17: You have really made a name for yourself. You are consistent with your personal brand, and have mastered the ways to make all the unique aspects of who you are work dynamically in your favor. Good for you!

18–25: It sounds like you are on the right track. Whether consciously or unconsciously, you are often leveraging your personal brand. If you harness the power of the brand you have already begun developing, you may be surprised at how much you can accomplish for yourself and your career.

26–32: At times you are able to harness the benefits of your personal brand, but often you are not. With the right focus and a little finesse, you can definitely make your personal brand work for you.

33–40 You may not be effectively communicating the fabulous combination of your unique components in a way that is advantageous to you and your career. But it's never to late—look at ways you can develop your brand and get started now!

PITFALLS

Creating a personal brand is not about manipulating yourself into something you are not or falsely influencing the opinion that others have about you. It is instead a way to leverage all of the wonderful characteristics that are uniquely you, and to contribute to your own success by using what you already are. Don't think for a moment that insincerity or dishonesty have anything to do with your own personal branding.

products and services that bring customers back again and again? Think about your own consumption of goods and services. Do you have a toothpaste you always use? How about a favorite cereal? Perhaps you have been going to get your hair done by the same person for 5 years or using the same real estate agent for 20. All of those products and service providers have one thing in common—your loyalty to their brand.

Brand loyalty is a consumer's tendency to purchase repeatedly the goods or services of another. The factors contributing to a consumer's brand loyalty are wide-ranging, and can be anything from perceived value to emotional attachment to lack of viable alternatives.[6] And brand loyalty is not just for products—people develop loyalty to personal brands as well. Think how devastated you were when your hairstylist moved to Austin or your plumber retired. The bottom line is that brand loyalty can work for you and your professional development: the same principles that keep people drinking Starbucks and wearing Nikes can be applied to you and your massage services. With your personal brand, loyalty is intertwined with establishing trust and developing relationships, not only with your employers, clients, or strategic partners, but with anyone you encounter.

Remember—in life and in your career, you are your own chief executive, the CEO of Me, Inc. You are the one responsible for your image at all times. The best part about building your personal brand and establishing personal brand loyalty is that it doesn't have to cost a thing. You don't have to launch an expensive ad campaign, do costly focus groups, or invest in posh marketing materials to hone your personal brand. Later in this chapter you will learn some free and inexpensive ways to leverage the Internet to build your personal brand as a therapist, professional, or even business owner, but in the meantime here are a few tricks to help you get started.

- *Be a connector.* Studies show that both extroverts and introverts can get a thrill out of bringing people together for the benefit of the other parties.[7] A **connector** is a person in a community who knows people across a wide array of circles and makes a habit out of connecting individuals that can mutually benefit by association. If you meet someone who has a problem that needs solving, draw from your pool of connections to offer them resources, and offer to make connections (virtual e-mail connections are fine).
- *Get involved in the community.* Get out there and participate in community events that will position you and your personal brand in a positive light. Love pets? Give chair massage at an ASPC fundraiser fun run, or volunteer for a charity auction for a local animal shelter. The more you participate in things that matter to you, the more others will come to associate you with your values.
- *Get fluent in your own skills.* You have accomplished a lot in your technical training and developed a unique skill set, but it doesn't matter if you can't let others know. Catalog your achievements and unique talents as a therapist, and practice tactful ways to get that information out confidently (hint: elevator pitches and mirror rehearsals work well).
- *Become an expert in your field.* Nothing gives credibility to a personal brand more than demonstrated expertise. You can give talks, teach classes, or write articles for local papers or massage publications touting the benefits of bodywork. Just as with any other profession, people want to employ or get a massage from someone who is a demonstrated expert in his or her field.
- *Be consistent.* Don't present yourself as cheerful and gregarious at one event and than somber and serious at the next. Of course moods will change and you don't want to be false, but projecting different personalities confuses people and dilutes your personal brand. Also, make it a point to fulfill all commitments you make. If you say you're going to call, call.
- *Build relationships.* At the heart of all business you will find relationships. That's the point of networking. Begin to regard your every interaction as an investment in the vital activity of building and maintaining relationships. The true test of any brand is how it makes people feel when they interact with it. When people are around you, how do you make them feel?
- *Keep polishing.* Ongoing education is a prime part of personal branding and continues to add value to what you have to offer to others. Many massage associations require you to take continued learning courses as part of membership, but even if they don't, approach it as a contribution to your professional development or to your own business. If cost is a consideration, look for free or inexpensive classes through a trade association or community center.

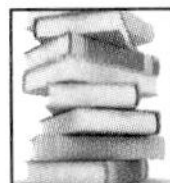

HELPFUL RESOURCES

If you'd like a few more tips on developing your own brand, reference *The Brand Called You* by Peter Montoya and Tim Vandehey (2003, Personal Branding Press) or *Be Your Own Brand* by David McNally and Karl Speak (2002, Berret-Koehler Publishers) for some helpful ideas.

GETTING ORGANIZED
Networking Cheat Sheets

It can be very helpful to create a "cheat sheet" to reference or bring with you when you head out to network. As you go through the "dos and don'ts" of networking below, take notes on the points that seem most helpful to you and keep them on file.

THE "DOS AND DON'TS" OF NETWORKING

Let's face it, when it comes to networking functions, very few people actually look forward to participating. Even the most outgoing extrovert can dislike networking. There can be a lot of social and mental gymnastics involved in networking events, and it can be intimidating to meet new people in new situations. There is a reason that *work* is the root of the word that describes this activity. Networking is more of an art than a science, and there is no one "right" way to do it effectively. However, if you understand a few key principles about networking, you can minimize discomfort and maximize results. The following "dos and don'ts" should give you a basic guideline.

First the "Dos":

- *Always think of how you can benefit another person.* This may sound counterintuitive since your goal is to advance your own career or build your business. But people respond to those who have their best interest at heart. Chances are good that you are someone motivated by helping others (or else you probably would never have gravitated towards a holistic career in the first place)—it feels wonderful to help someone. And when you help someone else, chances are they will want to return the favor by helping you.
- *Solve a problem, fill a need.* If you express genuinely a desire to provide a solution to another's problem or connect them to helpful resources, you position yourself as a solution provider that people react to positively. Whether the problem is an aching back or a leaky roof, people appreciate solutions to problems. Jess Dushane, owner of Awaken Within, suggests an innovative response to the inevitable question "What do you do?". Rather than respond with a flat and vague "I'm a massage therapist," Dushane suggests replying with the *benefit* you provide to clients: "I help people overcome their chronic pain," or "I help athletes perform at optimal levels," or "I help people find comfort in the final stages of their life." This can be much more meaningful and memorable than "I'm a massage therapist."
- *Treat everyone you meet like a VIP.* At the death of a great and wise spiritual teacher, one of his students asked of the teacher's closest friend, "Who was the teacher's favorite?" The friend responded "Whoever he was with in that moment." When you network, always treat everyone as though they are incredibly important. There are two reasons for this. First of all, everyone you meet *is* incredibly important, just by the virtue of being a human being. And second, you never know who someone is, where they have been, who they know, or where they will one day be. As evidenced by the "golden rule," treating everyone like a VIP in turns makes you a very important person.
- *Get creative in your networking venues.* Networking doesn't only happen at organized events over hors d'oeuvres and cocktails, but can happen virtually anywhere—at the local farmer's market, the coffee shop, your cousin's party, your high school reunion. Because your personal brand is being established even when you forget about it, start thinking of every interaction as a way to build that brand and start getting creative about where else you can network.
- *Network strategically.* Because there are so many opportunities to network at any given moment, it helps to be intentional and strategic with your precious energy. Plan a networking strategy that supports your goals and is compatible with your unique professional path or distinctive business model. Identify the kinds of people that you would like in your professional life, whether as employers, clients, coworkers, or just friends. Target the events where these people can be found.
- *Organize your contacts.* Whether in a spreadsheet, Microsoft Outlook, a business card organizer, or a good old-fashioned Rolodex, find a system to help you organize the contacts in your network. This way, when someone tells you of a need they have, and you know just the person to solve their problem, you can find the contact information for them immediately. It may be helpful for you to jot down notes on people's cards to remind you of where you met and the conversations you had for follow-up (such as "from Mary's party, needs chiropractor" or "Sumner's half-marathon, send article on muscle spasms").

> *A single act of kindness throws out roots in all directions, and the roots spring up and make new trees. The greatest work that kindness does to others is that it makes them kind themselves.*
>
> —Amelia Earhart

Now the "Don'ts" of Networking:

- *Don't treat networking as a business-card marathon.* When you are meeting people and growing your network, don't rush out to collect as many cards as you can while thrusting your card into as many hands as possible. Take time to make a connection with people, and really listen to what they are saying. Focus on the quality of contacts over the quantity any day.

- *Don't be pushy.* When someone chases you, don't you feel like running? Even if people like buying, they rarely care to be sold.[8] If you are overly pushy and shove your skills and services down someone's throat, they are most likely going to want to get away from you—it's human nature.
- *Don't be false.* When someone is being insincere or faking interest, people know it. When you are networking with others, present the genuine you, not a facsimile of what you think people want you to be. And when you listen, actively engage in what people are telling you.
- *Don't go anywhere without your business cards:* You never know when you might meet someone who is in need of your services, and it can appear less professional to not have a card when asked. Nothing looks more amateur than scrawling your phone number down on a scrap of paper (which is likely to get tossed anyway). If you work for someone, ask your employer to make you business cards on company stationery so you can promote both yourself and the company while you are networking.
- *Don't forget to say thank you.* In this busy world, people's time is very valuable, and when someone takes the time to answer questions for you, connect you to a resource, or just chat with you, acknowledge it. If you get someone's contact information after you meet, immediately follow up with an e-mail expressing the pleasure of meeting them and thanking them for their time. If you have a meeting, informational interview, actual interview, or any other face-to-face meeting in which someone took time out of their schedule, send a handwritten thank-you card or letter. Do this immediately so you don't run the risk of forgetting about it; you will also be fresh in the other person's memory (see Chapter 2 for more on follow-up). Saying thank you may seem like a small gesture, but it goes a long way.
- *Don't forget that the person you are talking to is human, too.* Think you were nervous walking in to the networking event tonight? Chances are the person in front of you is just as (if not more than) nervous as you. Always be kind, compassionate, and considerate. Remember, your network is ultimately your community. Look for a true connection rather than just the exchange of information between two networking automatons.

PITFALLS

Whether building their career or their business, Marilyn O'Leary of the Holistic Business Network says that there are five common mistakes that holistic practitioners make in the networking arena:[9]

1. Waiting for the opportunities to come to them rather than pursuing the opportunities
2. Being unclear on their goals for networking
3. Holding back for fear of appearing pushy, demanding, or "sales-y"
4. Not having a well-developed or informative "elevator pitch" and confusing the listener
5. Showing up to events unprepared and without doing their homework

Can you relate to any of the items above? Are there areas you might like to strengthen in your own networking strategy?

IT TAKES A VILLAGE: CONNECTING AND CROSS-PROMOTING WITH OTHER MASSAGE THERAPISTS

> *Our premise is that there are going to be a lot of winners. It's not winner take all. Other people do not have to lose for us to win.*
>
> —Jeff Besos, founder of Amazon.com

When considering places to network, there are several standard venues such as chambers of commerce and small business associations. It can be very helpful to connect with people who are not necessarily in the wellness industry themselves, as you may be able to connect your clients to unrelated businesses, or even develop new client relationships. However, it makes sense to network with people within the holistic industry as well; here you will find people who understand your specific market conditions, potential collaborative partners, and possible employers.

In many ways massage and other holistic practices are just like any other business, but in many ways they are not. Networking is a common practice in the corporate world, and as a result networking functions are commonplace and ever-present for some professionals. However, it may be hard to connect with concentrations of other healing professionals due to insufficient venues or lack of developed communities. This can be especially difficult when you are just getting started, working from home, or relocating to a new area and away from your established network.

Ask around for holistic networking resources. Massage schools might be able to point you in the right direction, as can trade associations such as AMTA or ABMP. You may find networking opportunities in local holistic magazines and publications, or even advertised on community bulletin boards. Online resources such as Meetup and Craigslist can help you locate existing holistic networking opportunities.

Even with these resources, many therapists find that they are still unable to find any cohesive group of like-minded professionals in their area. So what if you can't find an existing network of holistic practioners? Create one! Host an informal gathering at your house or business, inviting like-minded individuals to come and help build the local holistic community.

Make a list of all the holistic professionals you know, be they classmates or individuals that you go to for treatments, and call or send them invitations. You might even call other practioners that you don't know personally but have heard of (through word of mouth or local directories) and invite them to join in your event—even if you consider them to be "competition". Some people balk at the idea of networking with and promoting their competitors. Others find that developing relationships with "the competition" can be incredibly rewarding for both parties and contribute to mutual success. As one massage therapist put it, "There are certainly enough aching bodies to go around." No two therapists are the same, and you may connect with someone who could benefit your clients in ways that you cannot (and vice versa). The more practitioners you have in your network, the more ways you are able to ultimately benefit your clients (see Figure 6-2 ■).

As your network grows, you might have members start hosting events at their homes or businesses, which gives them the chance to promote their own businesses on their home turf. You might also invite members to give presentations or demonstrations on their various modalities. This gives an added value to all participants, who receive an education on services that might be beneficial to themselves or their clients. It also allows participants the opportunity to present themselves as experts in their field, which helps them develop their personal brand. Be sure to announce upcoming holistic networking events to keep the momentum going, and elicit volunteers to host the next event. Sharing the responsibility, creativity, and organization of the holistic network helps bring forth ownership and collaboration among the members.

There are so many benefits to being the creator of a holistic group. First of all, and most obviously, you get to be proactive about creating a community and advancing the massage and wellness industry. Second, you get to help other people advance their businesses or professional careers, and that feels wonderful. Third, you get to grow your network data by gathering e-mail addresses, business cards, and business addresses, which can be very helpful for building your subscriber list (see Chapter 15 for more on this). Creating a networking venue also contributes to your personal branding, and positions you as a proactive, well-connected professional. What other benefits can you think of?

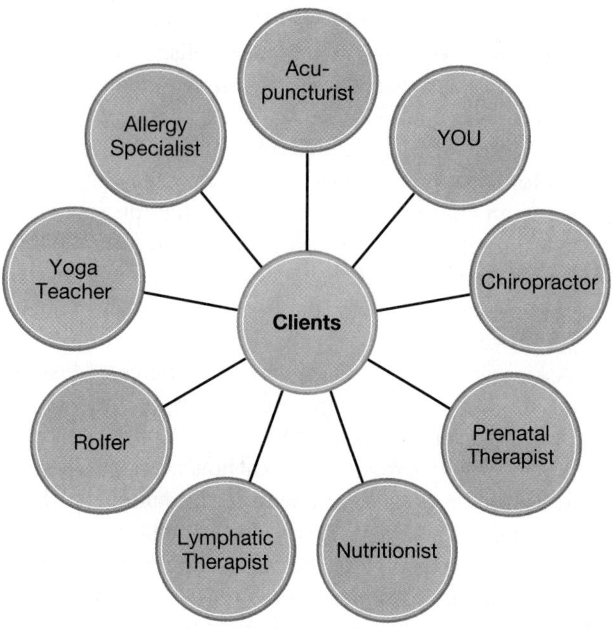

FIGURE 6-2

A strong network of skilled practitioners can be a great benefit to both you and your clients.

USING THE WEB TO BUILD *YOUR* WEB

In Chapter 15, you will learn how to use the Internet to develop your own business. In this section, you will explore how to use the Internet as a tool in your professional development and social networking. **E-networking** leverages the tremendous possibilities of the Internet into the techniques and goals of traditional networking. E-networking opens you up to virtual contacts you might never meet otherwise who may be able to provide knowledge on industry trends, job leads, client referrals, or other career boosters.[10]

So where do you go for this virtual networking? More and more people are using online forums and social networking sites to advance their personal and professional lives. **Online forums** (also known as chat rooms or discussion sites) provide a virtual platform where individuals can come together to ask questions, share knowledge, and discuss various topics. Often individuals form bonds with one another around mutual interests, and online communities begin to form.[11] **Social networking** refers to using online sites to connect with other individuals through virtual communities. Similar to online forums, social networks provide outlets for people to come together, associate, and communicate around shared ideas and interests. Popular social networking sites in the United States include Facebook, Twitter, MySpace, and LinkedIn.

Although the social aspect of these sites is inherent in their description, more and more professionals are discovering ways to leverage informal relationships into great professional opportunities. Networking online allows you to connect with people from the comfort of your home, which can minimize anxiety considerably (and no will ever know about your sweaty palms!). The Internet also allows you to take the time to compose your thoughts, craft responses, and present yourself the way you would like to. With so many discussion groups and community forums, the Internet also provides a wealth of knowledge while offering you an unlimited venue to position yourself as an expert and build your personal brand. And many recruiters search the Internet for potential employees, so your presence there might land you a great job as well!

However, the Internet can be a double-edged sword, particularly if you do not use it to network strategically. Because so much of human communication is nonverbal, you can be at a great disadvantage when stripped of your body language. It is much more difficult to control how your words are perceived by other people when you don't have eye contact and nonverbal clues. This can also make it more difficult to create real relationships with people. Moreover, once you put something into the ether, it stays there. Unlike a face-to-face faux pas, which is awkward but usually forgotten quickly, virtual blunders can spread exponentially and linger, damaging your reputation indefinitely (see Chapter 2 for more on nonverbal communication and "digital dirt").

Because of this, it is imperative to always use good "netiquette" when networking online (or doing anything online, for that matter). **Netiquette** refers to the collective standards for interactions online, and the expectation for well-mannered comportment by Internet users. Some forums and online communities have their own netiquette rules for what can and cannot be posted, or terms of consequences of abuse.[12] However, there are some general netiquette rules that apply across the board.

Without the help of verbal cues, you will want to be very conscious of your tone in e-mails, chats, and posts. Although you may never see them, remember that you are interacting with humans, and be very conscientious and respectful. Always try to learn the cultures and the behaviors of various sites. If you are new to a discussion group, check the FAQs before posting a question—you don't want to be the person to post the same question for the millionth time. Just as in person, always try and be helpful and offer solutions to others. Of course, netiquette requires that you behave online the same as you would in your regular life; always behave ethically and legally.[13]

GOING GURU: THE VALUE OF MENTOR RELATIONSHIPS

> *Ask not the sparrow how the eagle soars, for those with little wings have not accepted for themselves the power to share with you.*
>
> —A Course in Miracles

Professionals across industries have long known the benefit of developing relationships with mentors, or even being mentors themselves. A **mentor** is an experienced individual who imparts knowledge, skills, and wisdom to someone less seasoned. What distinguishes a mentor from your average network connection is the long-term goal and commitment to the relationship.[14] Mentors often have the experience, position, or career success that you would like to achieve yourself.

A mentor can be a teacher, an advisor, a sponsor, or a colleague. Mentoring is a great way to encourage personal and professional growth for both parties involved in the relationship. Conventional wisdom holds that "the best way to learn is to teach." Many mentors find that they benefit just as much from the relationship as those they are mentoring (Figure 6-3 ■). By sharing their acquired wisdom, opening up their networks, and imparting their insights, mentors can help you advance quickly in your massage career while reconfirming their own passion for their work.

At different times in your professional path, you may benefit from serving as both a mentor and a mentee. A **mentee** is one who is mentored, and is generally more of a novice in a profession or organization. Mentees are often younger than mentors, although that is not a hard-and-fast rule. The important differentiation between mentors and mentees is not age, but experience levels. Many massage professionals find that they serve as both mentor and mentee to various people at the same time.

The form of the relationships vary, but many mentors and mentees often formalize a meeting schedule. Whether biweekly, monthly, or every few months, the two parties come together at an agreed-on frequency. Because most holistic practitioners are givers by nature, you shouldn't have too much trouble finding someone with whom you can develop a mentor relationship. Perhaps a past graduate of your school, one of your favorite professors, or a seasoned veteran at your new job might be willing to work with you. You will ideally have good rapport with your mentor/mentee, and feel comfortable sharing openly with each other. At the same time, constructive criticism should have a

PUT IT IN WRITING
Netiquette
Networking online can be very beneficial if done properly. But if you do not engage good online manners, you could do more harm than good. Beyond the suggestions already listed, write out a few other ideas on safe, appropriate, and proper Internet behavior.

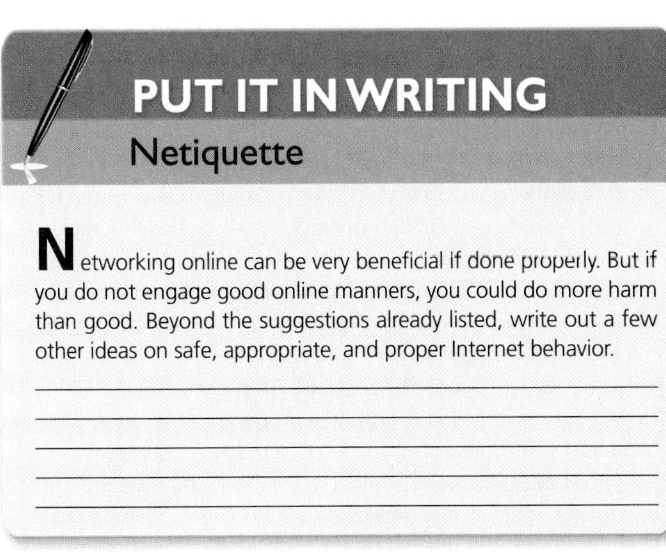

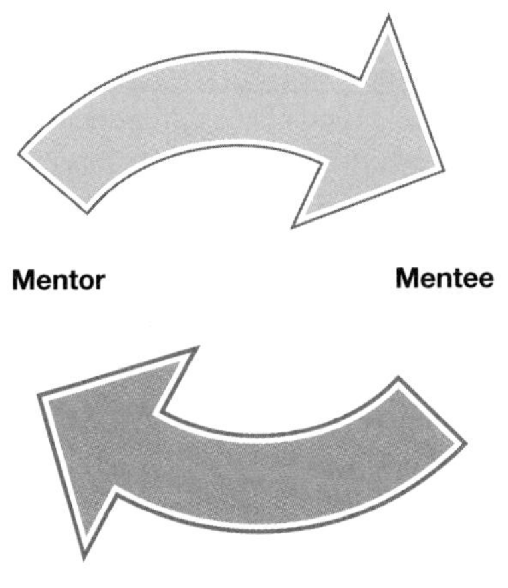

FIGURE 6-3

A mentor/mentee relationship greatly benefits both individuals.

PUT IT IN WRITING

Mentoring

1. Write down a few of your goals for a mentor/mentee relationship. What do you want to get out of your time together? Jot down a few ideas.

2. Who are some people you might consider asking to be a mentor? Write down five names.

3. What is it about each of the five people above that would make them a good mentor? Write the characteristics they possess that you would like to emulate or develop.

place in the relationship when necessary. While mentoring relationships should be comfortable, their objective is to advance you in your career. It helps to discuss your mutual desired outcomes. Both mentor and mentee should work together to establish goals for the relationship, both together and separately.

Always remember that your mentor/mentee is likely a very busy person. When they give of their time for you, remember to always be respectful of that. Keep appointments, be on time, and always remember to say thank you. It is very hard to quantify the value of mentor/mentee relationships, but if you are in one, you should always treat it as priceless.

While it is possible to be successful in your career without ever engaging the help of a mentor, working with someone who knows the industry can help you save time, minimize your learning curve, exponentially grow your network, and benefit from the experience of others. And beyond just the obvious professional propulsion, mentor/mentee relationships can provide the emotional support to survive the ups and downs of a career in massage therapy.[15]

STAY OPEN, BUT EXERCISE CAUTION

As important as it is to remain open, giving, and receptive to opportunities, you always want to put your own safety and security first. While it isn't necessary to be paranoid, it is important to keep your wits about you when networking, both online and off. There is a fine line between being open to the universe and making yourself vulnerable professionally or personally. Whether chatting online, sharing with a mentee, serving as the facilitator of a holistic networking group, or talking to someone in line at the grocery store, you always want to exercise common sense about how much you disclose and with whom you share your trade secrets. As sad as it is, not everyone is an ethical professional, and not everyone (even other holistic healers) has your best interests at heart.

If you can, spend a little time getting a good read of people and become aware of how you react. When you are in social situations, notice the people you are drawn to and those who are drawn to you. At the same time, pay attention to people who make you uneasy. While many first impressions can be proven wrong and many great relationships have been born of uneasy beginnings, it is always good to have faith in your instincts. If you don't trust someone or genuinely get a bad feeling, you are not required to talk with them or give them your information. You can politely disengage by smiling, shaking their hand, saying "lovely to meet you," and excusing yourself. Then go find someone to talk to who makes you feel great. In networking and in the rest of the world, life is too short for bad associations.

As you have already seen, it is not always easy to control the information that circulates about you online. This is true for anyone, but takes on another dimension for massage therapists due to the solitary nature of treatment and the lingering misdirection over the strictly therapeutic application of the work. No matter how much the industry legitimizes, there are still people out there who just do not get it and will always equate massage with sex. Even if you will never develop client relationships from your online networking, you still want to be incredibly cautious of the contacts you make as a massage therapist.

First and foremost, protect yourself by monitoring and censoring what you yourself put "out there." Emphasize your professionalism by using words like "therapeutic," "professional," and "specialist," and list your hard-earned credentials, licenses, and professional affiliations. When you are networking online, be selective about the people you engage with and the e-mail messages to which you respond. If someone tries to contact you, it is completely okay to do a little virtual background checking on them. Perhaps you can find similar professional or organizational affiliations, or maybe some friends or colleagues in common. Or maybe you find some off-putting digital dirt. If you do make contact with people online but feel uncomfortable with the virtual relationship, you can always ask to move the communication offline to phone calls or face-to-face meetings. This often makes the connections feel more "real" and possibly more secure.

Just as in person, listen to your instincts when dealing with anyone online. If someone is asking for too much information or you feel like a boundary has been crossed, you can terminate contact immediately. While the vast majority of Internet users are upstanding, ethical people, it is naïve to ignore the reality of Internet fraud and scams. A **scam** is deception of an individual or group with the intention of developing trust and confidence in order to defraud. In early 2009, the National Certification Board for Therapeutic Massage & Bodywork alerted its members to a scam targeting massage therapists and bodyworkers, and many similar scams continue to persist.[16] Several variations of fraudulent e-mails were sent to NCBTMB members, allegedly enlisting their massage services but really trying to get financial information. Confidence scams are illegal, and even the most intelligent individuals have fallen for them. If you think you have been the victim of a scam, contact the authorities immediately.

One of the most difficult concepts presented in this chapter for massage therapists (and most professionals, for that matter) to accept is collaborating with "the competition." Therapists feel that sharing any information with others can minimize their own accomplishments or cannibalize their clients. While success is not a zero-sum game, and there really are enough aching bodies out there for limitless lucrative massage careers, you do still want to protect yourself professionally when working with other holistic practioners. You don't need to reveal your secret sauce recipe, expose your trademark PNF technique, or open up your financials to other professionals in order to network. If you do operate from a belief in abundance and collaboration, it is completely possible to partner with others while still protecting yourself professionally.

CHAPTER SUMMARY BY LEARNING OBJECTIVES

1. **Define networking** Networking is the art of connecting with other people and building strategic alliances that benefit you, your career, and your business. The beauty of networking is that that benefits can exponentially spread to everyone with whom you network as well. Your network is a collection of all the people that you know, and consists of personal, professional, educational, and community contacts.
2. **Name the three key ingredients in networking success** Many career experts agree that there are three essential ingredients to success: skills, image, and exposure. Skills are the unique talents you have that generate value for your clients, employers, or others. Image is the combination of aspects (physical appearance, confidence, etc.) about yourself that you project to others and that becomes instrumental in the perception others have of you. Exposure refers to the frequency of contact you have with others.
3. **Explain the importance of networking for your career and the importance of networking authentically** In your career, networking is an ongoing process that helps to ensure a constant flow of customers, partners, and opportunities. Networking is important in any profession, though arguably more so in a field like massage therapy, where the service offering is more intimate and the ebb and flow of clientele can be dramatic. Businesses, like communities, are interdependent ecosystems, and they rely upon one another. Everything is interconnected, and when you look at networking from this perspective, you can't help but be authentic in your efforts to connect.
4. **Define personal brand and the function of brand loyalty** Personal brand is the unique combination of the components that make up who you are and what you have to offer others. A brand consists of all the factors that make you stand out as the unique and incomparable person that you are—your personality, your appearance, your skills, your humor, your individual style. Brand loyalty is a consumer's tendency to purchase repeatedly the goods or services of another. The factors contributing to a consumer's brand loyalty are wide-ranging, and can be anything from perceived value to emotional attachment to lack of viable alternatives,
5. **Identify ways to build your own personal brand** There are many ways to build a personal brand, such as getting involved in the community, being a connector for others, being an expert in your field, and committing to ongoing education; all these can make you and your personal brand stand out.
6. **Demonstrate some of the "dos and don'ts" of networking** While networking is not a science, there are some basic rules to follow that will contribute to your networking success. Commit to be of service to others by helping to resolve a need or problem, and

always treat everyone like a VIP (no matter who you *think* they are). Don't forget to engage authentically, don't be pushy, and don't treat networking events like business card marathons.

7. **Illustrate ways to connect with other healing professionals to promote one another collaboratively** Ask around for holistic networking resources. Massage schools might be able to point you in the right direction, as can trade associations such as AMTA or ABMP. Online sites like Craigslist and Meetup can be useful for finding holistic networking groups in your area. And if none exist—create your own!
8. **Explore the usefulness of the Internet, online forums, and social networking for your career** E-Networking leverages the tremendous possibilities of the Internet into the techniques and goals of traditional networking. E-Networking opens you up to virtual contacts that may be able to provide you information on industry trends, job leads, client referrals, or other career boosters.
9. **Illustrate the value of mentor relationships** Professionals across industries have long known the benefit of developing relationships with mentors, or even being mentors themselves. A mentor is an experienced individual who imparts knowledge, skills, and wisdom to someone less seasoned. Working with someone who knows the industry can help you save time, minimize your learning curve, exponentially grow your network, and benefit from the experience of others. It can also help you navigate the ups and down unique to a career in massage therapy.
10. **Discover how to protecting yourself professionally** As important as it is to remain open, giving, and receptive to opportunities, you always want to put your own safety and security first. While it isn't necessary to be paranoid, it is important to keep your wits about you when networking, both online and off.

ACTIVITIES

Quiz: Networking Review

1. What is a personal brand?
   a. The line of jeans you've been commissioned to design for Macy's.
   b. Your private-label massage products.
   c. The unique combination of the components that make up who you are and what you have to offer others.
   d. The things you always buy at the store.
2. Sheila is one of your classmates who has told you that she met someone online who wants to become a client. This person vows to visit once a week and to directly deposit $2000 into Sheila's account if she will just give him her checking account and bank routing number. She says she just gave him her information this morning and is excited. You tell Sheila that this sounds like a ______________ and she should immediately ______________.
   a. great deal, go shopping
   b. scam, contact the bank and the authorities
   c. a good business move, find out where they got her listing so you can get involved too
   d. suspicious situation, cancel the appointment
3. The three interdependent ingredients of career success are:
   a. timing, foresight, and expertise
   b. location, logo, and likeability
   c. skill, image, and exposure
   d. mentors, social networking, and talent
4. An introvert is someone who ______________.
   a. feels energized alone and drained around others
   b. lacks social skills
   c. always loves to network
   d. has panic attacks around others
5. Someone who feels energized around others but fades energetically when alone too long is likely ______________.
   a. codependent and insecure
   b. to be president
   c. self-absorbed
   d. an extrovert
6. ______________ are individuals or businesses with which you can ally to enhance one another's success. They can fortify your toolbox and augment the value you can bring to your clients and your company.
   a. Employers
   b. Strategic partners
   c. Mentors/mentees
   d. Online forums
7. Which of the following should you *not* focus on at networking events?
   a. Thinking of ways you can benefit the other person
   b. Being a connector for others that bring one another mutual assistance.
   c. Being compassionate and authentic with any individual before you
   d. Getting as many business cards as humanly possible. After all, it's a numbers game.

8. People may love to buy, but they hate to be sold. When most people are chased by a pushy salesperson, how do they typically respond?
   a. By signing on the dotted line as quickly as possible.
   b. By referring all of their friends.
   c. By running away and not doing business with her.
   d. By calling the Better Business Bureau.
9. _____________ refers to the frequency of contact you have with others. This can be either direct, like when you meet someone face to face, or indirect, such as when someone reads an article you have written or hears about you through word of mouth.
   a. Exposure
   b. Exchange
   c. Public relations
   d. Popularity
10. You have just moved to a new town and want to find a way to connect with other holistic practitioners in your new area. Where might you look?
   a. Meetup or Craigslist
   b. Trade sssociations such as AMTA, AMBP, or NCMTMB
   c. Local massage, chiropractic, acupuncture, or nutrition schools
   d. All the above
11. True or False: If you are going to be an authentic and holistic networking, you need to share as much information about your career or business as you can with others.
12. True of False: Businesses, like communities, are interdependent ecosystems, and rely upon one another to survive and to thrive.
13. True or False: Nothing gives credibility to a personal brand more than demonstrated expertise. Giving talks, teaching classes, or writing articles help to position you as an expert.
14. True or False: A connector is typically an antisocial person with a very small network.
15. True or False: A professional can be both a mentor and a mentee simultaneously.

Discussion Questions

1. What has been your experience with networking at this point in your life? Perhaps you have had many opportunities through a previous career, or perhaps you have not had the chance to network before. Discuss your experiences.
2. Do you know any great networkers? Perhaps you know someone who is a great connector across industries, ages, or social classes. Or perhaps you have a friend who just seems to *know everyone!* Explain what you think it is about this person that has helped him or her build such a large network.
3. Do you think it is realistic to work collaboratively with other massage therapists to promote your career and/or your own business? Do you think that it is a good idea to share information, pool resources, or join forces with someone who may take clients or opportunities from you? Share your thoughts.
4. You have heard that skills are one of the cornerstones of a successful career. Even if you know what you are good at, it can be challenging to articulate your skills and talents to other people. Take some time to articulate the skills you possess to a classmate or friend. Remember to try and frame your explanation in the context of benefits you provide to others, and not just technical skill. Having a succinct description of your abilities can be very useful in networking circumstances.
5. Brand loyalty can be an important part of professional success for service professionals such as massage therapists. Think of other professionals to whom you have developed a strong loyalty and whom you visit regularly. What is it about them that has earned your loyalty? How might you be able to do that for your future clients?

Beyond the Classroom

1. Find a networking event in your area that you would like to attend. Ask a friend, classmate, or a colleague to accompany you. Together you can approach the networking event as empirical observers of this phenomenon called networking. Before you go into the gathering, take a moment to discuss your authentic goals for the evening. When the party ends, sit down and compare notes. Whom did you meet? How did it feel? What would you do the same or differently next time?
2. Write out a personal brand description. What are your unique aspects? What do you have to offer people? Write out as many things as you can, and continue to refine your description until you arrive at something that you feel really fits you. If it helps, use images to communicate the brand that is you.

CHAPTER 7

Internal Abundance: Personal Financial Planning Basics

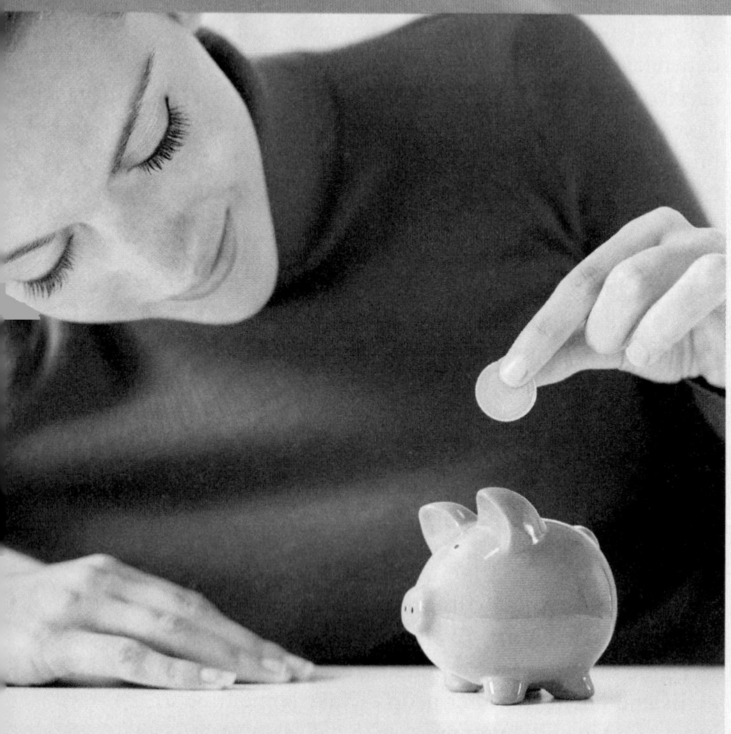

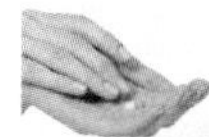

CHAPTER OUTLINE

LEARNING OBJECTIVES

1. Explain the importance of personal financial planning
2. Define assets and liabilities
3. Distinguish good debt from bad debt
4. Explore what money and wealth mean to you
5. Learn how to align money with values
6. Understand financial literacy
7. Create a financial plan
8. Explore compound interest and the time value of money
9. Understand the importance of an emergency fund, insurance, and estate planning to build your financial "house"
10. Discover the benefits of creating a financial community (*sangha*)

KEY TERMS

In all realms of life it takes courage to stretch your limits, express your power, and fulfill your potential . . . it's no different in the financial realm.

—Suze Orman

MONEY AND THE MASSAGE THERAPIST: PERSONAL FINANCIAL PLANNING

By now you fully understand the importance of self-care for the helping professional. Massage therapists cannot effectively and consistently help restore another person to good health and balance if they do not have good health and balance themselves. But good health exists on many levels: physical, mental, spiritual, emotional, creative, financial, and so forth. Think back to the Wheel of Life exercise you did back in Chapter 1. If you are neglecting the health of your financial self, how smooth can your ride be? **Personal financial planning** is the application of financial principles towards one's goals, and the crafting of a workable plan to achieve those goals.

In order to create and grow a flourishing, successful practice that promotes health and healing in others, it is vital to examine your relationship to your personal finances. How can you hope to have a flourishing career or expect to run a strong business if you cannot manage your own money? Many massage therapists that leave the field cite financial hardship as one of the main reasons for their career departure. But it need not be that way. In this chapter, you will explore the significance of your personal **financial health**—the way you relate to money and the development of constructive financial practices and positive money management. The recent excesses in credit card debt and consumption, record-low savings rates, followed by the harrowing decline in global markets, have made it more important than ever to take charge of personal finances. Tools to proactively manage your money are always important; in these uncertain financial times, they are essential. In Chapter 13, you will apply your holistic financial health to your business and learn how to navigate professional finances. But if you hope to have any form of career that flourishes financially, it is important to establish a firm foundation for your own monetary well-being.

For many helping professionals, there is an unspoken disconnect between the call to minister to another's well-being and the very real need to be paid for it. But money is just an exchange of energy, a mechanism to achieve your goals and live your values. Reduced to its essential purpose, money is a form of communication and interaction. It facilitates relationships, expedites adventures, advances causes, and provides a source for celebration. What you do with your money is an outward manifestation of your inner truths and values as a helping professional. Moreover, money has always had a place

PITFALLS

The information in this chapter is meant to be a very cursory overview of financial planning and is in no way meant to be instructive of choices nor substituted for sound consulting by a financial professional. Find a good financial planner in your area to help you craft your own financial plan and meet your goals.

PUT IT IN WRITING

Penny for Your Thoughts!

People hear messages about money and the abundance or lack or it all the time. From countless sources—parents, friends, the news, movies, religious sources, music, advertising—you may have absorbed some beliefs that continue to influence your relationship with money. When you think of sayings or messages about money, what are some of the phrases that come to mind? Here are a few examples to jog your memory:

1. A penny saved is a penny earned. ____________
2. Money is the root of all evil. ____________
3. It is easier for a camel to pass through the eye of a needle than for a rich man to enter the Kingdom of Heaven. ____________
4. Easy come, easy go. ____________
5. Money's just something you need just in case you don't die tomorrow. ____________

Now you. Try and fill as many phrases and messages as you can remember into the spaces below. Have fun with this one!

____

____

____

____

____

____

____

____

____

____

at the curative table. In ancient Rome, the goddess of health and fertility was named *Moneta,* and it was in her temple that the first money was ever minted.[1] From time immemorial, money was a sacred connection to the celestial, and was directly connected to the healing energy with which humans were entrusted.[2]

In today's American society, money seems to have an inflated magnetism. Love it or hate it, it is an inescapable facet of everyday life. Gone to extremes of adoration and clinging to money, it is easy to become fixated, anxious, or greedy. Gone to the extremes of money avoidance, however, one can opt for the ostrich approach, but this negates your power and zaps your energy. You may say "I just don't care about money," but you cannot deny the reality of the electric bill, the need to pay rent or buy groceries, or the rude shock of reaching retirement without a financial cushion to ease the descent.

Ignored or mismanaged, money can zap the creative energy force because your attention is focused on "paying the bills" or getting out of debt, not upon nurturing yourself and others. When a person is out of financial balance, he or she may have constant problems with debt and late payments. Or that person may go shopping unnecessarily and excessively to avoid painful feelings. If one is at the mercy of money, concerned only with the bottom line, a massage practice can be compromised and a healing canvas tainted.

> *Don't tell me where your priorities are. Show me where you spend your money and I'll tell you what they are.*
>
> —James W. Frick

Just as with so many other sections of the book, financial health starts with taking an honest inventory of where you are now. By being exceptionally truthful with yourself about your relationship to money, you can begin to uncover old beliefs and patterns while you discover areas of constraint and unintentional limitations. Financial planning really begins with your thoughts and beliefs.

It is not uncommon for obstacles, both internal and external, to get in the way of financial success (for a list of

PUT IT IN WRITING

Money Vitals

It's time to do some internal probing of your financial health. Free yourself from external distractions and clear your mind as you respond to the following questions. Be receptive to the answers that arise.

1. What is my truth about money?

   ____

   ____

2. What do I know about myself and money that I don't like to admit?

   ____

   ____

3. How much debt do I have right now?

   ____

4. What does financial abundance look like to me?

   ____

   ____

5. What are the stories I tell myself about money?

   ____

   ____

6. What things did I hear about money when I was a child?

   ____

   ____

7. Does my relationship with money harm me or anyone I love?

   ____

   ____

8. When I spend money, do I feel energized or drained?

   ____

   ____

9. What area of my financial life do I feel most shameful about?

   ____

   ____

10. What area of my financial life do I feel most proud of?

    ____

    ____

11. Are there things about my relationship with money that I hide from myself?

    ____

    ____

12. Are there things I hide from others?

    ____

    ____

Take some time with this. It might feel strange and uncomfortable to ask yourself these questions, but it is worth it. Remember, it is always best to explore where you are currently before you begin mapping where you want to go.

some of the most common ones, check out Appendix B). As you become more aware of your financial self and take stock of your current financial health, it is important to take a moment to examine some of the hurdles, both internal and external, that may lie before you. You may be sitting on well-cultivated gardens of personal and emotional monetary issues. You may possess some authentic and very real fears that are whipped into a frenzy whenever the subject comes up. As mentioned earlier, many helping professionals draw a conflicting line between curative pursuits and any semblance of economic pursuits. You may have seen your parents argue endlessly about money, and thus have an association with money as being the root of discord and anger. Or you may fear that grasping for money will make you selfish, greedy, and not a "good person." You may even fear your own financial success. Or you may have no conflictions at all and be ready to make a mint with your skills! Regardless of what your personal psychological landscape is, it is imperative that you really hold it in your focus, gaze at it with great compassion, and ask the question: "Does this belief still serve me? Could it, in fact, be harming me?"

Another issue you may encounter as you look over your internal financial/emotional landscape is blame.[3] Are you systematically pointing a finger, outwardly casting culpability for your subpar financial health? Even as you come to identify your messages or erroneous beliefs as coming from your parents, family, friends, or society, it does no good to remain wallowing in blame. This blame may not just extend towards the past either; you may blame a poor economy, an overspending partner, a miserly boss who doesn't pay you what you know you are worth. Although it is wonderful to acknowledge your thoughts and your beliefs, to hand the reigns of your holistic wealth over to any other party (especially with anger or blame) is the most detrimental thing to do. Find the places you can respond compassionately to any of these self-limiting beliefs. You might sit down with your parents, if they are still living, and ask them what their relationship is to money, and how you've interpreted their beliefs. You might find creative ways to minimize spending in that poor economy, find alternative solutions with that partner, or discuss a raise with your boss. The point is, you have limitless power to achieve your goals, and that power gets drained when you start to succumb to the undertow of anger, guilt, and blame for your financial situation. Turn those very human emotions into something productive, and watch what happens. Reach for the wonderful, rich aspects of a financial life; it's certainly better than the alternative.

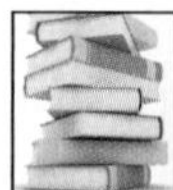

HELPFUL RESOURCES

If you are interested in exploring more of your subconscious relationship, as well as connecting your spiritual self to your financial self, check out *It's Not About the Money: Unlock Your Money Type to Achieve Spiritual and Financial Abundance* by Brent Kessel (2008, Harper One) and *The 9 Steps to Financial Freedom: Practical and Spiritual Steps So You Can Stop Worrying* by Suze Orman (1997; Crown Publishers).

UNDERSTANDING ASSETS AND LIABILITIES

If asked if they would like to be wealthy, most people would invariably say "yes." But what does that ultimately mean? Some might define wealth as nothing short of a $50 million portfolio, while another might say it is having $5000 in the bank. Another might say it is having a financial picture that allows enough time with friends and family on a regular basis. Another might say it is living in a certain neighborhood. Someone else might say having the freedom and resources to travel the world. Clearly, wealth is a fairly relative concept. A generally accepted and generally applied definition of wealth is the accumulation of assets and the minimization of liabilities. **Assets** are items of monetary value that are owned by an individual or a company, and typically can be converted to cash.[4] Examples of assets include savings, equity on a home, equipment, stocks, real estate, and so forth (Figure 7-1 ■). **Liabilities** are financial obligations that you owe to another person or company in exchange for capital, products or services you have used or consumed. Liability is just another word for debt. Examples of liabilities include credit card debt, school loans, mortgages, taxes, bills, and so forth (Figure 7-2 ■).

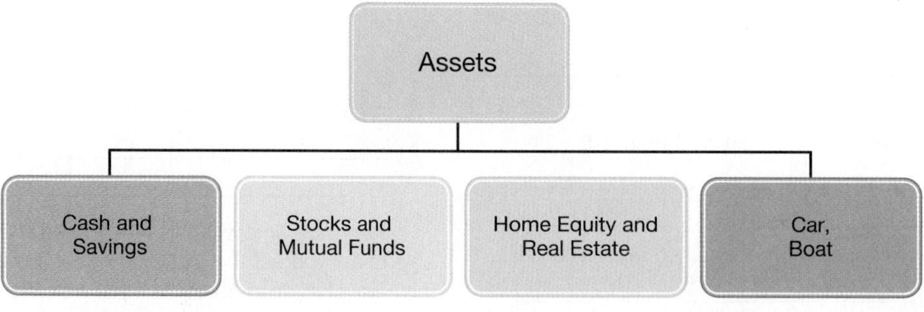

FIGURE 7-1

Assets are things of value that you own, such as your home, your savings, and stocks.

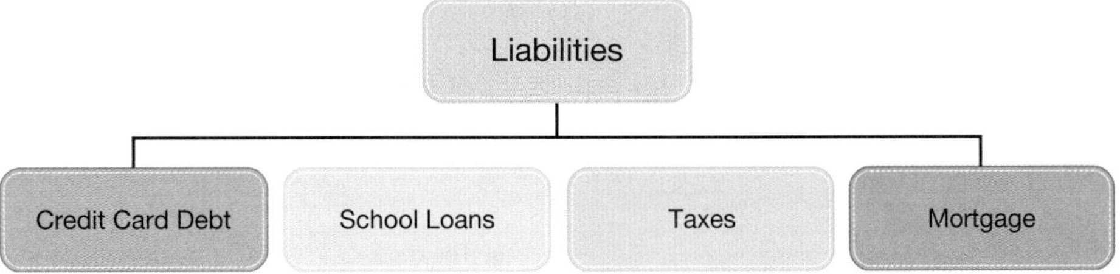

FIGURE 7-2

Liabilities are debts that you owe, such as mortgages, school loans, or credit card balances.

> *Money is better than poverty, if only for financial reasons.*
>
> —Woody Allen

Liabilities may automatically seem like a bad thing, and people often have negative associations when they think of debts. Not all liabilities are created equal, however, and it is important to understand the difference between "good" and "bad" debt. **Good debt** is money that is borrowed in order to obtain something that will ultimately increase in value. If in the long term the purchase will contribute to your overall financial health, it is usually good debt. Examples of this include taking out a school loan to pay for college (which will hopefully return a higher salary and better opportunities) or taking out a mortgage to buy a home (which will hopefully appreciate in value over time), or getting a loan for your business (which is going to go through the roof after you read this book). **Bad debt**, on the other hand, is money that is borrowed to purchase things that do not appreciate in value or contribute to your financial health. Typically you incur bad debt when you borrow money to purchase something you ultimately do not need and cannot afford without using credit. Some examples of bad debt include putting a new wardrobe, new jet skis, or a vacation to Bermuda on your credit card. In fact, even necessary things like groceries can convert to bad debt if purchased with a credit card. Because the interest rates on credit cards are so high, many financial planners insist that anything you buy with a credit card is automatically bad debt.[5] If you can finance things another way, do it. As a rule of thumb, it is always better for your financial health to purchase things you can afford without borrowing, but for many people it isn't practical to buy a house with cash. Understanding the differences between types of debt and leveraging the relationship between your assets and your liabilities is a big step to achieving wealth.

DEFINING WEALTH

> *It's the mind that makes the body rich.*
>
> —William Shakespeare

So now you are starting to understand more about the steps to achieving wealth. But what is wealth, and more importantly, what does it look like to *you?* By now you know the difficulty of obtaining anything without having clear definitions of your goals. Defining prosperity and understanding your financial objectives is the first step in achieving them. If you don't truly identify with another's definition of prosperity or don't have a firm one yourself, how hard are you really willing to work to achieve it? Really examining definitions of true wealth and abundance is something that few people do. But it is a very important part of your financial plan. Not only will it help you

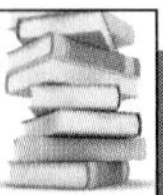

HELPFUL RESOURCES

Consumer credit card debt is a very hot topic, and one that has millions mired in a seemingly endless cycle of owing money. If you are someone with very large credit card debts, it is vital to get out from under it if you are really going to achieve optimal financial health. You can turn to a number of resources for help. Skip the too-good-to-be-true "experts," and seek out help from a reputable credit counseling service such as Consumer Credit Counseling Services (www.cccservices.com). These services can help you understand financial planning and connect you with local resources to get you on track.

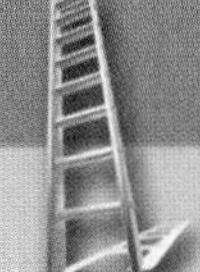

FIRST STEPS

Look at the people in your network: friends, family, coworkers. Choose someone you admire for the way they handle their financial health. Ask yourself what he or she does with money that you might like to emulate. You might even consider approaching that person and asking her to be your financial mentor. Many people are excited to share what they know about financial success with others. Refer back to Chapter 6 to learn more about mentor relationships.

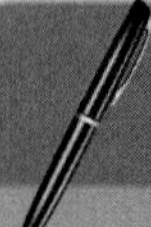

PUT IT IN WRITING

Healthy, Wealthy, and Wise

In Chapter 2, you explored your own definitions of success, which is an entirely relative concept. Now take a look at how you define wealth, which also has an elusive and subjective connotation. Complete the following sentences and/or answer the following questions.

1. As a wealthy person, I see myself doing ______________.
2. When I achieve my prosperity goals, I will no longer have to ______________________________.
3. The idea of obtaining real wealth feels ______________.
4. If I had wealth, would I get involved in philanthropy? If so, how? ______________________________
5. If I were truly wealthy, my family situation would be ______________________________.
6. The distance between my current financial situation and my dream financial situation is ______________________.
7. When I reach my financial goals, what will I do for friends and family? ______________________________.
8. As a wealthy person, what will my day look like? ______________________________.
9. Having achieved my goals for prosperity, where will I live? ______________________________ ______________________________.
10. Is travel part of my abundance package? If so, where will I go? ______________________________.

clarify and obtain your financial goals, it will help keep you true to your own trajectory and preempt any derailments. Moreover, it will deflect the temptation to fall into the trap of "keeping up with the Joneses." It is easy to let society's or someone else's definitions of wealth usurp your own, which ultimately zaps your power and handicaps your process. Having a clear and personal description helps you stay dedicated to your end goal and accountable to your values as you build your financial plan. And that clear vision and written goals for your financial trajectory will help you focus your efforts and motivate you to work hard to achieve your objectives.

PITFALLS

Because this chapter is about money and financial planning, wealth is often discussed in terms of the material. However, don't lose sight of the very real truth that a desire for material wealth must be balanced with a desire for emotional, mental, and spiritual wealth. Aligning these external and internal riches is key to ultimate fulfillment.

ALIGNING MONEY WITH VALUES

> *People will work hard for money but they will give their life for meaning.*
>
> —David Pottruck, CEO, Charles Schwab

You did a lot of work to identify your values in Chapter 2. Now connect your values about the way you live your life and the way you want to run your career or business to the way you interact with money. Are you spending in ways that reflect those values? One of the greatest benefits of money is its quality as a means to a higher end. Money can be the way in which you actualize the life you want to live and demonstrate what you value. This is a great opportunity to assess and renegotiate the outflow of your dollars. Take a moment to see, without judgment, how much you're currently supporting your values and places where you can do more. For example, if family is at the top of your values list, but most of your money is going to buy new clothes, re-evaluate ways you could channel that money towards what you truly value. If you value the health of the environment, yet have investments in companies that engage in harmful resource extractions, consider putting your money in earth-friendly corporations instead. If you value having fun,

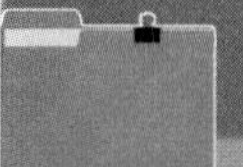

GETTING ORGANIZED

After all that hard work you just did in the above and following "Put it in Writing" exercises, you want to ensure that you stick to your plan. Make two copies of the goals you just created for yourself. One of the copies is for your files. The other one, and this is important, needs to go somewhere you can *see it*. Put it above your desk, on the door of the closet where you keep your massage sheets, or on your bathroom mirror. This will serve as a gentle reminder and a steady enforcer to keep you committed to your goals (see Chapter 8 for more tips on goal setting).

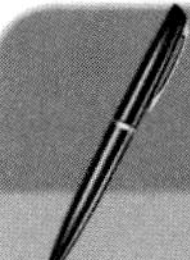

PUT IT IN WRITING

My Money, My Values

You will do a lot of exploration of your values in Chapter 8. For now, look at the list of values in Appendix B, and choose the ones that are most meaningful to you. Chose your *top five values* from the list, and write them out here.

1. ______
2. ______
3. ______
4. ______
5. ______

Now assign *a financial goal* to each to each of those values. For example, if your number one value is independence, make a goal that supports that value. "I will start a Roth IRA with automatic monthly investments by March 18 in order to ensure my independence from the government in my retirement." For more examples, see Appendix B.

1. ______
2. ______
3. ______
4. ______
5. ______

For each of the goals above, anticipate an *obstacle* you might face in achieving it. You may want to increase your revenue by 10 percent, but the economy may take a downturn. Or you may want to build a sizeable emergency fund but foresee the temptation to use the money for other things. Write out some of the challenges that might arise.

1. ______
2. ______
3. ______
4. ______
5. ______

The best thing about identifying potential obstacles is that it gives you an opportunity to proactively preempt those. That way when those challenges do arise, you are prepared. For example, if you want to grow your business 10 percent in a bad economy, acknowledge that all kinds of businesses still experience growth in slowed economies. Commit to ramping up your marketing plan so that more people can hear about you. Look again at the obstacles you anticipated above, and write out a creative solution for each one.

1. ______
2. ______
3. ______
4. ______
5. ______

Fantastic! You have figured out some actionable ways to align your values with your finances. You also boosted your chances of achieving your goals by foreseeing things that could derail you.

create a **joy account**, an account that is completely designed for playing and nothing else. The above "Put it in Writing" will help you connect your values to your financial planning.

FINANCIAL LITERACY

Financial literacy is the ability to understand and manage your financial health and plan for your financial present and future. As the onus of financial responsibility falls more and more to the individual, educating yourself about finances is more imperative than ever (to test your financial know-how, check out the quiz in Appendix B).

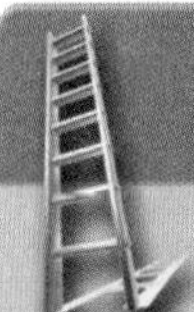

FIRST STEPS

Even after doing the work to examine your money messages and align your values with your finances, you may still feel uncomfortable getting yourself started. That is completely okay, and may be a sign that you need to do some clearing work or affirmations. If you think that may be the case, see Appendix B for some more exercises.

Tradition has held that a financial education was only really warranted and granted to those with considerable money to manage—the landed gentry, the corporate executives, the stock tycoons: in short, the rich. To educate the masses about money was not only unnecessary, it was in poor taste. Financial urban legend tells that John D. Rockefeller once overheard the conversation of two blue collar workers discussing their stock portfolios in an elevator in New York. Believing that the involvement of the working poor in the stock market was portentous of a dire situation, he withdrew all his money shortly before the market crashed and the Great Depression began. Regardless of that tale's veracity, those cultural roots run deep. Only recently is the pendulum shifting and the importance of everyone's financial literacy becoming apparent. In 2002, the U.S. Treasury established the Office of Financial Education. A year later, the U.S. Congress created the Financial Literacy and Education Commission under the Financial Literacy and Education Improvement Act. By 2006, the Commission had adopted a national strategy for financial literacy to help all individuals access information, gain knowledge and tools, and take ownership of their financial futures.[6]

History shows that it is not only the irresponsible or the financially imbalanced who find their money situations to be grim; the recent subprime mortgage crisis in the United States has left innumerable people's homes in foreclosure and many fiscally responsible people in bankruptcy. Just as you have seen throughout this book, the solution to avoiding financial hardships and obtaining your financial aspirations is, quite simply, to prepare. Even though there is always the possibility and risk of external circumstances, the best way to navigate the financial landscape is to educate yourself and plan accordingly. In order to achieve the wealth you desire you need to plan for it. No one ever got rich by simply wanting to have an abundance of money—everyone needs to do a little financial planning in order to reach personal monetary goals.

CREATING A FINANCIAL PLAN: BASIC PRINCIPLES

Just like building a massage practice, financial literacy and health take time, patience, and strategic planning. You must devote time and energy to your process, and most of all maintain compassion with all the aspects of the journey—compassion for where you currently are financially, compassion for where you may have been or what you do not know, and compassion for your goals, whatever they may be.

Many people who have been in the massage industry for several years will tell you that it can be a "feast or famine" career. It is important to be prepared for both the highs and lows of the business. When the economy takes a downturn, people usually continue to buy standard items such as toothpaste and toilet paper, yet will decrease paying for things they regard as discretionary spending. **Discretionary spending** is money that is spent on nonessential items such as movies, vacations, or luxury items. Obviously you know the intrinsic and essential value of massage therapy, or else why would you be starting your massage career? However, many people regard massage treatments and other healing modalities as discretionary spending items. Part of succeeding as a massage therapist and as a helping professional in general is to understand the often volatile economic landscape of the industry, and to prepare accordingly.

As you may have anticipated, a successful financial process is enhanced and advanced by a financial plan. Like a business plan or a marketing plan, a **financial plan** outlines your goals and objectives and delineates your strategy for achieving your financial ambitions. A financial plan can be used in your personal life and for your business; these two plans may be quite similar or very different depending on factors such as size and scope of your business endeavor. You will learn more about specific elements of a financial plan for your business in Chapter 13.

You may have the good fortune of a friend, family member, or educator who has taught you the ropes of financial planning. Or perhaps you've already done extensive research to teach yourself. But many people are paddling in the financial world without even the most rudimentary of oars. This section will give you a very brief overview of some of the common financial principles, products, and terms that will help you get started. Remember, this chapter provides only an overview, so consult with a certified financial planner and continue to learn more from other resources.

IT'S NOT JUST ABOUT MAKING MORE

Many people erroneously believe that the secret to wealth accumulation is having a very large salary. They believe that the only thing holding them back is their limited income. This is a misleading, incomplete, and inaccurate assumption. Earning more money is not a guarantee to having better financial health. In fact, typically the larger your income, the more costs are associated with maintaining your lifestyle. Examples abound of people who make six-figure salaries yet have no assets and huge debts. At the same time, many people have developed million-dollar fortunes with incomes of less than $25,000 a year. Understanding that there is no amount of income that cannot be outspent, you can see that it isn't about *making more* but *spending less.* Any personal trainer will tell you that the secret to weight loss is expending more calories than you consume. The same principle, when inverted, is true in financial planning: the secret to amassing wealth is the ability to expend less money than you earn. Simple perhaps, but few people elect to live below their means and will readily opt instead to use credit and debt to live well beyond their means.

Explore ways to cut back, and allow your creativity in alternatives to flow. Can you delay the instant gratification of a dinner in a fancy restaurant or an expensive trip to Fiji for the bigger picture? Why not experiment with a gourmet recipe at home and invite some friends, or head off with your partner for a day at the beach, a hike in the mountains, or a discount backpack trip instead? There are literally thousands of ways to live inexpensively, and with your brilliant mind, you'll harvest some wonderful alternatives as well.

PUT IT IN WRITING
Penny Pinch

There are so many creative ways to save money without feeling like you are sacrificing. The possibilities are endless. Take a look at your daily, weekly, monthly, even yearly expenses and purchases and see if you can come up with five changes that will save you money. If you could use a little nudge or would like to explore some other tips on thriftiness, see Appendix B.

1. ______
2. ______
3. ______
4. ______
5. ______

Becoming wealthy is not a matter of how much you earn, who your parents are, or what you do. It is a matter of managing your money properly.

—Noel Whittaker

YOU FIRST!

When asked where their paycheck goes, most people can come up with a litany of the bills they pay out every month: rent, groceries, credit card bill, phone bill, medical expenses, and so on. If they do put anything into savings or investments, that money is usually culled from whatever is left after everyone else is paid. More often than not, people will say that they'd like to save and invest more money, but there simply isn't anything left after the bills have been paid. But when you stop to think about it, who are you ultimately working so hard for? Certainly not your bank, the grocery store, or the oil companies, but rather for *you and your loved ones*. Therefore many financial planners tout the importance of always **paying yourself first**. The idea behind this concept is that you always come first in your line of expenditures. Paying yourself first is the financial planning and wealth building precept that maintains that the first bill you pay is always to yourself.

Although putting off the creditors and obligatory monthly bills to pay yourself may feel counterintuitive, if not downright perilous, paying ourselves first is one of the most important concepts in exercising a fit financial body. And it can be very easy to do. Nearly every retirement account or savings account offers you an automated deposit option. This means that without even having to think about it, your money will be systematically saved for you. And, if you're putting this money into a 401(k) or a traditional individual retirement account (or individual retirement arrangement), or IRA (more on these things later), your investment is tax-deductible.[7] Here's the beauty part of **tax-deductible contributions**—you actually pay fewer taxes while you save more money. Your taxes on this money is deferred until a later date, typically when it is withdrawn. In the meantime, that money is able to work for you (see the next section on compound interest). Here is an example: Imagine that you took $300 and deposited it monthly into your traditional IRA or 401(k) retirement account, which, again, is tax deductible. By doing this you are reducing your taxes by $100, and your $300 contribution only costs you $200.[8] In other words, the government has actually created a way for you to legally avoid taxes so you can pay yourself first. As for the amount of money you pay yourself first, this correlates directly with the goals you have set for yourself. Standard financial wisdom usually suggests tucking away about 10 to 15 percent of your **pre-tax income**—the money you make from work, businesses, or investments before any income taxes are deducted.

Happiness is not in the mere possession of money; it lies in the joys of achievement, in the thrill of creative effort.

—Franklin Delano Roosevelt

Beyond the tax advantages, paying yourself first enforces the notion that you are the most important person, and, after all, the one for whom you're working to earn the money. Not the government, your landlord, the grocery store, but you. After a very short time, you will be amazed at how little you even notice that automatic deduction from your paycheck, and how easily you adapt to the change.

MAKE YOUR MONEY WORK FOR YOU: THE POWER OF COMPOUND INTEREST

One secret that many wealthy individuals know is that very few people get rich by simply working hard for their money. That can be part of it, of course, but real exponential prosperity happens when your money *works really hard for you*.[9] What does that mean? Consider **interest**, the money paid on borrowed resources as a fee to use those resources. Interest is paid upon **principal**, the original amount invested or borrowed. When you put $500 of your money into a savings account, for example, the bank pays you interest on those funds. Why? Because in essence, the bank is borrowing the capital you are giving them in the form of a deposit. **Capital** refers to resources (typically financial) available to create new resources. It takes money to make money, and using other people's money is how a bank survives. The bank pays you interest because it is lending out your money at a higher interest rate in the form of loans.

But not all interest is created equal, and two of the most common types are explored here. **Simple interest** is calculated only on the principal, and is not applied to the principal. So if the bank gave you a 2 percent return on your $500 deposit, you would have $510 at the end of the time period ($500 × 2% = $10; $10 + 500 = 510). With **compound interest**, on the other hand, the interest you are paid goes back into your account and gets applied to the principal, so both are earning interest together. So, if you put your $500 into an account that has its 2 percent

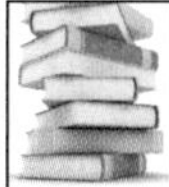

HELPFUL RESOURCES

Some great books on generating prosperity on modest incomes are *The Automatic Millionaire* series by David Bach (2004, Broadway Books), *The Wealthy Barber* by David Chilton (1997, Three Rivers Press), *The Total Money Makeover* series by Dave Ramsey (2009, Thomas Nelson), and *The Millionaire Next Door* by Thomas J. Stanley (1996, Longstreet Press). Check them out and see if you can learn some new tricks.

TABLE 7-1 Compound Interest

YEAR	5%	7%	9%	10%	12%
1	$1228	$1239	$1251	$1257	$1268
5	$6800	$7159	$7542	$7744	$8167
15	$26,729	$31,696	$37,840	$41,447	$49,958
25	$59,551	$81,007	$112,112	$132,683	$187,885
30	$83,226	$121,997	$183,074	$226,049	$349,496
40	$152,602	$262,481	$468,132	$632,408	$1,176,477

interest compounded every month, at the end of the first month you would have $510. Interest is then earned on $510, and next month you would have $520.20 ($510 × 2% = $10.20; $10.20 + 510 = $520.20). By putting your money into investments that bear compound interest, the money that you pay yourself first is working for you by earning money exponentially.

Compound interest also applies to investments, where your interest becomes dividends and returns and can be variable due to market conditions. Say you have a beginning balance of $0 but invest $100 every single month ($1200 per year) into an IRA account, and believe that your investments have a 5–12 percent return potential. Adjusting for inflation, the U.S. stock market's historical average return has been 10 percent, so a 5–12 percent return is within the realm of possibility for returns.[10] Though there are always many mitigating factors and *never any guarantees,* Table 7-1 ■ illustrates of the power of compound interest.

By staying in the market and letting your money work for you, you could turn your $48,000 principal investments into nearly $1.2 million by the time you retire. But that will never happen unless you make a habit of always paying yourself first!

UNDERSTANDING THE TIME VALUE OF MONEY

Like a snowball that gets bigger and bigger as it rolls down a wintry hill, compound interest helps your money grow. The real magic of compound interest occurs when a vital ingredient is mixed in: time. In finance, the **time value of money** incorporates a series of valuation calculations of money, but for the purposes of this chapter, it simply refers to the exponential benefit of compound interest over time. Consistent contributions and time are the key to building your financial wealth.

Table 7-2 ■ tracks the lives of two different massage therapists, Rachel and Kate, who have both just turned 25 and have just finished massage school together. Rachel decides that, though her business is slow, she will commit to investing $150 a month, or $1800 a year, in her Roth IRA. She does this consistently every month for the next 10 years, but stops when she turns 35. Rachel does not make another contribution to her IRA again, and retires at 65.

After massage school, Kate feels like she really needs to get her business turning substantial profit before she can even think about investing anything, and puts off her savings for 10 years. At 35, she opens a Roth IRA and commits to contributing $300 a month until she retires at 65. Both women put their money into a Roth IRA account with an average 10 percent return. Take a look at what happens to both women's money at the end of each year.[11]

Remember, Rachel stopped investing at 35, while Kate began at 35 and faithfully made monthly payments until the end of her 65th year when she retired. In other words, Kate contributed $108,000 over those 30 years of investing, while Rachel only contributed $18,000 over ten years of investing. And Rachel still had more money at retirement than Kate. Even though Kate contributed six times more money than Rachel, she still was not able to save as much money. Rachel was using the power of compound interest and the value of time to secure her financial health. This powerful illustration is why many financial planners will tell you it is *time in the market,* not *timing the market.*

PITFALLS

Do not panic if you are older and are just beginning to start saving. You are not the only person who has waited to begin preparing for the future. You may have to take more extreme measures and make more sizable contributions to meet your goals, but you can absolutely still make them. Many people do not leverage the power of compound interest until later in life and still acquire their financial goals—even exceed them. Don't be dissuaded from getting involved, because it's never too late to take care of your financial health.

TABLE 7-2 Earnings Versus Age

Age	Rachel	Kate
25	$1884	$0
26	$3967	$0
27	$6267	$0
28	$8808	$0
29	$11,616	$0
30	$14,717	$0
35	$35,829	$3770
40	$58,950	$29,434
45	$96,991	$71,658
50	$159,580	$117,900
55	$262,559	$217,212
60	$431,991	$380,612
65	$710,758	$639,456

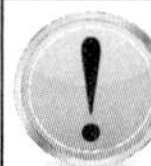

PITFALLS

A common mistake that many people new to financial planning will make is to entrust all of their money to a financial planner hastily and then walk away. Don't relegate all your power to someone just because they are a professional—ask lots of questions of prospective advisors. Find out how they are compensated for their work, if they profit from your selection of financial products, or if they have any conflicting interests. Shop around—talk to lots of different individuals to find someone whose style is aligned with your values. Once you've found a person who you'd like to work with to be a financial guide, remember the importance of your inner guide and continue to be an active part of the process. After all, the person most qualified to be your financial planner is you!

NUTS AND BOLTS OF A PERSONAL FINANCIAL PLAN

It is beyond the scope and purview of this book to go into all the details and nuances of all the facets of comprehensive financial planning. Moreover, with the multitude of financial products available and the ever-shifting landscape of the financial markets, it is advised that you speak with a qualified financial advisor or planner before you invest your money in any market vehicles. A **financial planner** is a professional who has been certified with a reputable national organization such as the National Association of Personal Financial Planners, Certified Financial Planner Board of Standards, and the Financial Planning Association. You can contact any of the above organizations for names of reputable financial advisors in your area.

In the meantime, this section will introduce you to some of the basic elements of a personal financial plan and some basic investment terms. A personal financial plan can include your goals for retirement, monthly savings allocations, tactics for debt alleviation, and a personal budget. A **personal budget** is the intentional plan for how much money from your earnings you will allocate for your personal expenses and outlays, and can help break down those expenses by percentages of income. Remember to use your after-tax (or net) earnings, not your pre-tax (or gross) earnings. For example, say Aurelie makes $3,400 a month after taxes from her massage business. She has several different expenses every month that she must pay (of course she pays herself first!) Table 7-3 ■ is Aurelie's budget (see Appendix B for a blank budget worksheet you can fill out to create your own budget).

By now you undoubtedly understand the importance of knowing where you are currently before you can begin planning; take a moment to figure out your personal present net worth. **Net worth** is what you have left over when you subtract all of your liabilities (debts) from your all of your assets. This is your **personal balance sheet**, which summarizes your financial position at any given time. You will explore this same concept as it applies to your business's balance sheet in Chapter 13. Let's take a look at Aurelie's personal balance sheet (Figure 7-3 ■).

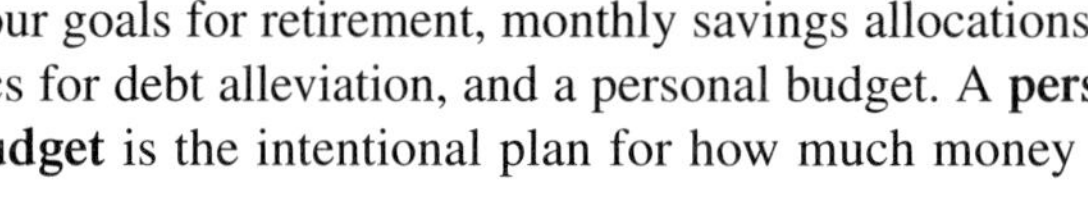

HELPFUL RESOURCES

If you are older and just getting started with saving and preparing for your future, there are a lot of resources out there to help people just like you. Check out *Start Late, Finish Rich* by David Bach (2005, Broadway) or *It's Never Too Late to Get Rich* by Rich and Jim Jorgensen (2003, Fireside).

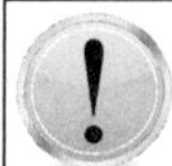

PITFALLS

The term *net worth* is used in this text because it is a generally accepted and widely used term in accounting, personal finance, and small business. However, never make the assumption that your inherent worth has *anything* to do with the money in your possession. Your intrinsic worth is always incalculable.

TABLE 7-3 Personal Budget

Category	Monthly Amount	Yearly Amount	Percentage of Income
Total income	$3400	$40,800	100%
Savings/investments	$375	$4500	11%
Rent/mortgage	$750	$9000	22%
Food	$450	$5400	13%
Transportation costs	$150	$1800	4%
Insurance	$340	$4080	10%
Debt repayment (loans, credit cards)	$425	$5100	12%
Entertainment	$120	$1440	4%
Clothing	$120	$1440	4%
School/childcare	$370	$4440	11%
Miscellaneous	$300	$3600	9%

Aurelie's Assets		Aurelie's Debts	
Home equity	$75,000	Mortgage	$60,000
Checking account	$ 1,500	Credit cards	$ 5,500
Savings account	$ 4,000	School loans	$22,000
Mutual funds	$ 8,000	Medical bills	$ 7,000
401(k)	$10,000		
Cash	$ 500		
Total Assets	$99,000	Total Debts	$94,500

Aurelie's Net Worth

Total Assets	$99,000
Total Debts	$94,500
Net Worth	**$ 4,500**

FIGURE 7-3

A personal balance sheet helps summarize a person's financial position at a given point in time.

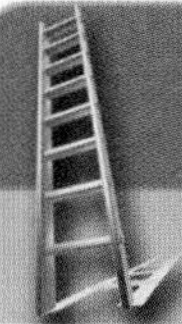

FIRST STEPS

Dig out everything that pertains to your current finances: your bank statements, credit card statements, insurance policies, investment portfolios, mortgage, recent check stubs, retirement accounts, and so on. What you're going to do now is to calculate your net worth. Remember, net worth is the balance after your liabilities have been subtracted from your assets. Liabilities are what you have that take money from you (mortgage, taxes, car payment, rent, etc.), while assets are things that are of value or bring you money (cash, stocks, savings, rental properties, etc). In short, net worth is the difference between what you own and what you owe. Quite obviously, wealth is achieved by widening the gap between the assets and liabilities, owning more and owing less.

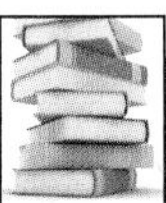

HELPFUL RESOURCES

There are lots of resources out there to help you maximize your financial health. Mint.com is a free online money management site that helps you track your spending, prepare a budget, and helps you save. It is quick to set up and very user friendly. This site has won many awards and been spotlighted in many publications.[12] They are able to maintain the site for free due to revenue generated by advertisers. Though most sites like this are secure, always do research and use common sense when putting any personal or financial information online.

CONSTRUCTING YOUR FINANCIAL HOUSE

Many financial advisors employ the analogy of constructing a pyramid or building a house to illustrate the interdependent components of a sound financial plan (see Figure 7-4 ■). Just as your physical house provides you shelter from external elements, so too will a well-built financial house help protect you from financial conditions beyond your control.

BE PREPARED FOR THE UNEXPECTED: INSURANCE

The best-laid financial plans can be pulled asunder by unexpected circumstances; thus, insurance is an important part of any financial plan. **Insurance** is a way to guarantee your financial protection against possible losses. An **insurance policy** is a contract in which an individual or business receives a designated financial protection or compensation against loss from an insurance provider. For many people, the idea of insurance can be very off-putting. It can be seen as unnecessary, complicated, fear-laden, a demurral to the elephantine insurance fat cats, and about as exciting as, well, an insurance seminar. In spite of all these associations, insurance is a very important component in the construction of your financial plan. Failing to invest in insurance can cost you and your loved ones a devastating sum and can wipe out entire fortunes.

GETTING ORGANIZED

Create a personal finance section in your *Business of Massage Therapy* notebook. After you have completed a personal budget and personal balance sheet, put it all into your notebook, as well as all the journaling work you did about your money beliefs. In a few months, do these exercises again, and see if your answers differ at all with time.

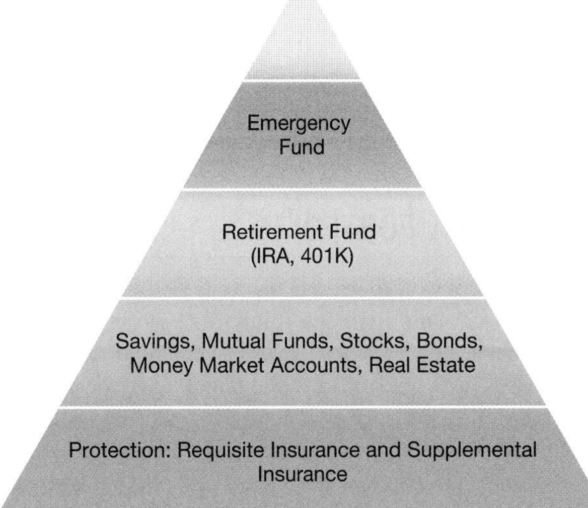

FIGURE 7-4

A strong financial plan includes many elements, such as savings, insurance, a fund for emergencies, and retirement planning.

There are many kinds of insurance products on the market, and the types of insurance will correlate with your situation. You will want to talk with a licensed insurance provider to explore your unique needs. Below is a short list of some of the most common types of insurance you will encounter. You will learn more about business-specific insurance in Chapter 10, "Organizing and Legal Structuring."

- Automobile insurance
- Health insurance
- Home insurance
- Disability insurance
- Fire and theft insurance
- Liability insurance
- Life insurance (Term, Whole Life, Universal)
- Product liability insurance
- Renter's insurance
- Worker's compensation

Insurance on your largest assets represents the *first floor* of your financial house. Many of these kinds of insurance, such as car and home insurance, are compulsory—required by law—so most people have them. In the interest of saving in the short term, many people will opt for the minimum coverage required, but fail to consider the potential effects upon their financial houses. The key is having enough to adequately protect you, and calculating that for yourself may be difficult. A rule of thumb in financial planning is to have coverage that is greater than, or at least commensurate with, your net worth.[13]

You will also want to fortify your foundation by protecting assets for which insurance is not necessarily required by the government—assets that are much more difficult to quantify. This type of insurance shelters such things as your health, potential disability, or even your life. Many people fail to insure these aspects of their lives, thinking perhaps that they aren't really relevant to their situation. In fact, the number one reason for bankruptcy and foreclosure, second to debt mismanagement and credit card bills, is lack of adequate health or disability insurance.[14] And the disability or death of a financially contributing member of your family can have a devastating impact on the wealth you worked to build.

CREATING A PORTFOLIO

The *second story* of your financial house is built with asset accumulation. This includes things like savings, mutual funds, stocks, bonds, money market accounts, real estate, and so forth. This level of financial planning is one that gets a lot of attention, as wealth accumulation is strongly emphasized in this culture. However, it is just one aspect of the entire picture. The assets you acquire are only as strong as their foundational support and future protection.

PREPARING FOR THE FUTURE

You are almost done building your house, but you are going to need an attic. The rest of your house protects you from things that could happen today or in the immediate future, while your attic provides a place to position your long-term financial goals. With Social Security attenuating to possible extinction and company-offered pension plans becoming a thing of the past, the importance of retirement planning is at an apex. If you don't plan for your retirement, who will?

EMERGENCY FUND

One of the top suggestions of financial planners and advisors alike is to have an **emergency fund**, or a monetary cushion to catch you should you fall. As the name implies, this is money that you devote to emergencies only—a sudden loss of income, unexpected home repair, or unforeseen car repairs. Emergencies, by definition, are usually unanticipated events, and so how do you know how much to have in your fund? There is wide variation on the exact amount suggested as a safety net, ranging from one month to one year's worth of expenses. To figure this out for yourself, calculate your monthly expenses (rent/mortgage, food, car payments—essential expenses, not the discretionary stuff), and then start with three months' worth in your savings. And then decipher your exact needs, and the reality of how long you could face unemployment should your job be suddenly terminated, your business closed, or any other such calamity befall you. Find the number that will help you sleep at night should the bottom fall out of your current income quotient. The important thing about an emergency fund is that it be safe and have high liquidity. **Liquidity** is the degree to which an asset is convertible to cash. Savings accounts, checking accounts, and mutual funds are usually very liquid. If you have an emergency, you will probably need the money quickly. Because of this, emergency funds are usually kept in savings, money market, or checking accounts.

UNDER ONE ROOF

The structure of your house needs something to cover and encapsulate all its parts. In your actual house, the roof provides shelter for the entire building. In your financial house, the roof is your estate plan. This can include wills, trusts, establishing power of attorney, and designating beneficiaries. Although an "estate plan" sounds like it could only possibly pertain to the most affluent of individuals, don't be deceived—it is for everyone. **Estate planning** ensures that your financial house passes to the people you wish. These are your **beneficiaries**, the people who receive your money, assets, or other benefits. **Your beneficiaries can be anyone you choose.** Good estate planning can help minimize taxes and minimize the involvement of **probate court**, which has as its primary purpose the distribution of the assets of the deceased.[15]

One of the main goals in estate planning is to make sure that all of your assets (the stuff you worked so hard for) are directed in a way that is aligned with your values when you are no longer here. Even if you have $10 to your name, you are entitled to have that money distributed as you wish.

BUILDING A FINANCIAL COMMUNITY

Before concluding your exploration into your personal finances, take a moment to consider the role of community in achieving your goals with money. In Buddhism, *sangha* is the word used to describe a spiritual community, and its importance in the journey is one of the tenets of the faith.[16] In Chapter 6, you explored the importance of community building and networking for the strength of your business. It is important to understand the power of financial community when working towards your financial health. A **financial community** is a network of people that come together for the common goal of financial health. Many people grew up with the message that money is an extremely private matter, and that to discuss it with others is not only distasteful, it can be dangerous. Nothing could be further from the truth. Just as with other aspects of health, financial health can be augmented by the sharing of information and the leveraging of relationships that are found in any community.

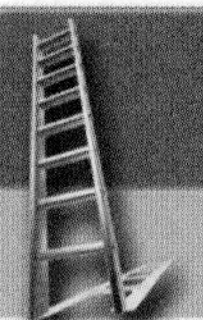

FIRST STEPS

Even if your assets are simple, navigating the right choice for you may be more complex. Tax codes shift and legal nuances may prove overwhelming. Enlist the help of a professional. Many estate planning attorneys will do a free consultation, and your financial planner can help you plot a course that is right for you.

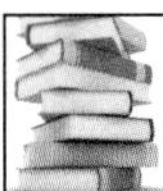

HELPFUL RESOURCES

If you would like to be better informed before taking the step to talk with a lawyer or consult with a financial planner, you might start with a trip to the library to learn more about estate planning. Look for books like *Estate Planning Basics* by Denis Clifford (2007, NOLO), *60 Minute Estate Planner* by Sandy F. Kraemer (2007, AMACOM), or *Estate Planning for Dummies* by Jordan Simon and Brian Caverly (2003, Wiley).

If the people who make the decisions are the people who will also bear the consequences of those decisions, perhaps better decisions will result.

—John Abrams

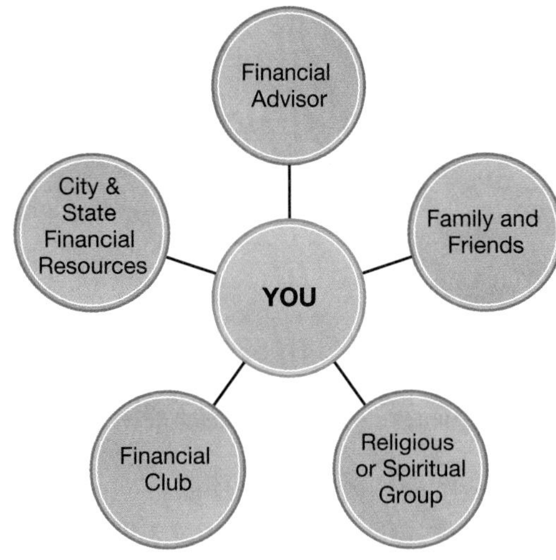

FIGURE 7-5

It can be very beneficial to develop a financial community to help you attain financial success. Engage people who will help you stay accountable to your plan and reach your goals.

Chances are pretty good that there is an investment group or financial support group in your area. Websites like Meetup can help you identify such groups of interest. Type your city and phrases that relate to your interest, such as "massage therapists financial planning" or "women's investment group" in the search engine, and see what comes up. You might check with your local government to see what resources it offers for financial education and support. People that you already know, such as family, friends, religious groups, or other people in your life, can become part of your financial community as well (Figure 7-5 ■).

If you can't find a money group or financial community that piques your interest online or within your existing network, get a recommendation from a financial planner or even a debt alleviation counselor. The important thing is that you want to make sure you surround yourself with positive people who will help you achieve your goals.

Still can't find a group? Start one! Invite friends, family, massage therapists, and other helping professionals from your network to join your financial community. Together you can set out your goals, your agreements, and your group's structure. The focus in the group need not be fixated on financial strategy or stock market fluctuations—it can be about gaining clarity, storytelling beliefs, and anything else that supports the members.[17] The form and content are up to you.

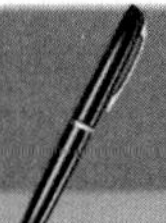

PUT IT IN WRITING

Strength in Numbers?

You have been asked to initiate a financial group for helping professionals in your area. The goal of this group is to empower all members to achieve their financial goals. Make a list of 10 people that you would like to include and think might be interested.

1. ____________ **6.** ____________
2. ____________ **7.** ____________
3. ____________ **8.** ____________
4. ____________ **9.** ____________
5. ____________ **10.** ____________

Groups have the most impact when they are interactive and engaging. Activities could include inviting speakers to come and talk to the group, doing financial book studies, watching movies with financial themes and having a discussion after, or taking field trips to places like real estate auctions or banks. What are some things you would like to do in your group?

____
____
____
____
____
____

CHAPTER SUMMARY BY LEARNING OBJECTIVES

1. **Explain the importance of personal financial planning** Personal financial planning is the application of financial principles toward one's goals and the crafting of a workable plan to achieve those goals. In order to create and grow a flourishing, successful practice that promotes health and healing in others, it is imperative to examine your relationship to your personal finances.
2. **Define assets and liabilities** Assets are items of monetary value that are owned by an individual or a company, and typically can be converted to cash. Examples include savings, equity on a home, equipment, stocks, and real estate. Liabilities are financial obligations owed to another person or company in exchange for capital, products, or services you have used or consumed—in short, debt. Examples of liabilities include credit card debt, school loans, mortgages, taxes, bills, and so forth.
3. **Distinguish good debt from bad debt** Good debt is money that is borrowed in order to obtain something that will ultimately increase in value. Examples of this include taking out a school loan to pay for college, a home mortgage, or a business loan. Bad debt is money that is borrowed to purchase things that do not appreciate in value or contribute to your financial health. Typically bad debt happens when money is borrowed to purchase something you ultimately do not need and cannot afford without using credit.
4. **Explore what money and wealth mean to you** Defining prosperity and truly understanding your financial objectives is the first step in achieving them. If you don't truly identify with another's definition of prosperity or don't have a firm one yourself, how hard are you willing to work to achieve it? Really examining definitions of true wealth and abundance is something that few people do. But it is a very important part of your financial plan.
5. **Learn how to align money with values** One of the greatest qualities about money is its means to a higher end. Money can be the way in which you actualize the life you want to live and demonstrate what you value. By being clear on your values, you can align the financial choices you make to be in step with what matters most to you.
6. **Understand financial literacy** Financial literacy is the ability to understand and manage your financial health and plan for your financial present and future. As the onus of financial responsibility falls more and more to the individual, educating oneself about finances is more imperative than ever.
7. **Create a financial plan** A successful financial process is enhanced and advanced by a financial plan. Like a business plan or a marketing plan, a financial plan outlines your goals and objectives and delineates your strategy for achieving your financial ambitions. A financial plan can be used in your personal life and for your business; these plans may be quite similar or very different depending on factors such as size and scope of your business endeavor.
8. **Explore compound interest and the time value of money** With compound interest, the interest you are paid goes back into your account and gets applied to the principal, so both are earning interest together. By putting your money into investments that bear compound interest, the money that you pay yourself first is working for you by earning more money exponentially. The longer an investment is able to leverage compound interest, the more exponential growth—this is the time value of money (simplified).
9. **Understand the importance of an emergency fund, insurance, and estate planning to build your financial "house"** Just as with building a house, there are many interdependent components of constructing a solid financial plan. An emergency fund is money that is set aside only for extenuating circumstances: a sudden loss of income, unexpected home repair, and unforeseen car repairs. Insurance is a way to guarantee your financial protection against possible losses, and areas of coverage can range from your house to your car to your health to your very life. Estate planning is a method of ensuring that your assets continue on in a manner consistent with your wishes.
10. **Discover the benefits of creating a financial community (*sangha*)** A financial community is a network of people that come together for the common goal of financial health. Just as with other aspects of health, financial health can be augmented by the sharing of information and the leveraging of relationships that are found in any community.

ACTIVITIES

Quiz: Financial Planning Basics

1. Ginger has just been told that she needs to cut back on her discretionary spending by her financial planner. If she were to follow his advice, which item might she forego?
   a. Rent
   b. Groceries
   c. New iPod
   d. Toothpaste
2. Matteo wants to start an emergency fund, and he knows that he wants to keep it liquid. This means:
   a. His money is in a secure place and cannot be accessed.
   b. His money is easily converted to cash.
   c. His money is not insured by the government.
   d. His money is soaking wet.
3. There are many challenges to obtaining wealth. Four of the most common obstacles to achieving personal financial goals include:
   a. Spouse, parents, friends, and your boss
   b. A bad economy, government, predatory lenders, the Fed
   c. Not planning, overspending, consumer credit, not planning for retirement
   d. Bad information, impossible-to-understand terms, bankruptcy, medical bills
4. In ancient Rome, the goddess of health and fertility was named ______________.
   a. Venus
   b. Athena
   c. Angie
   d. Moneta
5. Therese is just starting out in her massage career and does not have a lot of extra money. However, she knows that if she commits to putting a small amount of money into her retirement account each month starting now, she will easily be able to reach her financial goals for her future. She understands that if she waits even a few years, she will have to invest more to achieve the same amount. Which of the following principles is Therese applying in her financial planning?
   a. *Time in the market* rather than *timing the market*
   b. The power of compounding interest
   c. Consistent contributions
   d. All of the above
6. Pok is working on his personal financial statement, and has gathered all of his relevant documents to help him calculate all of his debts and all of his assets. Next he subtracts his debts from his assets, which tells him his______________.
   a. Net worth
   b. Intrinsic value
   c. Cash flow statement
   d. Common stock
7. Caitlin wants to start saving and is interested in ways to pay herself first. She talks with a financial planner, who tells her that a great way to start is to cut discretionary spending. If she follows this advice, which of the following things should Caitlin NOT buy?
   a. Gas for her car
   b. Groceries
   c. Health insurance
   d. New ski boots for her Aspen vacation
8. Manny has worked really hard to build his massage business, buy a home, and invest in his future. He does not have a will or a trust, or any other estate plan. In the event that he dies, what is the most likely thing that will happen to Manny's assets?
   a. They will go directly to the beneficiaries Manny would have wanted.
   b. His estate will go through probate court, which will decide how to distribute his assets.
   c. They will be seized by the government to pay for a bailout.
   d. They will be donated to science.
9. Laura has had a really rough month professionally and personally. Laura's friend CJ wants to cheer her up and suggests the two of them go on a weekend getaway into wine country. Laura has not been making any extra money lately, but really wants to take the trip with CJ. If she wants to stay true to her financial plan and not undermine her financial house, what is the account she should use to fund her trip?
   a. Her joy account
   b. Her emergency fund
   c. Her retirement fund
   d. The money she got from refinancing her house
10. Which of the following is not a liability?
    a. School loans
    b. Credit card debt
    c. Equity on a home
    d. Taxes on income

Case Study

Jean's Personal Financial Statement

Jean has decided to take a look at her current financial standing. She has pulled out all of her financial statements to get a good idea of her position. Grab a calculator and help her sort it out.

Jean has a lot of assets. She bought a house two years ago for $200,000. Jean made a down payment of $40,000 and has been putting another $1000 per month towards her equity in the house. With interest payments accruing on the principal, she still has $142,000 on her mortgage. Jean does have a checking account, and her current balance is $800. Her statement shows that her savings account, which has been growing exponentially over the years, contains $3000. She also has an emergency fund, which has a balance of $8000—enough money to get Jean through 6 months of expenses should anything happen. Jean has also been growing her retirement account since her late 20s, and has managed to accrue a balance of $94,500 for her retirement in a Roth IRA account. Jean doesn't like to keep too much cash, and only has about $40 in her wallet.

Jean also has a lot of debt. As you saw earlier, she is still carrying a $142,000 mortgage on her house. Jean also has a considerable amount of credit card debt, though she has been working to pay it off. Her collective balance on her two credit cards is $12,000. Jean took out $10,000 in student loans to pay for massage school, and consolidated that loan with the $25,000 she still has to pay off on her undergraduate studies. She has no medical bills, and no other outstanding debts.

Now calculate Jean's assets and Jean's debts in Figure 7-6 ■. Then figure out her overall net worth. Look at the sum, and reflect on what this means for Jean. If you were Jean's financial planner, what would you tell her to do?

Jean's Assets		**Jean's Debts**	
	$		$
	$		$
	$		$
	$		$
	$		
Total Assets	$	Total Debts	$

Jean's Net Worth	
Total Assets	$
Total Debts	$
Net Worth	**$**

FIGURE 7-6

Personal balance sheet.

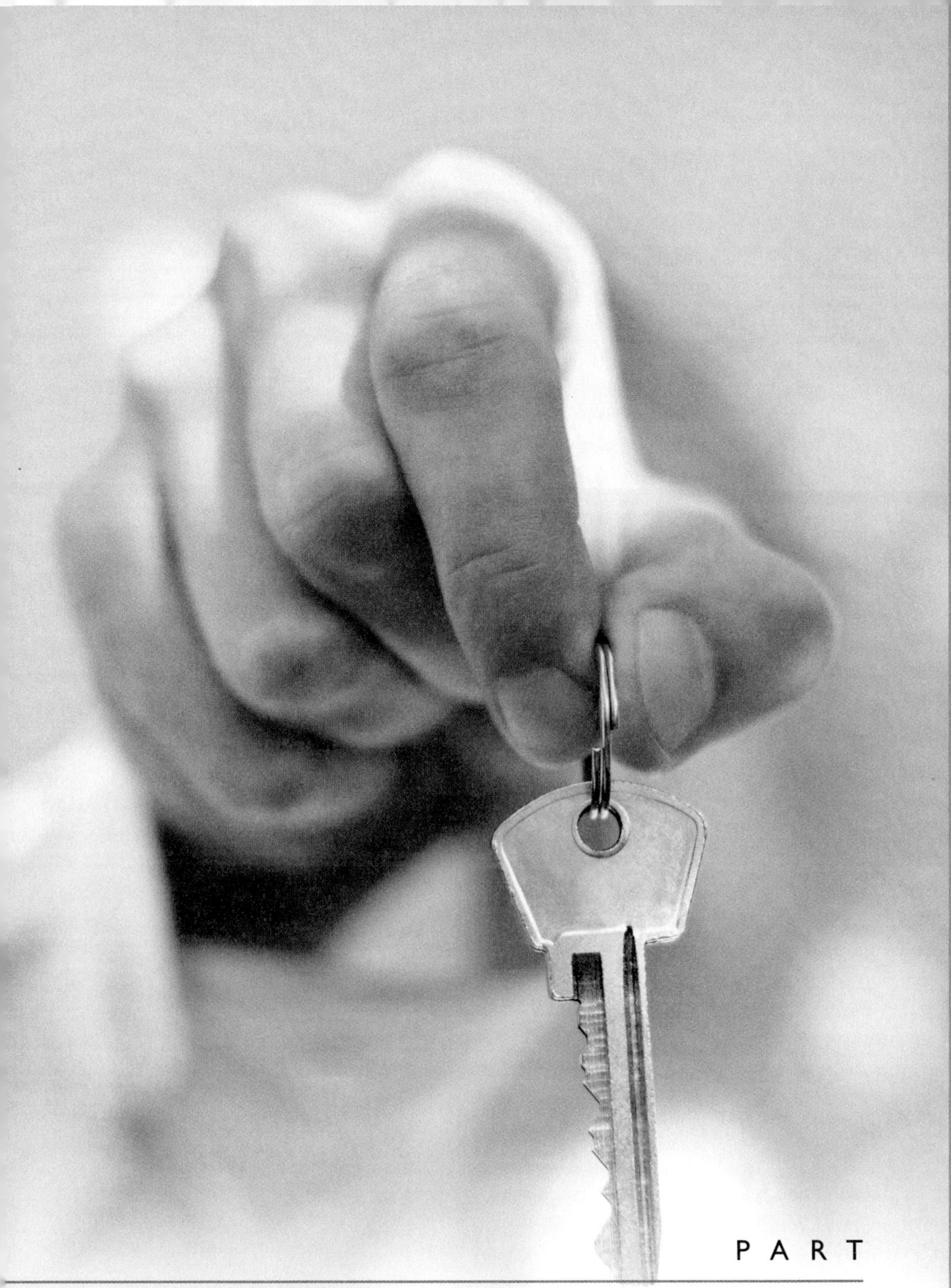

PART

2

A Thriving Massage Business to Call Your Own

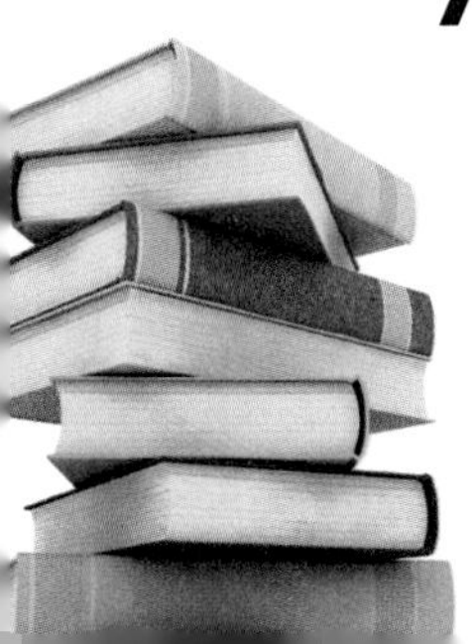

CHAPTER

8 Your Own Practice: Getting Started

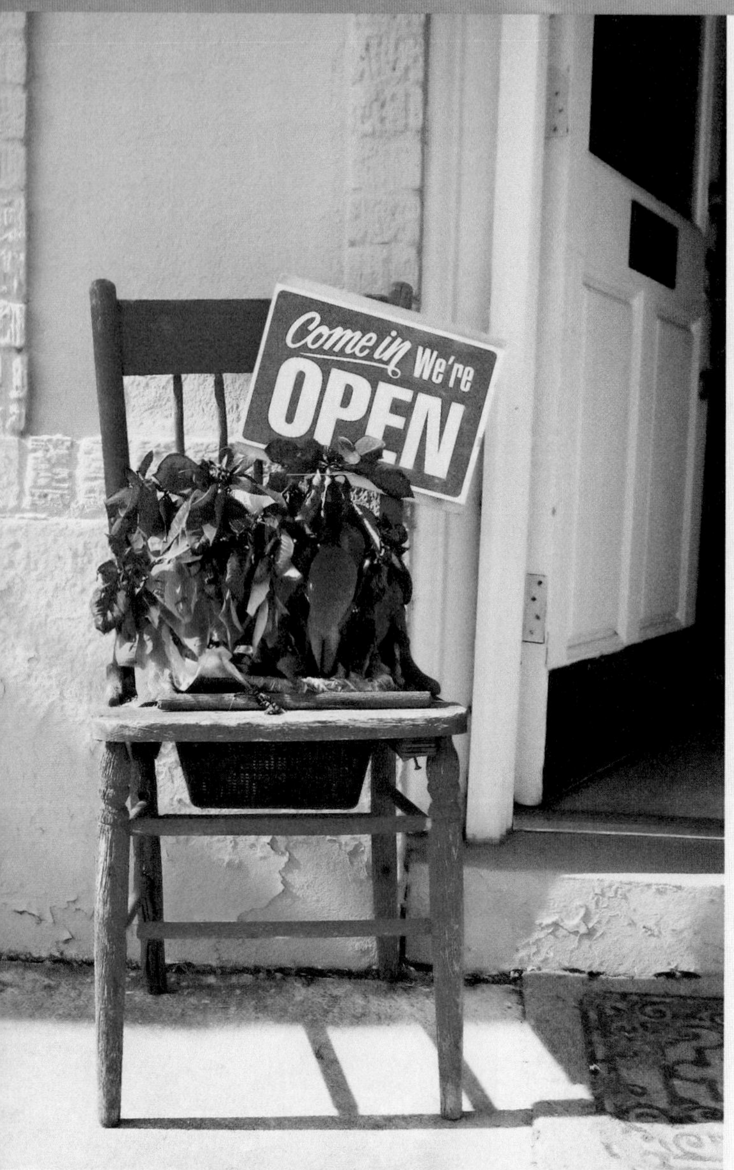

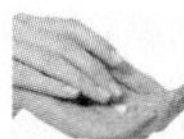

CHAPTER OUTLINE

LEARNING OBJECTIVES

1. Create your own definition of success
2. Describe barriers to success and self-imposed limitations
3. Evaluate the applications of creative visualization, affirmations and gratitude lists
4. Identify the challenges in getting started with a new business
5. Uncover the importance of setting goals
6. Examine the components of a plan and a time line
7. Incorporate values, purpose, and vision into your plan
8. Discover ways to anticipate obstacles and create solutions
9. Create a two-year plan and a time line

KEY TERMS

Success is not the key to happiness. Happiness is the key to success. If you love what you are doing, you will be successful.

—Albert Schweitzer

WHAT IS SUCCESS?

If asked, most people will say that they want to be very successful in life. But being clear on one's definition of success is a very large part of obtaining it. While the dictionary defines success as both the degree of one's succeeding and the attainment of wealth, favor, and eminence, success is a concept relative to each individual. In a general sense, **success** is a person, group, project, or event for which an intended purpose is attained.

Success is a very fluid concept, and can mean very different things to different people. Its ultimate definition is relative to the individual's own goals and values. One person may gauge a successful life by the amount of money he or she earns or the number of lucrative possessions acquired, while another may feel successful if he or she earns enough to sustain a very simple life. Others may thrive by surrounding themselves with family or friends. Some may find success in creating something that endures after they are gone, such as a body of writing or a work of art. There is no monopoly on the definition of success, and it is imperative that you explore your own definitions before you set out for that ever-illusive finish line. Understanding your own definition of success will help you set goals more effectively, and will help you recognize and celebrate your accomplishments.

Those who try to do something and fail are infinitely better off than those who try nothing and succeed.

—Lloyd Jones

Creative visualization is the practice of envisioning the future you want in very specific detail. It can be a very imaginative and pleasurable part of goal setting and achieving success. Creative visualization can work for you, and your successful massage career, and can help you to envision and create the business you would like to have.The idea behind creative visualization is that envisioning things a certain way and connecting to that vision with as many senses (sight, sound, smell, taste) and details as possible can help manifest that reality. For example, if a man wants to succeed in losing 30 pounds, he can creatively visualize his life and his body 30 pounds lighter. By closing your eyes and imagining yourself in a swimming pool, you can "see" yourself in your suit, feel your muscles contracting as you move through the

PUT IT IN WRITING

How Do I Define Success?

Take a few minutes to write out your feelings about success and what it means in the context of your own life. Look at the questions below, and write out your answers.

1. To me, I am the most successful when I
____
____
2. When I look back, some of my most important successes include
____
____
____
3. I consider these successes important because they represent
____
____
____
4. In the past month, what has been my biggest success? What goals did I set in order to achieve this success, and how did I implement them?
____
____
____
5. Who is the most successful person that I know, and why do I think so?
____
____
____
6. What one thing would I like to accomplish but have never tried? What has prevented me from doing this?
____
____
____
7. If I were to achieve my ultimate definition of success, how would my life look different than it does now?
____
____
____

Take some time to reflect on your responses, and try to keep these ideas in mind as you go through the rest of the chapter. Remember, the only person who can determine whether you have been a success in your life is you!

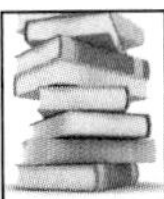

HELPFUL RESOURCES

If you're new to creative visualization and would like to explore it further, check out Shakti Gawain's book *Creative Visualization: Use the Power of Your Imagination to Create What You Want in Life* (2002, Nataraj Publishing).

water, smell the chlorine in the water, hear the splashing sound as you swim—you're doing a creative visualization. It doesn't matter if you do visualizations with your eyes open or closed; the important part is engaging your imagination to experience your success internally to attract and expedite the success externally. Just as many of us don't understand the intricacies of gravity but still function under its principles, you need not understand or even believe in it to have the principles of creative visualization work for you. Not believing in gravity doesn't mean you suddenly are weightless!

Goal setting and success are ultimately not final destinations; it is a mistake to think that once a goal is set or even obtained, it need not be maintained. There are several tools for both manifesting and maintaining goals. Affirmations and gratitude lists are two powerful techniques to help you get started and keep moving in the right direction.

Affirmations are a very helpful tool on the road to success, and can help you stay on that road when things get tough. Affirmations are positive assertions about the way things are that help manifest a positive reality. Typically, they are declarations of things that you want to create in your life, spoken as though they already were so. Affirmations are always personal (I, my) statements and always in the present tense. Even if the statement may not yet be true or may not be what you have previously believed about yourself or a situation, say it as though it were. For example, to support a weight loss program, a man might use the affirmation "I have a strong and healthy body, and I shed weight easily." Affirmations have various purposes: they help route new positive pathways into your mind, and they take the place of the negative thoughts that have spent years digging ruts in the psyche. Affirmations help retrain your thought process into a more supportive one, paving the way for real changes[1]. Affirmations are the foot soldiers for the adage, "If you can believe it, you can achieve it."

In holistic thought, what you focus on expands. This can be true of wealth, family harmony, illness, or anything toward which you direct your attention. By expressing gratitude for the things you already have and the goals you've already achieved, you open yourself up for more abundance and success. Writing gratitude lists is a great way of targeting your focus on the positive and priming yourself for more of the good stuff. **Gratitude lists** are another tangible tool for

PITFALLS

It is not uncommon to feel self-conscious or uncomfortable with many of these techniques, especially if you've never done them before. Many people experience resistance in the form of skepticism or doubt and cast many of the techniques by the wayside. Of course, only use what works for you, but give these a try for a while before you decide. You may just find yourself pleasantly surprised at how much you can manifest when you put your mind to it.

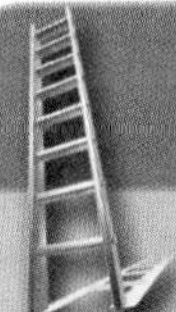

FIRST STEPS

Take a little time each day to say your affirmations. You can choose some from the list below, or make some of your own.

I am okay even when I am scared
I am very loveable
I always attract quality people into my life
I am successful at work and relationships
I am a powerful individual
I am creative and intuitive
My body is strong, healthy, and beautiful
My work is deeply fulfilling
I take responsibility for my success and my happiness
I welcome new experiences and embrace the unknown
I am limitless in my creativity
I am healthy in my body, mind, spirit, relationships, finances, and every other area of my life.
I always have time for the things that matter to me
My life is a manifestation of joy, love and abundance
I deserve to achieve my goals

Your affirmations:

1. ______________________
2. ______________________
3. ______________________
4. ______________________

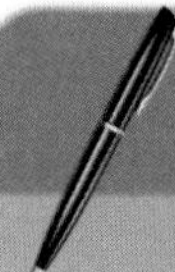

PUT IT IN WRITING

Gratitude Lists

The following is an example of a gratitude list. Use it as a guideline to create your own. See if you can think of five things each day. Each time you do the exercise, see if you can come up with five new things for which to be grateful.

Today I am grateful for:

1. My strong and healthy body
2. My great education
3. Soup and sweaters on a cold day
4. My wonderful life partner and our warm and welcoming home
5. The smell of my baby's hair

There is absolutely no right way to do this—write whatever arises in your mind. Now you try:

1. __________
2. __________
3. __________
4. __________
5. __________

achieving your success by focusing on all the things that are going right. As you begin to pay attention to the positive things in your life, you will find you have more and more things for which to be grateful. When you get started, gratitude lists help you to see how much you already have going for you, and as you progress along they help you to appreciate how far you've come. Affirmations and gratitude provide technical support for success.

BARRIERS TO SUCCESS AND SELF-IMPOSED LIMITATIONS

Even when our vision of success is crystal clear, it is not uncommon to find the path to that success impeded by many things. External circumstances may present challenges to achieving your success. The economy may be very poor, a parent could get unexpectedly ill and need caretaking, or a competitor may open shop next door. All these things can affect your success no matter what you do.

However, more often than not, it is the internal barriers that are the true culprits for inhibiting success. **Self-imposed limitations** are ways that people hinder themselves from going forward and achieving what they want. It is often part of the complex human psyche that people sabotage their own desires and limit their own accomplishments. This can be done in many ways: "forgetting" to keep an appointment, not paying bills on time, not following through with a client, procrastinating, miring in addictions, quitting just before the finish line, etc. This can be rooted in so many things: fear of failure, feelings of inadequacy, apprehension about leaving the familiar and heading into the unknown, or quite simply a fear of success. Understanding the myriad reasons behind self-sabotage is beyond the scope and purview of this book, but it can be very powerful and clearing to simply acknowledge and explore ways in which you may be standing in your own way. And it is a very important step to take *before* embarking on the journey towards your holistic business.

> *There are two great tragedies in life: the first is to lose your heart's desire. The second is to obtain it.*
>
> —George Bernard Shaw

As the old adage maintains, the best indicator of future behavior is that of the past and the present. Before understanding the ways you may consciously or unconsciously obstruct your path to success in the future, let's begin by looking at your past.

> *Whether you think you can or you think you can't, either way you're right.*
>
> —Henry Ford

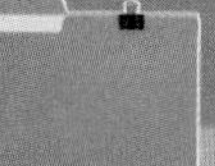

GETTING ORGANIZED

Keep your responses to the "What Came Before" exercise in your *Business of Massage Therapy* notebook, and come back to these responses from time to time. It might be quite telling to return to do this exercise again as you progress with your business, and see how the answers evolve.

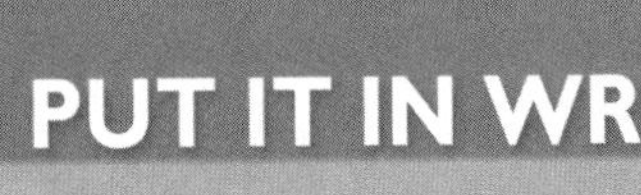

PUT IT IN WRITING

What Came Before

It's time to jog your memory and look at ways that you may have impeded your own progress or success in the past. Pay attention to the feelings that come up as you delve into your past. As best as you can, release all criticism and judgments about the way things have been. This is merely an exploration, not a time to self-deprecate.

Copy the following sentences, completing them with as much detail as you can muster.

1. When I was little I dreamed of becoming ______________. I did/ didn't because ______________. This makes me feel ______________.
2. The last project I started but did not complete was ______________. I didn't complete it because ______________.
3. When I think about starting or taking the next step with my massage business, I feel ______________.
4. I have set many goals in my life. The ones I have achieved are ______________. The ones I still have to accomplish are ______________.
5. When I think of achieving ultimate success with my business I envision ______________. On the upside, this success will mean ______________. On the downside, this success will mean ______________.
6. When it comes to following through, I see myself as ______________.
7. When it comes to following through, others see me as ______________.
8. What happens if I achieve success as I define it? ______________
9. What happens if I don't achieve success as I define it? ______________
10. The things I am willing to do to reach my goals are ______________.
11. The things I refuse to do to reach my goals are ______________.

PITFALLS

Many people suffer from a condition called "terminal uniqueness," in which they believe that they are the only ones to suffer from insecurities, procrastination, fear of failure, or other human imperfections. It is very important to understand that self-sabotage is a large part of the human condition, and to proceed with great compassion for yourself as you explore the terrain of your past in order to move forward into your future. Everyone has been there!

Behind most self-sabotaging behavior is fear, pure and simple. **Fear** is a very natural emotion that can be quite functional in many situations of danger, whether real or perceived. In our Western culture we often try and conquer fears, or deny them altogether. However, just as with so many things, fear is usually the most powerful when unexamined. Attempting to deny or destroy your fear can actually be counterproductive; the truly brave and constructive approach is to be open to the fear and to act in spite of it. The root of the fear, or why it exists or what it means, ultimately don't matter. It simply matters that you acknowledge it. Like germs in sunshine, fear is dispelled when put under the light. The "What Came Before" exercise helps explore some of the ways fear plays into your path to success. The next exercise, "Then What?" will help you shine some light on those fears.

> *Courage is not the absence of fear; but the judgment that something else is more important than fear.*
>
> —Ambrose Redmoon

In spite of all those fears, you have still managed to succeed in innumerable ways already. Take a moment to look at all the ways you've already been successful. Have you completed high school, college, or other levels of higher education? Have you met financial goals that you have set for yourself by saving for a new home, a vacation, or a new car? Have you sustained a loving long-term relationship with a friend, partner, or family member? Perhaps you have trained your body for a marathon or have committed your time to volunteer for something important for you. Look at places in your life where you have set goals and accomplished them. Celebrating your successes is an important part of the process, and helps to set the stage for future success. Confidence breeds confidence and appreciation for what you've already achieved makes room for new achievements. Take a moment to pat yourself on the back!

Now that you've acknowledged self-limiting behaviors in your past, recognized the role of fear in your process, and taken a moment to congratulate yourself on the many successes you have already accomplished, you possess a better understanding of where you are starting from. Now it is time to explore where you are going and how to get there. Another mistake that many make when starting a new business is forgetting to look at the details

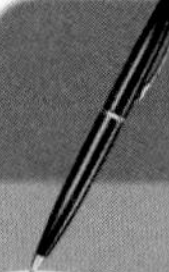

PUT IT IN WRITING

Then What?[2]

- When you succeed, what will the benefits be? Then what?
- What will this achieve for you? Then what?
- What can you do then? Then what?
- What will you get then that you really want? Then what?
- Who will be excited about these outcomes? Then what?
- Who will be threatened or unhappy about these outcomes? Then what?

Often it is the consequences or outcomes of actions rather than the actions themselves that can make you afraid to move forward. This is a nice exercise to help relax the grip that fear can sometimes have on you. In your *Business of Massage Therapy* notebook, write down three things that really scare you. Underneath each one, write what would happen if that scary thing actually occurred. And if that thing happened, then what? And if that next thing happened, then what?! You'll often find that if you follow the chain of events to a logical conclusion, the outcome might not be that scary after all. Here is an example:

My fear: I am of afraid leaving my current job to start my own business.

Then what: If I leave my job, I won't have the financial security I've known the last five years.

Then what: I will stay up late worrying that I cannot provide for my family.

Then what: I may have to borrow money from a bank or my parents to have an extra cushion.

Then what: I'll owe the bank or my parents money.

Then what: I'll have an extra incentive to work twice as hard at my new business, which I have had to do anyway whenever I start something new. I'm not a stranger to hard work.

Then what: If I worked that hard at a job I hated, then maybe I'll be even more successful jumping into my own business with both feet and my whole heart.

Then what: Then I will know that I tried my best and took a chance. In time I will pay the money back plus interest!

of their desired destination. Many thrust themselves into the work of starting a business so enthusiastically that they forget to make strategic plans based on what they really want. A massage therapist might set a goal by saying "I'm going to make $70,000 my first year in business," without considering the hard work, sacrifice of family, friends, free time, and other life changes that will go along with such a goal. Moreover, he may fail to consider what making $70,000 may truly mean in his life—what will that look like as far as taxes are concerned? What was he making before? Is the $70,000 the representation of success, or the number of clients he is able to attract to make that much? How will that amount of money inform and affect his financial goals down the line?

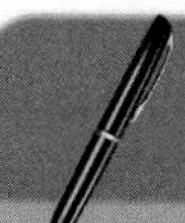

PUT IT IN WRITING

Celebrate Your Success!

It's time to acknowledge and celebrate as many successes as you can recall. You've worked hard for your accomplishments, so relish in them! A few examples are given below; now see if you can't think of 10 things you can applaud.

1. Traveled 26 percent of the world—over 25 countries
2. In a healthy relationship
3. Learned another language
4. Sustained several close friendships for more than two decades
5. Kept my business going for two years

Now you:

1. ____________________
2. ____________________
3. ____________________
4. ____________________
5. ____________________
6. ____________________
7. ____________________
8. ____________________
9. ____________________
10. ____________________

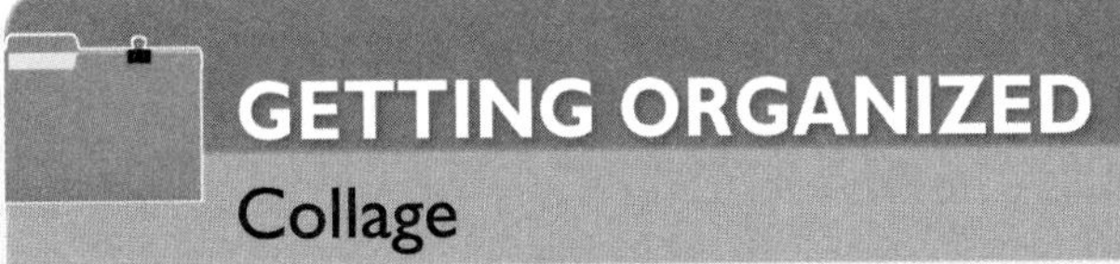

GETTING ORGANIZED
Collage

Creating visual representation of your goals for success can be a very powerful approach to achieving those goals. One helpful exercise is to create a collage. Grab a handful of old magazines, a piece of construction paper or cardstock, some scissors, and some glue or tape. Go through the magazines and cut out any images that represent your goals to you. Reference the Wheel of Life exercise you did in Chapter 1 so that you remember to incorporate all of the aspects of your life that are important to you. Now glue the images together in a collage and put it somewhere where you can see it often. It may sound like kindergarten—but it works!

GETTING STARTED

So often, the most difficult part of beginning anything new is simply getting started. Whether beginning a new exercise routine to lose 20 pounds, going back to school to get that degree, or putting out a personal ad to find a new relationship, taking the first step towards something new can be very daunting. This is often the case when starting a new business, particularly for those with little past business experience. "Where to begin?" "What if I do it wrong?" "What if I can't make enough money?" "What if I don't succeed?" Sometimes considering all of the many things that can go wrong in a new venture feels like being nibbled to death by minnows.

> *The journey of a thousand miles begins with one step.*
>
> —Lao Tzu

For helping professionals and holistic practitioners, starting a new business can be even more challenging because of the personal element intertwined with their services. Rather than being in business to sell an impersonal product, a massage therapist's service is intensely personal as it is an extension of his or her energy. In essence, massage therapists are selling themselves when they sell their massage skills. This can make the first steps even more overwhelming. Often therapists take one of two unsuccessful approaches when starting a business: *Fire Ready Aim,* in which a therapist jumps headfirst into a practice without doing adequate preparations or planning. This hasty approach can cause innumerable problems down the road, and being ill-prepared for the reality of the business causes many people to leave the massage profession completely. The other extreme is *Ready Aim Ready Aim Ready Aim,* in which a therapist spends countless hours researching and planning and investigating, but never takes any action. Many therapists fall into this category when starting out, uncertain how to actually get started.

When starting any new business, of course there are the very pragmatic steps to take such as analyzing your market conditions, assessing financial requirements for a start-up company, evaluating potential customers and competitors, and getting all the appropriate licensure and paperwork filed (and don't worry—all these skills will be covered in this book). But before any of the external assessments and actions should take place, it is incredibly important to take the time to do some internal self-assessments. This is an often overlooked consideration in the business world. Regardless of the nature of the business being started, at the end of the day all businesses are created, administered, and controlled by people. If the personal human elements are not taken into consideration, businesses rarely thrive.

As was mentioned earlier in the chapter, one of the imperative steps to getting started in any business is knowing the point from which you are starting. If you're trying to find your way to Kuala Lumpur, it really helps to know that you are starting in New York! How can you set a weight loss goal without knowing your current weight? It may sound like an oversimplification, but so many people start new business ventures or embark on new goals without taking the time to really grasp their current reality. They believe that having a goal and having passion is enough to deliver them to the doors of success, only to find that they miscalculated (or never thought to calculate) the distance between where they were and where they wanted to be. Because you have taken the time to do the exercises in this chapter and really understand aspects of yourself as an individual, you will likely be more successful in your goal setting and goal attainment for your business and for yourself in general.

GOAL SETTING

Throughout the chapter, you have been laying the groundwork for goal setting. **Goal setting** is the intentional positioning of an ambition and the implementation of actionable steps towards actualizing that aim. Your goals can relate to any aspect of your life: personal, physical, spiritual, community, relationships, education, career, and so forth. Goal setting is the practical action that converts wishes into real life, the alchemical process that turns a dream into a reality. It's the "how-to" stage of envisioning your ideal life.

> *If you can't predict the future, you must prepare for it.*
>
> —John W. Bachmann

To be truly effective, goals must be specific. It is not enough to say "I want to make more money this year." What does that ultimately mean? Is an additional $5 enough? Or $10,000? To get specifically what you want, be specific in what you ask for. Don't just say you want more clients in your practice—set a realistic number and a date you want to achieve the goal. Decide which measure will demonstrate success for yourself. The most successful goal setters know that their goals need to be actionable and quantifiable; they need to be SMART goals. SMART is a helpful acronym for effective and concise goal setting. **SMART goals** are Specific, Measurable, Attainable, Realistic, and Timely goals (Figure 8-1 ■).

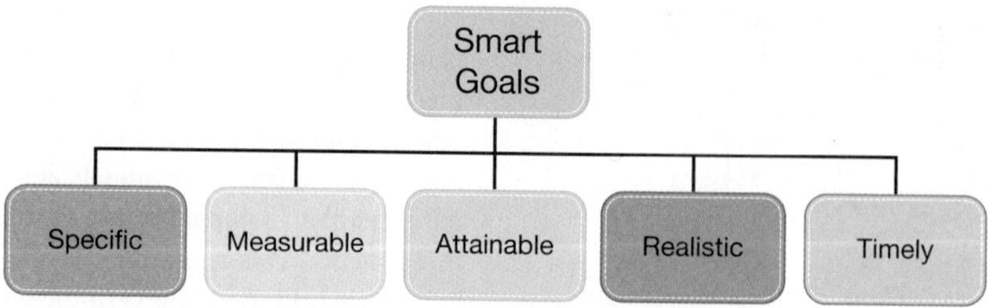

FIGURE 8-1

Making your goals SMART helps ensure their achievement.

First, *write it down!* The written word is incredibly powerful in achieving goals. In 1979, a survey was done of the graduating MBA class at Harvard.[3] The students were asked, "Have you set clear, written goals for your future and made plans to accomplish them?" Thirteen percent reported having goals in mind, but never committing them to writing. Surprisingly, only 3 percent of those surveyed had any written goals . . . and 84 percent of the graduates of one of the most sought-after training programs in business claimed to have no specific goals at all. In 1989, when a 10-year follow-up study was conducted on these same participants, it was found that the 13 percent with clear but undocumented goals made twice the salary of the 84 percent without them. And what about those students who had written out their goals in a clear and measurable way? They were, on average, earning as much as 10 times more than the other 97 percent combined.[4] This famous story is a perfect illustration of the importance of not only clarifying your goals, but recording them.

One great way to formalize your goals in writing is to create a contract to yourself. In this contract, write out specifically and precisely what your goals are. Include step-by-step actions and the deadlines you set for each one. Sign and date this contract just as you would a contract with someone else. It can be helpful to include rewards for yourself for every goal you make: a bar of chocolate, a massage, a new book. Sometimes it helps to share this contract with someone whom you trust: a sibling, a spouse, a friend. Make sure to put it somewhere you can see it and where you will be reminded of the agreements you have made with yourself. And, just as with any other contract—stick to the obligations and commitments you have made!

DEVELOP A PLAN AND A TIME LINE

A plan can be written for any length of time: a week, 6 months, 10 years. When starting something new, it is often most helpful to consider a digestible amount of time so as not to become overwhelmed. For the purposes of this chapter, start with a **two-year plan**. Of course, if you are more of a long-term or short-term person, you can adapt the length of time that is comfortable for you. The time frame ultimately doesn't matter—the specifics, measurability, attainability, realism, and timeliness do (SMART, after all).

Once you've completed all the "Put It in Writing" exercises that follow, compiling a two-year plan is a snap. It's really just a compilation of your values, your purpose, your vision, the step-by-step plan to bring your vision to fruition, barriers or contradictions you foresee in achieving your goals, and a time line for achieving them. Below are the ingredients

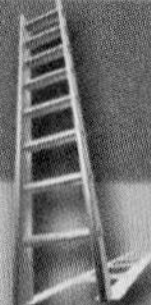

FIRST STEPS

Making SMART goals is a very helpful thing, and can actually be quite fun. Try it out! Come up with a simple goal for today. It can be something as simple as "I want to get the laundry done by 8:00 tonight" or "I will buy new drapes for the massage studio before my 10:00 am appointment tomorrow." With that goal in mind, fill out the spaces below.

Goal: ______________________________

Now, make sure your goal passes the SMART test. Is it specific (doing laundry, buying drapes)? Is it measurable (will you know the goal is met when the laundry is folded or when the drapes are hanging)? Is it attainable? Realistic? And how about timely?

Now try a larger goal, something that is a bit more complicated than doing a load of laundry or going shopping. For example, "I will have saved $3000 to start my own business by Thanksgiving 2012." Think of something you would really like to accomplish within the next year or two, and write it down. Remember, you are just getting started so make sure you set a goal that you have a good chance of fulfilling.

Goal: ______________________________

Run this longer-term goal through the SMART test, reworking it if necessary. When you have a goal you feel good about, put it somewhere you can see it. When your deadline comes, compare your progress to the goal you set for yourself.

(to find a two-year plan template and a completed two-year plan, see Appendix B).

I. Goals
II. Values
III. Purpose
IV. Vision
V. Obstacles
VI. Solutions
VII. Time line

You will begin your two-year plan by plotting out a life plan that is supported by many large and small goals. Incorporate as many goals as you would like to accomplish, but not too many that you minimize your chance of overall success with your plan (see Figure 8-2 ■). Your goals can be personal, professional, spiritual, physical, or relating to any area of your life that you choose. It might help to choose two or three small goals, and support these with smaller sub-goals. For example, if one of your large goals over the next two years is to save $3000 for your new business, some sub-goals might include starting a new savings account with monthly automatic payments, talking with a financial planner to streamline your financial management, adding another day onto your work schedule, or even finding a job that pays you better income so you can save the money without changing your lifestyle. Some of your sub-goals, like finding a new job, may require mini-goals for their own additional support (see Figure 8-3 ■).

You can include as many of these little goal branches as you need to for your plan (templates are included in Appendix B). You can also flesh out these goals and supportive steps when you create your time line. To optimize the impact of goal setting in your two-year plan, it helps to really understand what is underneath it. Take a moment to begin to dissect your goals down into their foundation and its structure. Consider the metaphor of a building. A building is the sum of many parts. Of course, every building needs a foundation to give it support. With goals, it is your **values** that are the foundation. Your values are your core beliefs that you hold most dear, giving you meaning and direction in life.

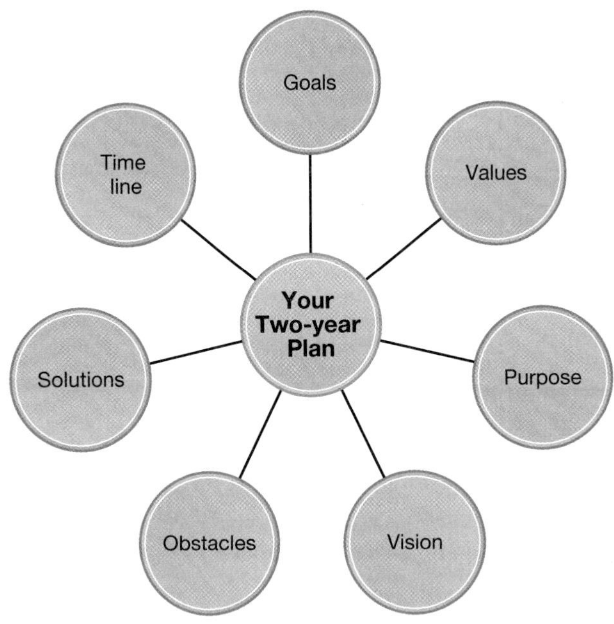

FIGURE 8-2

The elements of a good two-year plan include goals, values, purpose, vision, obstacles, solutions, and time lines.

> *We need to learn to set our course by the stars, not by the lights of every passing ship.*
>
> —General Omar Bradley

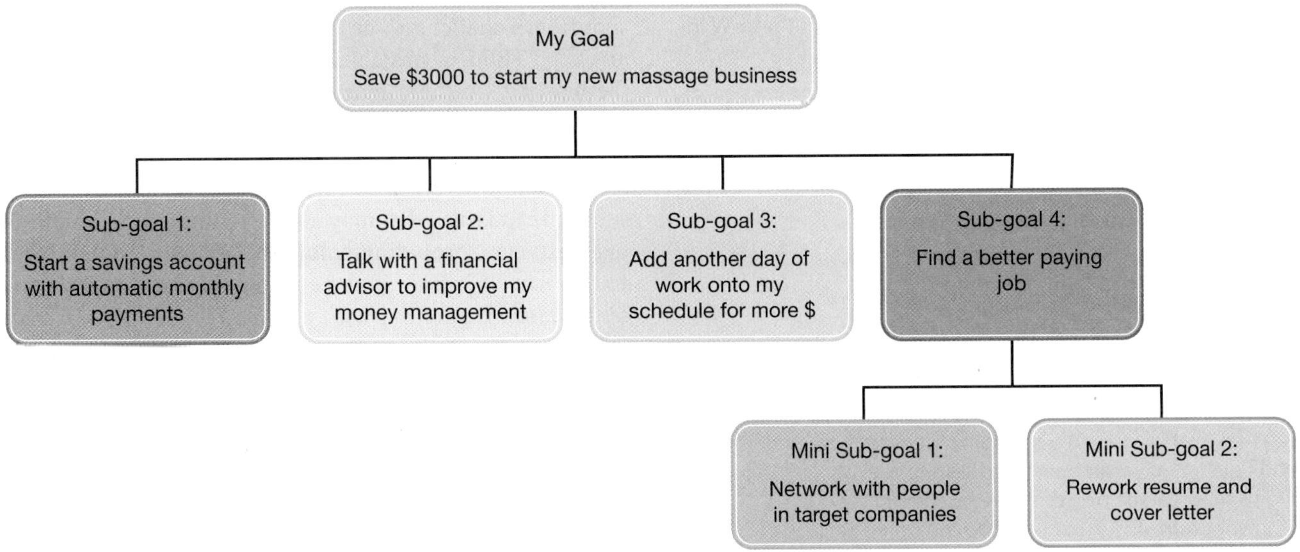

FIGURE 8-3

A sample goal chart, with sub-goals and mini-goals supporting the overarching goal.

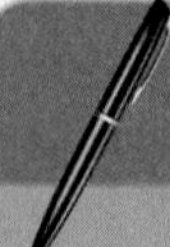

PUT IT IN WRITING

Values Exercise

Below is a list of 27 values. Some of the values may sound similar, but can have very different meanings for different individuals. From the list, choose 10 of the values that resonate with you.

Compassion	Acceptance	Adventure
Learning	Loyalty	Autonomy
Relationships	Health	Fairness
Exploration/openness	Family	Communication
Creativity	Sexuality	Travel
Spirituality	Empowering others	Community
Romance		Education
Diversity	Truth	Power
Harmony	Joy	Religion

1. ____________ **6.** ____________
2. ____________ **7.** ____________
3. ____________ **8.** ____________
4. ____________ **9.** ____________
5. ____________ **10.** ____________

Now pare your list down to the five most important values for you. Read through your list above and take a moment to reflect on how these values manifest in your life. Chose the five that feel most relevant to your life today.

1. ____________
2. ____________
3. ____________
4. ____________
5. ____________

Now the tough part: from those five, try and refine the list to the top three values, these are the foundation of your goals. It may be hard to distill your belief system into only three values, but take your time to prioritize what's most meaningful to you. This can really help you understand that upon which you set your course in life.

1. ____________
2. ____________
3. ____________

Purpose is the overarching culmination of your values. Your purpose is not a destination or something that you ever complete, but rather something that gives your life perspective and meaning[5]. Purpose is the frame for the building that rests upon the foundation and gives it its structure. This can be somewhat difficult to wrap your head around at first, so to get you started, look at the example in the "Put It in Writing" box.

PUT IT IN WRITING

Purpose

Example: The purpose of my massage career is to make optimal physical health accessible to communities that are underserved, and to utilize my compassion and skills to alleviate physical suffering so that I can be part of a healthy community.

Your turn: The purpose of my ____________ is to ____________ so that ____________.

Vision refers to the picture you have in your mind for the goal you want to achieve or the life you want to manifest. Vision is the blueprint for your goals. Refer to the "Perfect Day" creative visualization exercise at the end of this chapter. This will help connect you to your vision. **Obstacles** are the things that contradict your goals, present future challenges, or may interfere with your plan in any way. Think of obstacles as the intemperate weather or the big bad wolf that may try to blow your house down. This is the area where you can address the barriers and hurdles along the path that you explored earlier in the chapter and where you can anticipate problems and create solutions to issues that may arise. Setting goals, identifying obstacles, providing solutions, achieving goals, and setting new ones is a circular and ongoing process throughout life (see Figure 8-4 ■).

Obstacles can be both internal and external, and can exist along a continuum of scale and severity; however, there are almost always solutions for any challenge. **Solutions** are the creative ways you can develop to overcome your obstacles. For example, your ideal vision includes a lot of mention of abundance and prosperity, but you know that you have unresolved issues about lack and scarcity and that could present an obstacle in achieving your goal. Mention that here, explore it as much as you wish,

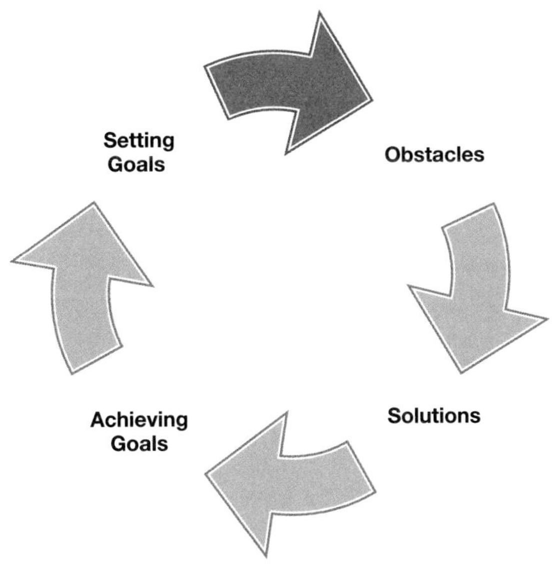

FIGURE 8-4

Because life is always evolving, setting goals, identifying obstacles, providing solutions, achieving goals, and setting new ones is a circular and ongoing process.

and brainstorm a few things you could do to counter those barriers. Examples to resolve the lack and scarcity issue could be working with a life coach or a therapist to uncover some of your deep beliefs about scarcity. Or you could surround yourself with friends and mentors who have created lives of real abundance for themselves. This way, when and if problems do arise as you and your business are getting going, you are better prepared to handle them.

A **time line** is the graphic representation of everything you've done in your plan thus far, and focuses on the time aspect of your goals, objectives, strategies and tactics. Remember the importance of putting deadlines into your SMART goals? Time lines illustrates the actions to take towards goal achievement upon a calendar of sorts, and helps you stay organized and focused. As you progress with your goal setting, a time line will help you visually see where you are, how far you've come, and how close you are to your goals. Notice the action orientation of time lines, and how following them propels you along. Time lines are where you are able to map out all of the

PUT IT IN WRITING

Obstacles and Solutions

If you can think of a challenge that might threaten your goal, chances are you can think of at least one solution to overcome it. In fact, you may be able to think of several solutions for every obstacle. Try this exercise to brainstorm any foreseeable bumps on your road as well as innovative ways to level the path. Here are some examples to get you started.

Goal: To take the National Certification Exam by September 20, 2012.

Challenge: I am very scared of standardized tests and afraid I might fail.

Solution 1: Form a study group with other students.
Solution 2: Take an exam prep course.
Solution 3: Practice practice practice! After all, I know this stuff so well!

Goal: To rent a space for my practice in the prestigious Woodlawn Shopping District by December 1, 2012.

Challenge: The rents are very expensive and I do not know that I will be able to build my practice quickly enough to support expenses.

Solution 1: Rent space from a holistic business in the area.
Solution 2: Hit the ground running with marketing and networking to build a solid client base more quickly.
Solution 3: Develop a strong financial plan to make sure I understand my monetary needs so I feel more in control of income and expenses.

Now you give it a try.

Goal:

Challenge:

Solution 1:
Solution 2:
Solution 3:

Goal:

Challenge:

Solution 1:
Solution 2:
Solution 3:

Goal:

Challenge:

Solution 1:
Solution 2:
Solution 3:

Expand this list out as far as you like, and try and be as detailed as you can. The more you support your goals with actionable steps, the more likely you are to reach your desired destination!

TABLE 8-1 Sample Therapist's Time Line for Accomplishing Set Goals

Action	J	F	M	A	M	J	J	A	S	O	N	D
Community networking		X		X	X	X	X	X	X	X	X	X
Vacation			X									X
1. Become licensed massage therapist										X		
1.1 Graduate from massage school by Aug.							X					
1.1.1 Complete required hours	X	X	X	X	X	X	X	X				
1.1.2: Complete courses and coursework	X	X	X	X	X	X	X	X				
1.1.3 Exit interview								X				
1.2. Take all requisite exams											X	
1.2.1 Register/schedule state/national Exams								X				
1.2.2 Study one month for each exam									X	X		
1.2.3 Take tests and ace them!											X	
1.3 Register for licensure with the state											X	
1.3.1 Online research for requirements								X				
1.3.2 Obtain/submit paperwork and licensure fees										X		
1.3.3 Submit all documents on time										X		

supporting activity that will ensure your goals are met. If you want to incorporate ongoing activities into your plan, such as networking, time with family, or vacations, include them in your time line. Table 8-1 ■ is a one-year time line for Phil, a new massage therapist. Phil's main goal is to become a successful therapist over the next two years. Notice that Phil has aspects of both his personal and professional life in his time line.

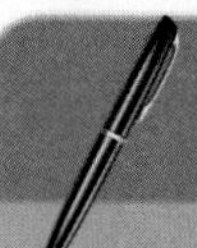

PUT IT IN WRITING

Your Time Line

Get started with your time line, using all the activities that will help support you in your goal. Remember to include the aspects of your life that are important to you but may not be business or career related: time with family, recreation, religious activities, and so forth. Remember the Wheel of Life exercise and the importance of balance. Table 8-2 ■ may not provide nearly enough room for all of your steps, so make your own chart if you need more room!

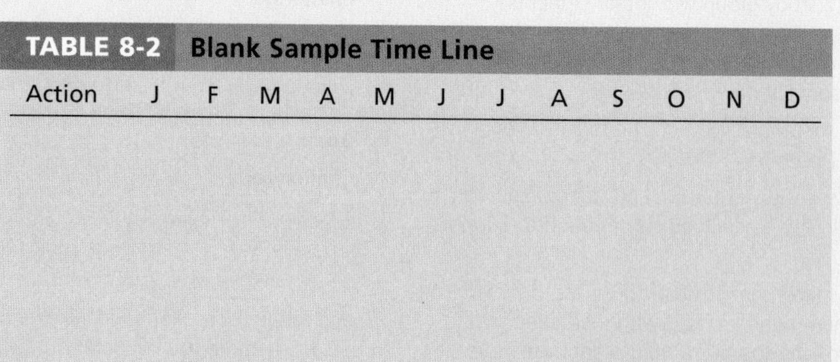

TABLE 8-2 Blank Sample Time Line

Action	J	F	M	A	M	J	J	A	S	O	N	D

GETTING ORGANIZED

Now put all of your exercises together in your *Business of Massage Therapy* notebook—the values, purpose, obstacles, solutions, and time line. Flesh out any of the details for the goals you have set for yourself over the next two years. Check out the two-year plan template and the sample completed plan in Appendix B. Congratulations! You have yourself a two-year plan!

CHAPTER SUMMARY BY LEARNING OBJECTIVES

1. **Create your own definition of success** Success is a fluid concept, and can mean very different things to different people. There is no monopoly on the definition of success, and it is imperative that you understand your own definition of success before you set out to achieve it.
2. **Describe barriers to success and self-imposed limitations** External circumstances may present challenges to achieving your success. However, it is also very common for the largest barriers to success to arise internally. Self-imposed limitations are ways that people hinder themselves from going forward to achieve what they want.
3. **Evaluate the applications of creative visualization, affirmations and gratitude lists** Creative visualization is the practice of envisioning the future you want in very specific detail. Affirmations are positive assertions about the way things are that help manifest a positive reality. Typically, they are declarations of things that you want to create in your life. Gratitude lists build on the principle that what you focus on expands; as you begin to pay attention to positive aspects of your life, you will find more things for which to be grateful.
4. **Identify the challenges in getting started with a new business** Taking the first step toward something new can be daunting. This is often the case when starting a new business, particularly for those with little past business experience. For holistic practitioners, starting a new business can seem even more challenging because of the personal element intertwined with their services.
5. **Uncover the importance of setting goals** Goal setting is the intentional positioning of an ambition and the implementation of actionable steps towards actualizing that aim. Goal setting is the practical action that converts wishes into real life, the alchemical process that turns a dream into a reality. It's the "how-to" stage of envisioning your ideal life.
6. **Examine the components of a plan and a time line** Whether a one-month, two-year, five-year, or hundred-year plan, most plans typically have the following components: your values; your purpose; your vision; contradictions; objectives, strategies, and tactics; and a time line.
7. **Incorporate values, purpose, and vision into your plan** Your values are your core beliefs which you hold most dear, giving you meaning and direction in life. Purpose is the overarching culmination of your values. Your purpose is not a destination or something that you ever complete, but rather something that gives your life perspective and meaning. Vision refers to the picture you have in your mind for the goal you want to achieve or the life you want to manifest. Vision is the blueprint for your goals.
8. **Discover ways to anticipate obstacles and create solutions** Obstacles are the things that contradict your goals, present future challenges, or may interfere with your plan in any. Obstacles can be both internal and external, and can exist along a continuum of scale and severity, but there are always solutions for any challenge. Solutions are the creative ways you can develop to overcome your obstacles.
9. **Create a two-year plan and a time line** By working through the above elements piece by piece, you can create your own two-year plan and develop a visual time line to keep you on track.

ACTIVITIES

Discussion Questions

1. When setting goals and making plans, a lot of emphasis is placed upon time lines and measurability. Why do you think that is? What do you think about the relationship between goal setting and time lines? Does emphasizing deadlines feel comfortable to you?
2. You took some time in the early part of this chapter to acknowledge and celebrate your successes in the past. Looking back, can you remember steps you took to ensure that success? Did you have a game plan, or do you think things just worked out in your favor? How will this impact your approach in a new massage business?
3. Goal setting and planning are important in any business. In Chapter 1 you explored some of the recent trends in the massage industry. What are some of the additional characteristics of a career in massage today that make planning especially important?
4. Some of the techniques in this chapter (such as clearing, affirmations, gratitude lists, and creative visualization) are becoming more and more common in small business coaching. However, not everyone is familiar with these methods and some people do not feel comfortable with them. Discuss your personal take on these kinds of exercises and how it felt for you to do them.
5. Not everyone is in agreement about goal setting and the road to success, and some even believe it can hinder it. In her book, *Making Pigs Fly* (1995, Phoenix Press), Judith Sinclair maintains that rigid adherence to a goal can encumber the flexibility and adaptibility needed to succeed in an ever-changing world. Discuss your thoughts on this. Which approach is more aligned with choices you have made in the past to get what you want?

Beyond the Classroom

Perfect Day Exercise

This guided creative visualization exercise will help you define your idea of success by fleshing out some details[6]. This can be done in many ways: you can go through the exercise below and jot down any responses in your *Business of Massage Therapy* notebook, or perhaps you can enlist the help of a friend to read the exercise to you as you envision it. Yet another highly recommended option is to get a tape recorder and record the exercise in your own calm voice, and then play it back as you visualize the answers. Take your time with this exercise and try and bring forth as much detail as possible. Enjoy creating your own success in your mind!

> Get in a comfortable position and relax. Close your eyes. Take several deep, cleansing breaths. In your mind, see yourself in your favorite tranquil place, all alone. Look around, and observe the sights and smells of the place where you are. Perhaps you are on the beach, listening to the waves roll in. Perhaps you are in the mountains, smelling fresh pine on the wind. Breathe deep. Stay here a few minutes.
>
> Now flash forward two years into the future from this very moment. Today is your perfect day, exactly the way you want it to be. This day represents the culmination of the success you have built over these two years. You are waking up slowly in your ideal home. What does the room look like? Now slowly see yourself getting out of the bed, and looking in the mirror. What do you look like? Is your hair long or short? Just observe your reflection and the look in your eye. Visualize yourself getting into the shower, dressing and readying yourself for the day ahead. What clothes do you wear? What are the parts of your morning routine? Who, if anyone, is there with you? As you eat breakfast, take a moment to look around your home. How is it decorated? What is the location? Do you have any pets? Who are your neighbors? What relationships are fostered in this home? Be in this space, and experience what it feels like in your life.
>
> As you leave the house, what kind of transportation will take you to work? A car? A bicycle? On foot? Picture your mode of transportation, and see yourself getting to your place of business. Is it far from your home, or very close? What is the journey there like? You arrive at work, and take a moment to look at the exterior. What is it like? Perhaps you see a tall office building, or a small cabin in the woods with only one room. Look at the windows, and the things that surround the building. What sounds do you hear?
>
> As you walk into your office, what are the first things you see? Is there anyone else there to greet you, or are you alone? Take a moment to observe the way the walls are decorated, the light in the room, the way it smells. This is your perfect workspace, and you can create it any way you like. Be here for a moment, observing the details.
>
> Take a few moments to see yourself going through your day. How many clients will you see? What kind of

clientele have you attracted to your business? Who are the people you will interact with? How much does each one pay you and how? How do you feel working with these people? Observe.

Now your work day is ending, and you close up your workspace. You go to meet with friends for a meal—who is there at the table? What is the conversation? How does it feel? When the meal ends, it is time for one of your favorite activities of the week—what is it? See yourself enjoying this activity and allowing it to feed your spirit.

As you return home by your chosen mode of transportation, you pick up the mail and see two things. The first is a statement from your bank that reflects your financial picture to you; look at it and see how much money you have. The second is a letter from a client you have worked with who wants to express what your work together has meant to them. Look at it and read the words. Then walk into your ideal home, sit down in your favorite chair, and reflect on the life you have created for yourself. Ask yourself: is this success? Witness the answer.

CHAPTER

9 Location, Location, Location

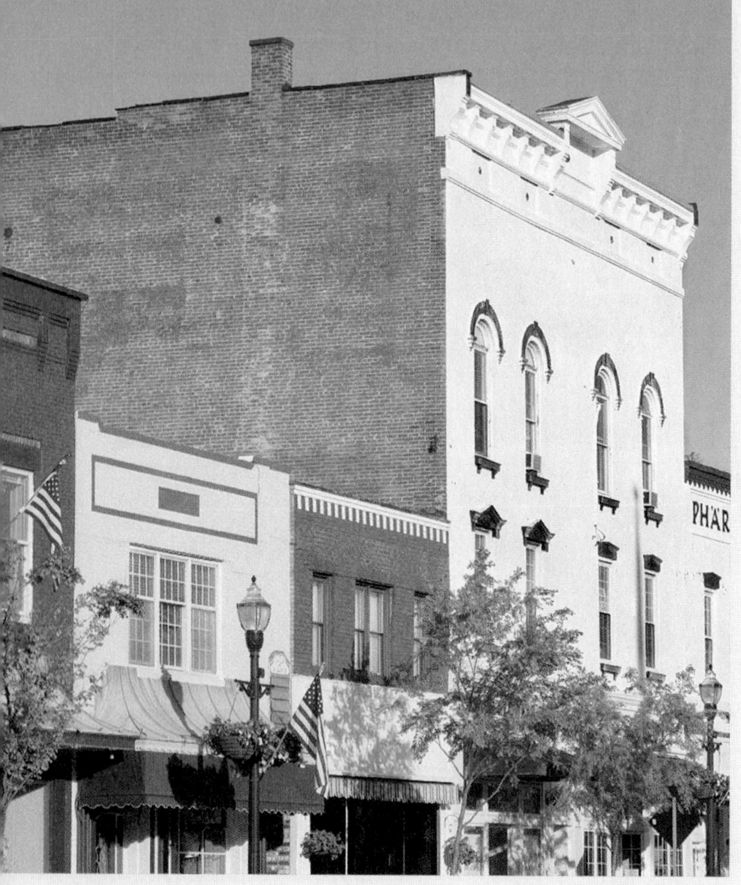

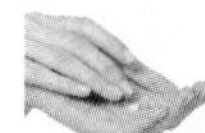

CHAPTER OUTLINE

Learning Objectives
Key Terms
Space Odyssey: The Importance of Location
All Shapes and Sizes
Eye Spy: Finding the Perfect Place
Keep It Moving: A Mobile Business
The Zoning Zone: Licenses and Permits
Exploring the Pros and Cons of Working from Home
The Benefits and Challenges of Collaborating with Others in Your Space
Retail
Discover How to Brand Private-Label Retail Products
Chapter Summary by Learning Objectives
Activities

LEARNING OBJECTIVES

1. Explain why location is so important to a business
2. Use creative visualization to conceive the right space
3. Examine different scopes and scales of massage businesses
4. Employ techniques to find the right place and identify equipment you will need in your massage business
5. Evaluate mobility
6. Define zoning, licensing, and permits
7. Examine pros and cons of working from home
8. Contrast the benefits and challenges of collaborating with others in your space
9. Explore the merit of retail sales in your business and demonstrate how to use retail to maximize customer service
10. Discover how to brand private-label retail products

KEY TERMS

brick-and-mortar business *140*
commercial real estate agent *143*
due diligence *143*
equipment *143*
leasing agent *143*
location mix *140*
overhead *145*
private-label retail *150*
vendor *150*
wellness and spa consultant *142*
wellness center *147*
zoning *146*
zoning variance *146*

The two most important requirements for major success are: first, being in the right place at the right time, and second, doing something about it.

—Ray Kroc, founder of McDonalds

SPACE ODYSSEY: THE IMPORTANCE OF LOCATION

It is often said that the three keys to success in business are: location, location, and of course, location. Where you choose to operate your business can be the determining factor in its success or failure. Unless you plan to do an exclusively mobile practice, you will need to think of ways to optimize your brick-and-mortar business. A **brick-and-mortar business** refers to any business that operates out of a physical location and offers face-to-face contact with clients and customers. This term has become an increasingly popular distinguishing phrase as more and more businesses turn online for e-commerce, service delivery, and nearly everything else (see Chapter 15).

Finding and selecting the right location for you and your business are some of the most important elements when getting started, especially for a service-driven enterprise like massage. Often this decision is given short shrift by business owners eager to get operations underway. Many entrepreneurs rely more on emotional factors (convenience to the therapist him/herself, lease price, proximity to home) than on logical factors that contribute to business success (convenience to clients, adequate parking, curbside appeal, proximity to other attractive shops). Many will argue that massage therapists need not worry about location as much as other businesses because of the "referral factor" (i.e., people will only seek out a therapist on a recommendation, not on location), but that simply isn't true. Just like any business, location is still key to attract and retain clients. It has to be convenient and comfortable for clients to find you; in fact, having a high-traffic location can minimize your marketing efforts.[1]

As a massage therapist, your location is often even more crucial than for those offering other goods or services. Beyond just a practical locale to administer products and services, your location is a prime ingredient in the experience that you create for your clients. And it is not just the geographic location that needs to be considered, but the entire location mix. Sure, being lucky enough to secure a spot at the intersection of Perfect Place and Location Location Location Lane helps, but many elements other than geography go into the right location. A **location mix** is the combination of all the factors that clients interact with sensorially at every direct point of contact with your business: locality, exterior, design, layout, aesthetics, retail sales offerings, even scents and sounds. It is the blend of factors that go into creating the experience for your clients. It is imperative that clients feel safe in your space, and that you provide an environment conducive to relaxation and healing. But before you start scouring the real estate section and hitting the streets in search of your dream locale, you must have a firm grasp on what you are looking for. Later in the chapter you will explore the pragmatic aspects such as budgeting and zoning regulations, but first get solid on the vision of your perfect spot.

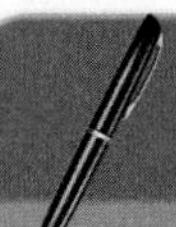

PUT IT IN WRITING

Think Like a Customer First

You may never have thought of yourself as a location scout or as any kind of interior decoration whisperer. But whether or not you know it, you already have qualifications due to your years of experience as a connoisseur of products and services. Think of five of your favorite places to spend your money, whether you are spending it on products or services (for the purposes of this exercise, forget about online venues and just focus on physical places you go). It could be your neighborhood restaurant, a sporting goods store in the next town, an upscale spa in Aspen, or the barbershop where you've been getting your buzz cuts since you were 10 years old. It doesn't matter. What *does* matter is why you chose those five. First, write them down:

1. ______
2. ______
3. ______
4. ______
5. ______

Now write as many positive things that you associate with the *location* of the businesses listed above. Think about obvious things like convenience, but also the "je ne sais quoi" of the place—that intangible attribute or memorable aesthetic that makes it stand out in your mind. Write those down here:

1. ______
2. ______
3. ______
4. ______
5. ______

Now as you begin to select and design your own location, you will be in a better position to see things from a customer's perspective, not just that of a business owner.

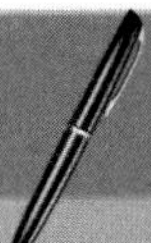

PUT IT IN WRITING

Visualizing Your Space

Knowing what you are looking for makes *finding* what you are looking for all the more manageable. You just identified things you like about other business spaces; now is the time to visualize your own. You already touched on creative visualization of your space when you did the "Perfect Day" exercise in Chapter 8. Refer back to the work you did there. Remember seeing yourself going to your perfect working space, and remember all the details that you imagined. If it helps, go through the exercise again and see if anything has changed or if any new details emerge . . . Is there anyone else there? What color are the walls? Is there a clock in view? Are there windows? Try and be as specific as possible about all the aspects of your working environment.

Now, after you've reviewed the journaling you did before or gone through the exercise again, jot down as many details as you can in the spaces provided. The more items you can specify the fuller your vision becomes.

ALL SHAPES AND SIZES

Many holistic business consultants actually tell clients that their location is not as important as those for other product and service providers. This advice is based on the premise that clienteles are built by word of mouth rather than brick-and-mortar exposure. And word of mouth is an incredibly important factor in generating client loyalty. Yet in the ever-shifting landscape of the massage industry, it is remiss to assume that your location is not as much a competitive advantage and marketing component (see Chapters 11 and 12) as any other business. Moreover, massage businesses come in all shapes and sizes, and your location needs and considerations will have a direct relationship to your scale and scope of operations. Not all massage therapists will have the same needs, of course, and you need to consider your unique blend of factors when approaching location. The following is a brief description of the most common types of massage businesses, and a few location considerations for each.

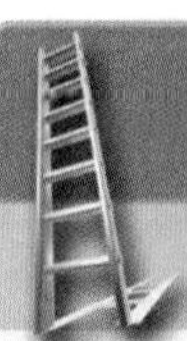

FIRST STEPS

Perhaps you find it difficult to visualize the perfect location or environment that you want to work in. This is often the case when starting out. Don't worry. It is not only permissible to draw ideas from other sources, it can be essential to sparking your own innate creativity. If you find yourself drawing a blank when it comes to details, do a little research on the ways that other spas, wellness centers, solo massage therapists, and holistic practitioners have created their spaces. Are there elements that you like that you could put your unique spin on and incorporate into your vision? If there are no wellness practitioners in your area, or if you aren't comfortable doing the research in person, go virtual. Look online, in books, and in industry magazines to get some creative inspiration.

- *Home practice:* Working from a spare room in your home can bring great benefits but also some considerable challenges (more on this in a later section).
- *Mobile practice:* A mobile practice could bring your business to corporate offices, hospitals, bridal showers, a farmers market, or to a public school for teacher appreciation day. All you need is a portable table and a reliable car to craft a successful mobile practice.
- *Office space:* Massage therapists have built their businesses out of offices in boutique districts, skyscrapers, office parks, carriage houses, strip malls, converted mansions, and airports. Think creatively when looking for office space.
- *Collaborative space:* Many massage therapists join with other wellness practioners to propel their businesses. Examples of professionals with whom to share collaborative space include chiropractors, acupuncturists, doctors, birthing coaches, counselors,

nutritionists, herbalists, yoga teachers, and personal trainers. These spaces will need to be fairly large, and with enough enclaves and treatment rooms to be conducive to private sessions.

- *Day spa:* Spas typically have unique considerations that are above and beyond the scope of most massage practices. Many new spas will require construction of a new facility or major rehabilitation of an existing building. While most massage students may never start a spa of their own, many will, as day spas are very lucrative in certain markets and the industry continues to grow.

If you are investing a sizeable amount of money in your new location, you might benefit from working with a professional who is highly knowledgeable not only about the demographics in your area, but also about the specifics in your industry. A **wellness and spa consultant** is an industry expert who advises holistic business and spa owners on all operational aspects of their business. Typical, these professionals have years of experience in creating, designing, marketing, and maintaining spas, wellness centers, and other kinds of holistic businesses. In recent years, these professionals have eked out an increasingly popular niche in the consulting field, and they can command a high price for their time. However, it can often be worth the upfront investment to avoid costly reworking down the road.

> *If you think hiring a professional is expensive, wait till you hire an amateur.*
>
> —Red Adair

EYE SPY: FINDING THE PERFECT PLACE

As you have seen, location matters. When asked about the most important factors in frequenting a massage therapist, many clients will report location as one of the top considerations. Even if you are an incredibly skilled therapist, choosing a location that is inconvenient and not conducive to your clients' needs could thwart your business. Of course, convenient and conducive are relative concepts, but there are some consistent things to look for when seeking space. Consider aspects such as neighborhood security, street noise, available (and affordable) parking, visible signage, and foot traffic when you are out looking for potential locations. If there is a high concentration of your target market in a neighborhood, clients could even walk to your office. Even with the perfect combination of convenience factors, a gut-check is an important part of the process. This may sound too obvious to even state, but it is of paramount importance that you really like the space. After all, you will be spending a great amount of time here and you need to feel at home, no matter how many parking spaces are available, how unbeatable the price, or how posh the other neighboring businesses.

There are many approaches to actually finding your dream spot. One of the most effective is to do it yourself. Target neighborhoods where you feel your business would be successful. Put on a pair of comfortable walking shoes and start pounding the pavement in search of signs of available spaces. This option can take a bit of time, but you get to experientially explore your options while getting a good feeling of what is available to you. It also gives you a good opportunity to scout out neighboring businesses to search for potential competition and collaborative partnership opportunities.

Another option for finding a great location is to ask around. So much of doing business occurs through your network, and finding a location is no different. Word of mouth and referrals are a great way to find a prime location for a massage practice. Chances are good that someone in your immediate network knows someone (or knows someone who knows someone) who has a space for rent or is looking to bring a holistic business into their office.

You can also go online to do some research (see the "Helpful Resources" box). People are turning more and more to online community boards and classified services such as Craigslist, OfficeList, and Oodle to advertise their available rental space. Even professional massage organizations such as ABMP and AMTA offer their members online classified listings for everything from office space to used equipment to continuing education.

If your scope of operations is more advanced and your needs are more complex, you may want to work with a real

PITFALLS

Facing the Competition

Many entrepreneurs will immediately rule out a premier location because it is swamped with competition. While it's true that high saturation of available massage services in your immediate area can pirate your business, don't be too quick to walk away. Generally there is a reason why practitioners are clustered in some areas and absent in others. Often there are higher concentrations of target markets in the area, or other factors that spell a good location. Many experts agree that being near competitors can actually be beneficial, as you can benefit from the education and marketing they have already done in that particular market.[2] You will need to evaluate this on a case-by-case basis and go with your instincts here. And who knows? You may find creative ways to collaborate rather than compete. Competition will always be a factor in your business, so be sure you know how to leverage it rather than run from it.

estate professional. A **leasing agent** is a professional who typically works for landlords to identify, attract, and retain quality tenants to occupy commercial space. They generally are the ones to handle all the aspects of a lease, and a good agent will be able to provide you with all the information on the building's history and the general area. Similarly, a **commercial real estate agent** is a professional who helps broker leases and sales of commercial property. They are often hired by commercial real estate owners to sell or lease property on their behalf, although they can be hired as a representative of the tenant (you) to scout out a prime location.[3] This can be of little or no cost to you because the agents make their money from the landlords. Keep in mind that because leasing agents and real estate agents have the landlords' interests at the forefront, you will have to be responsible for taking care of your own interests.

When considering a location, you will want to do your due diligence. **Due diligence** is the process of gathering relevant information, assessing risks, researching opportunities and threats, and thoroughly investigating potential investments or acquisitions for a business.[4] In short, doing due diligence is doing your homework. The term typically applies when buying or acquiring a new business or real estate, but for your purposes consider it part of evaluating leases as well. Even if you are only renting a space, you are making a contractual monetary commitment and that money is still an investment in your business. You need to investigate all the things that generate traffic in the neighborhood; this includes things such as demographics, schools, other businesses, community development, and so forth. Doing your due diligence in the beginning will help you make informed decisions, and can save you from innumerable headaches down the road.

Once you have identified and secured the perfect space, you will need to spend a little time evaluating the equipment you will need. **Equipment** refers to any tangible materials you will need to perform your service (massage) and run your business. The amount of equipment you will need to acquire depends in large part upon your scale, scope, and start-up budget (see Chapter 13 for more on budgets and financial management). Take a moment to look at three categories of equipment: standard, specialized, and optional/supplemental.

Standard: Regardless of your target market, your massage modality, or your location, there are a few pieces of equipment that are fairly standard in any massage practice. Standard equipment includes:

- Massage table
- Massage stool
- Linens
- Lubricants (oils, creams, gels)
- Bolsters/face cradles

What are some other standard items that you can think of that are not on the list? Write them here:

1. ______________________
2. ______________________
3. ______________________
4. ______________________

PITFALLS

Lease Fever

Many entrepreneurs are so enthusiastic about getting their businesses started. Add to that the euphoria of finding a location that seems like everything you ever wanted and the fear that someone else will snatch it up if you don't, and you can understand the common mistake of prematurely signing a lease. It is not uncommon for individuals armed with passion and a great idea to sign a five-year lease before any other factors are in place. Remember, a lease is a binding legal contract, and you are responsible for meeting all the agreed-on terms. You are entering into a relationship with the landlord, and you will want to approach discussions strategically. Find out as much as you can about the space: Why is it available? How has it been used in the past? Is it zoned for the work you want to do? What are the conditions of the lease, and how many rights will you have as a tenant? If you don't know or aren't reasonably certain that you can satisfy the lease payments from the profits on your business, you may find yourself in a very sticky situation down the road. Because leases are legal contracts, it is advisable to have an attorney look over the documents before you sign—the expense can be well worth it down the road. In the midst of all the excitement, remember your common sense and really make sure you know what you are getting into before you commit.

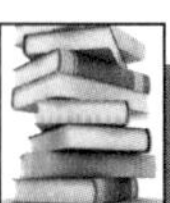

HELPFUL RESOURCES

Knowing where to begin due diligence when scouting locations can seem daunting, but there is a wealth of resources available to help you evaluate your options and make informed decisions. Online resources such as ZIPskinny and www.(yourzipcode).com (i.e., www.80218.com) provide demographic information by zip code, as well as information and reviews on local businesses by industry. The U.S. Census can also provide you valuable statistics on local economic indicators. Talk to local business associations, chambers of commerce, local small business development centers, and even the business desk at the local library to get all the information you need for informed decisions.

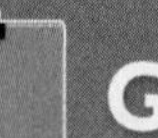

GETTING ORGANIZED

Location Checklist

If you are itching to get your location scouting underway, you would be wise to have a list of questions with you when you talk with realtors or potential landlords. Here is a brief list of questions that you should be able to get an answer to before making any decisions. Copy the list and keep it in your *Business of Massage Therapy* notebook for easy reference.

- Is the rent on this space within your budget?
- Is there enough room to operate and sufficient storage for equipment and supplies?
- What is the parking situation for you and your clients?
- Is it accessible for physically challenged clients, and does it meet all Americans with Disabilities Act (ADA) requirements (www.ada.gov)?
- Are the building and the area in line with the image you are trying to project for your business?
- Are you free to decorate or modify the interior?
- Are the current layout/utilities/appliances sufficient for your needs, or will you need to do any construction/rewiring/plumbing to make it suitable for your needs? If so, what are the lease parameters, and can you afford the changes?
- Are there security or safety issues in the neighborhood? If you plan to have evening hours, is there adequate external lighting?
- If your business grows, can that growth be accommodated in this space?
- Can you collaborate with your neighbors, or might they be a hindrance?
- Is it close to public transportation?
- Is the building quiet and removed from street noises?
- Are you able to have external signage for your business?
- What are the zoning regulations for this space?
- Can you sublease any space to other practioners?
- Do you have control of heat and air conditioning?
- How much of the building's maintenance are you responsible for?
- Is there a lot of competition close by?
- Is there foot traffic out front?

What other questions can you think of that need to be addressed before you can make a qualified decision on a location? Brainstorm a few ideas and list them here.

1. ______
2. ______
3. ______
4. ______
5. ______

Remember, it is better to take your time in the beginning rather than rushing in and having to relocate or make significant changes later.[5]

Specialized: Specialized equipment is specific to the particular modality/modalities that will be performed in your massage business. For example, if you are doing a lot of sports massage, you will likely want to invest in a hydrocolator for hot packs. If you will be doing raindrop therapy, you will need essential aromatherapy oils. Specialized equipment can include:

- Thai massage mat
- T-bars
- Hot stone set
- Aromatherapy oils
- Massage chair

Write some other ideas here:

1. ______
2. ______
3. ______
4. ______

Optional/Supplemental: These are items that are not necessarily essential to performing a massage, but can make the experience much more enjoyable for your clients. Optional equipment includes things such as:

- Music
- Table warmers
- Candles/diffusers/incense
- Hot towels
- Sa-wan herbal packs

Write some other ideas here:

1. ______
2. ______
3. ______
4. ______

The equipment you will need to run your business successfully will obviously not only be for the execution of a massage session, but also to cover your administrative and operational needs as well. Over time, you may find that your equipment needs will grow and expand. The above is by no means an exhaustive list, and you should feel free to use your best judgment and experimental curiosity to compile just the right equipment inventory for your business. Like so many things in business, this is an ongoing and evolving process.

KEEP IT MOVING: A MOBILE BUSINESS

Those with a passion for the open road and a change of scenery might consider fashioning their business into a mobile one, rather than signing a lease and setting up a stationary storefront. While many therapists may supplement their brick-and-mortar business with occasional on-site table or chair massage, a number have crafted an entire career out of making their therapeutic touch "to go." A good mobile massage entrepreneur knows the virtue of investing in reliable transportation, external signage on their car, and a lightweight table or chair that is easy to break down, set up, and carry from place to place.

There are many massage styles that are highly conducive to portable massage. Because they can all be performed with clients' clothes on and in more public venues, shiatsu, Thai, and chair massage are all popular for mobile massage sessions. Many successful massage therapists have positioned themselves as mobile therapists in resort communities, where locals and tourists alike will pay top dollar to have a massage in the comfort of their homes or hotel rooms.

But some people aren't satisfied with a 25-mile radius, and have thus cast their lot on an international scene. Some have done this by continuing their massage education with programs abroad and then surveying opportunities to get jobs or work independently once there. By hiring or contracting with hotels, resorts, or local communities, many therapists have made their portable massage careers world-class. Though many people do this kind of work "under the table," you would be wise to research local regulations on working as a foreigner.

Whether a mobile massage business takes you down the street or across the world, it is important to consider the benefits and challenges of this option. If you do use massage as a way to see the world, you could be opening yourself up to amazing experiences and meeting fascinating people from around the planet. Due to the physical exertion, transportation costs, and personal risk assumption of a locally traveling therapist, one can usually charge a premium for outcall massages closer to home. Because people appreciate the convenience and comfort of receiving a massage in their office, hotel, or home, they are typically happy to pay the higher price (see Figure 9-1 ■).

Many therapists are attracted to mobile businesses because of the lower overhead as well. **Overhead** refers to the continual operating costs associated with running any business, such as rent, electricity, wages, and so forth. In a strictly mobile business, you typically will have lower overhead than you would in a brick-and-mortar building. This ability to charge more per service yet have lower overhead can be attractive to many people. Even if your goal is to have a physical location for your business, on-site massages can help you get the capital together to start working from a permanent location.

Of course, there are challenges to mobile practices as well. If you are working as a massage therapist internationally, you will be responsible for satisfying all visa and residency requirements. You will also have the challenge of language and cultural differences to deal with; this can be enough mental gymnastics on its own, but when you factor in different cultural values and behaviors connected with massage, this can be a mental overload. Even if you stay close to home, you may have a lot of requirements to contend with. As was mentioned earlier, when it comes to regulating massage, local governments are not always uniform across the board. Driving to a client's home to give her a massage in the next town over may not be permissible by her local rules, and being caught could result in losing your license (remember: ignorance of the law is not a legal defense). A mobile practice demands that you have a workable knowledge of rules and regulations wherever you perform your service, and quite likely will require you to obtain a license or permit in any jurisdiction you set up your chair or table. In addition, your auto insurance costs might also be at a premium because of the amount of time spent in the car or the increase in risk assumed due to driving from site to site or house to house.

Low/no overhead
Adventure and new surroundings
Travel locally and inter-nationally
Premium pricing potential
Mobile Massage Therapist
Personal safety consid-erations
Meeting residency and licensure requirements
Physical exertion
Transportation and insurance expense

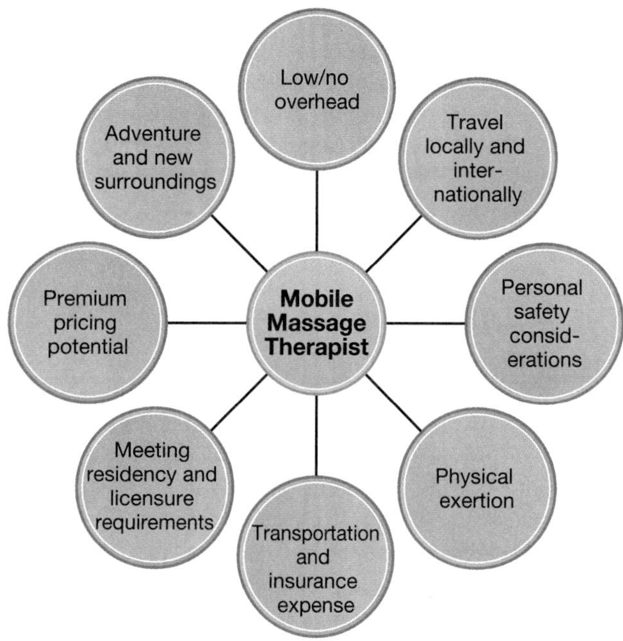

FIGURE 9-1

There are many benefits and challenges to being a mobile massage therapist, and many factors to consider.

Speaking of risk, the reality is that you can risk personal safety going into the home or personal space of another person, especially someone unknown to you. While the majority of clients are great people, it is always best to keep your wits about you. As with working from your own home or in other massage situations, some basic rules apply to preserve your personal well-being and safety. If possible, develop a referral-based clientele and/or develop a pre-screening process so that you have a modicum of control over the situation. Be clear about your therapeutic focus in all of your marketing and in all points of contact with potential and actual clients. Let others know where you are going, and carry your cell phone or BlackBerry with you in case of an emergency. And remember, if you ever feel unsafe, it is perfectly okay to hightail it out of there, even if you have to leave your equipment behind. Above all, trust your judgment and respect your own boundaries.

THE ZONING ZONE: LICENSES AND PERMITS

No business operates in a vacuum; government at every level tends to have something to say about business, and ways to regulate it. As excited and zealous as you are to start your new business, common sense dictates that you should always do your research on local ordinances, state laws, and federal rules before diving into any enterprise. Any business owner should always comply with city, state, and federal laws on everything from zoning to taxes (more on this in Chapter 10, "Organizing and Legal Structuring").

Before you begin your business, you will want to pay particular attention to local rules on zoning, licensing, and permits for both yourself and your business. **Zoning** is the designation for use of different areas by local governments. Zoning laws or ordinances dictate what types of businesses can and cannot be conducted in various neighborhoods and locations. For example, some streets are zoned for schools, others for businesses, others for residences, and still others might have a multi-use combination.

If you are considering operating a massage business out of your home, be sure to seek clarity on local zoning laws, as many municipalities restrict or prohibit this or other home-based small businesses (see the next section). You can check with your town clerk for information on zoning in your area. He or she may also be able to help you apply for a **zoning variance,** which is an exception to an existing zoning law for which businesses can apply.

Your geographic location will also dictate the kinds of massage business license and permits you will need to obtain in order to do business. Although some towns still do not have any laws regulating massage therapy, many do, and some are very involved in what you can and cannot do in your business. Auspiciously, these regulations originated to help crack down on prostitution and legitimize the profession, though many contend that they are a way for governments to cash in on the revenues from this lucrative industry. Regardless, the rules must be followed. Local governments vary widely on their laws and regulations for massage therapy, and you are advised to check with your town or county, as well as to stay abreast of any changes made in policies that could affect you. Some towns are very lax on regulation, while others can be quite strict. In fact, some areas are so strict that many business owners will elect to open up shop in another nearby town just to avoid the headaches and hoops.

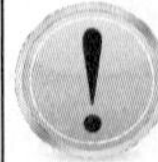

PITFALLS

Nothing can put a damper on a massage like a noisy office. Imagine how difficult it is to relax if sirens are wailing by, or if the sounds from the 2 pm aerobics class next door are blaring through your walls. Many people sign a lease on a space without visiting during various times of the day or even asking about noise levels. If possible, do as much research as possible on what you and your clients can expect to hear before signing on the dotted line.

In towns that have more stringent regulations for massage, it is not uncommon to need a license (or permit) to practice massage *and* a license or permit to operate a massage establishment. Separate paperwork, processes, and fees all apply to both kinds of licenses/permits.

Some towns' massage ordinances seem more directed at eradicating prostitution than regulating massage therapy; long lists of scandalous things one cannot do in practice can often be demoralizing and offensive to massage therapists who have worked hard for their education, credentials, and expertise. Rather than simply resent or even ignore the regulations, massage practioners are encouraged to work together with local officials for the equitable revision of regulations in order to reflect the therapeutic, health-related, and highly skilled nature of the industry and its professionals.[6]

EXPLORING THE PROS AND CONS OF WORKING FROM HOME

Like many service-based businesses, it is not uncommon to encounter massage therapists working out of a home office. With the affordability and interconnectivity of technology, home businesses are increasingly popular. In fact, *Inc. Magazine* conducted a study revealing that more businesses are started at home than in commercial venues.[7] There are certainly many advantages and challenges to this location option, and it is highly recommended that you consider them all before making a choice. On the plus side, working from home can be tremendously convenient and help you cut your operating costs considerably. If you are starting your business on a shoestring budget, there can be huge savings in working from home. Home-based practitioners also report that they benefit from being able to productively attend to things around the house between clients. With a home office you can typically have more control over the environment you are able to create for your clients, and can avoid the issues that often come along with negotiating remodels with landlords or other tenants. Working from home also provides more control over your own schedule, and can allow you more time with family. You

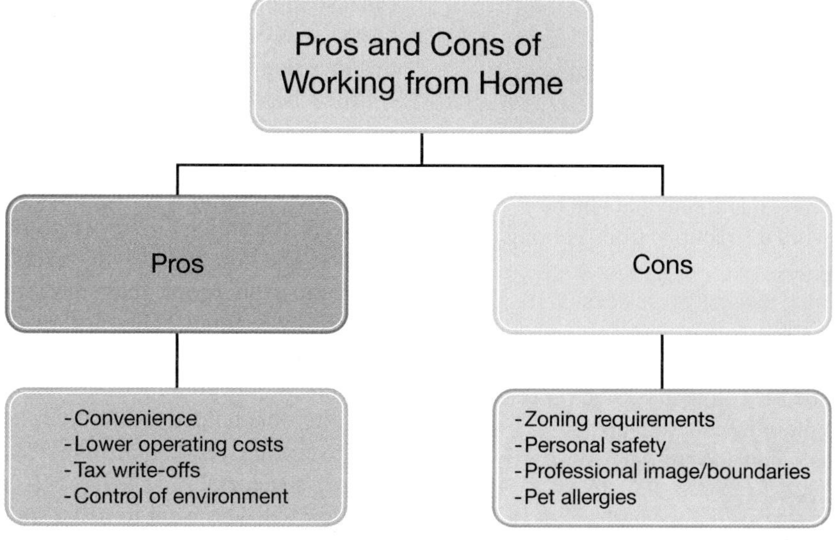

FIGURE 9-2

Some of the benefits and challenges of working from home.

can also get substantial tax write-offs for your home business[8] (see Figure 9-2 ■).

However, if you do elect to work from home, you will have unique challenges to consider. As mentioned earlier, some local zoning laws restrict or prohibit home-business activity. Check requirements with your local board of health, city administration, or your local licensing agency to see if it is even an option for you to work from your home. Inviting people into your home to do massage can present some security issues, so you will optimally want to build a referral-based business and have screening and security systems in place. You may want to revise and tailor your marketing plan if you don't want just anyone coming through your family's door. If you have household pets, these can present problems to clients with allergies or even animal phobias. If your home is in a hard to find, inaccessible, or out-of-the-way location, it may prove very inconvenient for clients to come to you. It can also be very difficult to delineate clear boundaries between your personal and professional life; even if you manage to do this well, others in your household may not.

THE BENEFITS AND CHALLENGES OF COLLABORATING WITH OTHERS IN YOUR SPACE

There can be tremendous advantages to working in a location with other massage therapists or holistic practitioners. Generally speaking, clients that seek out one kind of holistic therapy will be inclined to seek out another.[9] In other words, if someone is willing to pay for acupuncture, they will be more likely to pay for a massage, especially if referred by their acupuncturist. Collaborative marketing and referral networks are explored in Chapters 6, "Networking" and 11, "Marketing Fundamentals," but it might help you to get a review/preview of the benefits of collaborating with others when you are approaching decisions on your location.

Some of the most successful therapists are those who get involved in collective wellness centers. A **wellness center** is any location where multiple wellness services are offered for clients looking to reduce their risk of illness, increase their level of health and fitness, and improve their overall quality of life. Examples of services offered in wellness centers include massage, personal training, nutrition counseling, acupuncture, yoga classes, health education classes, mental health counseling, pre/postnatal care, and so forth. Some massage therapists find existing wellness centers, while others will bring together other holistic practitioners to create a new one. Although the business models and structure can vary significantly among centers, many are run as a collective of independent businesses renting or subletting space from one individual or entity. But cross-referrals from one health practioner to another across the hall can be incredibly effective business-generating. In addition, working with other wellness professionals has the added bonus of community and security you're rarely alone in the building. Working with other professionals also has the benefit of sharing resources and expenses such as reception areas, fax machines, and advertising efforts. And working closely with other business owners gives you the advantage of collective brain power, especially if ideas and creative capital are shared much more easily than when your office is isolated from others. Many practitioners cite the positive professional community as a primary reason for coming together in one physical location.

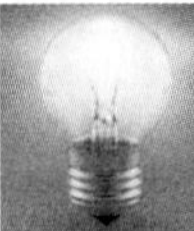

BRIGHT IDEAS

Tips for Maximizing a Home Practice

- Remember that a home business is still a business. All the same rules of the road apply.
- Keep it professional—make sure that you have a plan in place to avoid distractions from a crying baby or a barking dog.
- Don't put your home address on business cards; doing so can lend a less sophisticated air and can also present security concerns.
- Augment your time management skills; it is easy to slack on accountability and organization when working from home. Set a schedule and stick to it.
- Keep it clean; you will have to maintain a clean and aesthetically appealing home at all times. A cluttered or malodorous house can keep clients from returning.
- Communicate openly with others living in your home to make sure that everyone is clear on expectations and boundaries.
- Communicate with neighbors about the nature of your business, and work out any foreseeable parking issues *before* they arise.
- Make sure your professional insurance or your homeowners insurance covers your home business; if not, you may need supplemental coverage.
- Schedule activities away from home so you don't succumb to the homebound-prisoner syndrome.
- Stay connected; join local business groups and network heavily in your area. This can offset geographic disadvantages and lack of direct exposure to clients.
- Leverage the Internet strategically; you can still use the Internet to promote your business, but do it in a way that protects yourself and those in your household (see Chapters 13 and 15 for more information).
- Always consider the client's needs first. Continuing to view your home office from their eyes will help keep you sharp and professional.

On the other hand, there are challenges to consider when embarking on a location with others. As with many things, the more people involved, the more complex decision-making processes can become. Sharing space with others increases the stakeholders in the situation. Even if you are only sharing a small room with one other person, you will need to make sure that you both have a clear understanding on everything from schedules to payments to resource use. Sharing can also dilute the control you exercise over aspects of your business, as consensus may need to be reached by all the parties in a shared space. In addition, if there are personality conflicts between practitioners it can create a very unpleasant working environment.

The key to successful sharing is to have very clear communication, and to outline expectations up front. If you plan on subleasing space to other practioners, have very clear contracts on what each person is responsible for. Sara Vandergoot, massage therapist and founder of Vital Body & Mind Therapies, had regular team-building retreats with all of the independent holistic practioners from the very beginning of her wellness center. She maintains that this helped foster the relationships early on, so that everyone felt interconnected and invested in one another's success.

You will also want to make sure that your lease terms make sharing space with anyone else permissible; some landlords will only allow their location to be used by the individual whose name is on the lease. If you are considering subletting extra rooms or letting someone else use your office on days you aren't there, be sure that you are allowed to do this.

Of course, wellness centers or physical concentrations of holistic practitioners are not necessarily the best way or the only way to build your business collaboratively. If you want to work collaboratively, but not necessarily with other massage therapists or holistic practitioners, there are plenty of ways to do so. Lead generation groups, networking associations, and shared space in locations with high concentrations of professionals but few massage therapists can also help you build your business collaboratively. Your ability to share space and to work in partnership with others to build business is only limited by your imagination!

RETAIL

More and more massage therapists are incorporating retail sales into their business. Each therapist may have different reasons for this, but the benefits can be great for both your clients and your business, and expand your earning potential exponentially. If an entire business is service-based, revenues are limited to the amount of energy a service provider (i.e., massage therapist) can expend. If he or she cannot work for any reason, no income is generated. However, if products are sold, the income potential is greater and not reliant solely upon physical rendering (which, as you know, can be exhausting!). In addition, providing your clients with quality products can help them better meet their needs and solve their problem after their massage session has ended.

Many therapists feel conflicted about selling retail in their practice, as they are uncomfortable "pushing product" or playing the role of salesperson with their clients.

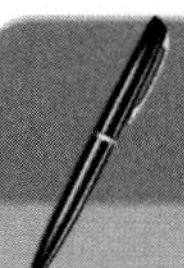

PUT IT IN WRITING

Retail Products

The following is a quick list of retail products that many massage therapists sell.

Hot/cold packs
Aromatherapy oils
Vitamin supplements
Self-massage equipment
Linaments/ointments
Salt scrubs
Herbal compresses
Candles
Books
CDs/videos

Think of retail products that would be supportive of your specific business. Brainstorm things that you might use yourself and would feel comfortable selling to clients. Write some ideas down here.

They are highly aware of the danger of dual roles and power differentials, and worry that incorporating sales into their service might be a conflict of interest. However, if you choose products that you truly believe in and that you feel will bring value and/or relief to your clients, you can consider your retail sales just another extension of the core of your business—helping people feel better and be healthy. Many clients are sincerely interested in buying supplemental products that enhance their wellness and can be incorporated into their everyday lives. Providing appropriate and quality retail products can be a cornerstone of excellent customer service and satisfaction.

In a brand new business, you may not want to invest a lot of money in a large inventory of retail products in the initial stages. Instead, conventional wisdom suggests starting out slow and small, and experimenting with different products to see which are well received by clients (see Figure 9-3 ■).

You always want to maintain boundaries on your retail ventures, however. While you can always recommend, you cannot prescribe. Because you are looked to as an expert of massage therapy, it is very important to be very clear with clients about the limitations of your training. Positioning yourself beyond your scope of practice by prescribing anything from your retail inventory is not only unethical, it can put you in a legal quandary as well.[10]

Before you dive in and start selling wonderful products to your clients, you will need to apply for a retail/resale license from your local government and a tax/employer identification number license with the Internal Revenue Service. You will also be responsible for paying retail sales tax for the items that you sell. To find out more information about the particular regulations in your area, contact your local departments of excise and license, as well as the IRS; many of these agencies allow you to gather the relevant information and apply for licenses and permits online.

If you are really serious about incorporating retail products into your business, the following tips will help you explore your options and expand your revenue potential.

- *Placement:* Have separate physical space for service and product sales if possible. Retail products should be displayed in a different area than the massage room, such as the reception area.

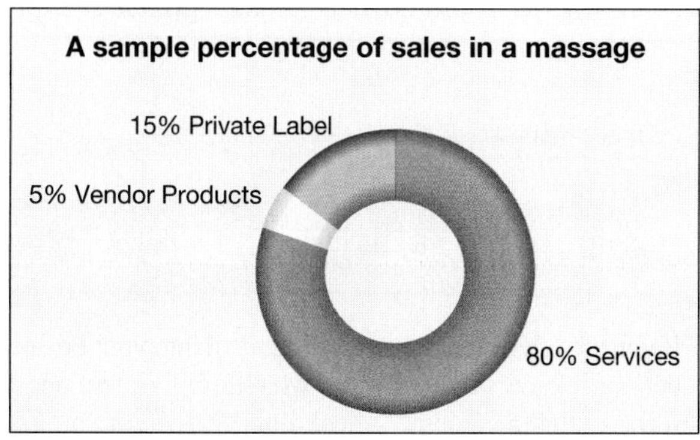

FIGURE 9-3

One massage business's percentage of private label, vendor retail, and service sales.

- *SWAG!:* Give your clients a small goodie bag of the samples of the products you sell. Giving people freebies has the double benefit of perceived added value for the client and direct exposure to your great products. And typically they cost your business very little. (If you are working in collaboration with other holistic practioners, you might develop your goodie bags together as a mutual marketing approach.)
- *Soft sell:* Do *not* be pushy or aggressive in your sales tactics. Doing so not only violates your professional ethics, it can also cost you clients. Many people will not return for another massage if they feel turned off by your sales tactics.
- *Educate yourself, your clients, and your staff:* Understand the advantages of the products you sell, and be able to answer any questions you may be asked about them.
- *Prove it:* If possible, incorporate your retail products into your service. If clients actually experience something, they are more likely to purchase it, especially if they solve a client's problem or meet a need. Integrate aromatherapy oils, paraffin treatments, or analgesic creams into your standards service. If you are selling CDs, play them during a session. If you sell it, use it.
- *Host an educational event:* Teach a couples massage or sports maintenance class, and introduce any supporting products that participants can buy and take home with them to continue what they have learned.
- *Tester test:* Place testers of soaps, hand creams, or aromatic spritzers in the bathroom, so clients can try them out while they are getting changed.
- *Literature:* Have supporting literature that communicates the properties and benefits of what you are selling. If you need to, create a brochure yourself and explain why you believe in the things you are selling.
- *Free gifts:* Include an added bonus gift with purchases to serve as an incentive to purchase products. Typically, clients are more apt to pay full price and get a free gift than to buy an item at a discount; the perception of value is greater if something is "free." Candles, soaps, aromatic spritzers, or a sample kit are good examples of free gifts given with the purchase of larger ticket items.

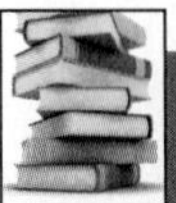

HELPFUL RESOURCES

If you are interested in introducing retail into your business, but don't know where to start, what to sell, or feel uncomfortable being "salesy," check out *1001 Ideas to Create Retail Excitement* by Edgar A. Falk (2003, Prentice Hall).

DISCOVER HOW TO BRAND PRIVATE-LABEL RETAIL PRODUCTS

When done correctly, selling retail is all about giving your clients what they want and helping them solve their problems. Finding just the right mix of products to achieve that goal can often be a lengthy process of trial and error, and many entrepreneurs find it cumbersome and time-consuming to not only find the right products to resell to their clients, but also to navigate the relationships and contracts with various vendors. A **vendor,** or supplier, is the company that provides the products to another company either for resale or for general operations.

Because many small business owners want to use products as a way to strengthen their relationships with their clients and as a way to enhance profitability, many companies sell private-label retail products. **Private-label retail** are products that are either created by a company for its own sales or manufactured by one company but sold under another company's brand. Examples of private labels range from Whole Foods' 365 label, virtually everything in Trader Joe's, and the organic, locally sourced soaps sold at a wellness center under its own logo. In many cases, private label can be a big part of a marketing strategy, as it can help a company differentiate on price, quality, or personal connection with the retailer.[11] Having your own line of holistic products to support your clients' health can be a real marketing advantage for you and your business. It can also help build the relationships between you and your clients, as you are custom-creating solutions to meet their needs.

Many holistic practitioners have taken hobbies such as making candles, soaps, oils, lotions, salves, potpourris, jewelry, and knitted items, and turned them into a nice stream of revenue through boutique private-label branding. If you are going to create your own private-labels product, make sure you know the regulations for manufacturing and distributing different items (this is particularly true if your items can be consumed or cause adverse allergic reactions). Even if you purchase a private-label product from another company, be sure to package it consistently with the look and feel of your business. If private-label marketing is something that sounds like it would be a great fit for you and your business, this might be a good reason to enlist the help of a wellness or spa consultant.

CHAPTER SUMMARY BY LEARNING OBJECTIVES

1. **Explain why location is so important to a business** Finding and selecting the right location for you and your business are some of the most important elements when starting your business, especially for a service-driven enterprise like massage. Client convenience is paramount for a massage business, so issues such as parking, public transportation, safety, foot traffic, noise control, and proximity to other stores can all be crucial to the success of a massage business.
2. **Use creative visualization to conceive the right space** Knowing what you are looking for makes *finding* what you are looking for all the more manageable. Creative visualization helps lay the blueprint for locating the right space, as it helps to clarify what you are looking for in a physical space that will best serve your business.
3. **Examine different scopes and scales of massage businesses** Massage businesses come in all shapes and sizes, and your location needs and considerations will have a direct relationship to your scale and scope of operations. Home practices, mobile practices, office rental, shared space, and day spas are some of the location scopes to consider.
4. **Employ techniques to find the right place and identify equipment you will need in your massage business** There are many effective ways of locating the best spot for your business. Physically exploring target areas on foot, asking around in your network, doing online research, and working with leasing agents are all good ways to find an ideal location for your practice. Detailed equipment needs vary from business to business, but items such as tables, linens, lubricants, and administrative supplies are typically standard for all startups.
5. **Evaluate mobility** Many therapists have built successful businesses without a brick-and-mortar location by developing mobile practices. Through on-site chair and table massage, mobile businesses have the advantage of less overhead and premium pricing; however they require a lot of energy, travel, and assumption of more risk than a stationary practice.
6. **Define zoning, licensing, and permits** Zoning is the designation for use of different areas by local governments. Zoning laws or ordinances dictate what types of businesses can and cannot be conducted in various neighborhoods and locations. Geographic location will also dictate the kinds of massage business license and permits you need to obtain in order to do business. Local governments vary widely on their laws and regulations for massage therapy, and you are advised to check with your town or county, as well as to stay abreast of any changes made in policies that could affect you. It is not uncommon to need both a license (or permit) to practice massage and another to own a massage business.
7. **Examine pros and cons of working from home** Benefits of working from home include convenience, reduced overhead, control over environment, tax write-offs, and time saved on commuting. Challenges include local restriction and zoning laws on home businesses, security issues, boundaries between personal and professional life, client allergies to household pets, and geographic inconvenience for clients.
8. **Contrast the benefits and challenges of collaborating with others in your space** By sharing space with other massage therapists or holistic practitioners, your business can benefit from shared resources, collective brain power, pooled marketing efforts, and a strong business community. The challenges can be difficulty with decision making, diluted control, personality conflicts, and limitations due to lease terms.
9. **Explore the merit of retail sales in your business and demonstrate how to use retail to maximize customer service** More and more massage therapists are incorporating retail sales into their business. Retail can increase business revenue substantially, and can be used to augment customer experience. Providing clients with quality products can help them better meet their needs and solve their problem after their massage session has ended. Professional ethics apply, and dual roles should be considered.
10. **Discover how to brand private-label retail products** Private-label retail are products that are either created by a company for its own sales or manufactured by one company but sold under another company's brand. Having your own line of holistic products to support your clients' health can be a real marketing advantage for you and your business. It can also help build the relationships between you and your clients, as you are custom-creating solutions to meet their needs.

ACTIVITIES

Quiz: Location Basics

1. Building exterior, geographic location, convenience, and interior decorating can all be part of the
   a. job
   b. location mix
   c. lease agreement
   d. leasing agent's responsibilities
2. Challenges to a mobile therapist include:
   a. deciding what to wear
   b. security screening clients
   c. travel time
   d. b and c
3. Home based businesses are:
   a. allowed everywhere
   b. more profitable than an office business
   c. can be very convenient and minimize operating costs
   d. always unprofessional
4. When working internationally, massage therapists:
   a. can gain professional experience that will be invaluable in their careers
   b. can gain amazing experience and education in bodywork modalities
   c. don't need to worry about local laws or residency requirements
   d. a and b
5. Which of the following would be the least effective method of finding a great location for your business?
   a. waiting for someone to ask you to join their wellness center
   b. looking at real estate online
   c. tapping your network to learn about available spaces
   d. working with a leasing agent
6. The term *due diligence* refers to:
   a. gathering relevant information
   b. evaluating risk
   c. researching opportunities and threats
   d. thoroughly investigating potential acquisitions for a business
   e. all the above
7. Which is the least important aspect of choosing a location from the items below?
   a. rental price and lease terms
   b. convenience for client
   c. already furnished
   d. noise pollution
8. When selling a product to a client, you prescribe her one of your signature oils, telling her that it is the only thing that can clear up her psoriasis. In doing so, you have violated both _____ and _____.
   a. salesmanship, retail best practices
   b. professional ethics, scope of practice
   c. honesty, respect
   d. retail licenses, business permits
9. True or False: Private-label products are only products that are made by the company selling them.
10. True or False: Working with commercial real estate agents is often the most expensive way to find a location for your business.
11. True or False: Leases can have clauses that explicitly prohibit the commercial use of anyone other than the leaseholder.
12. True or False: Wellness centers are the only way to successfully build your business in a collaborative way.

Case Study

Mirasol

Mirasol is very close to finishing her 1000-hour massage therapy program. Mirasol's dream is to start a spa, as she feels this niche of the market is the most suitable for her personality and her experience. She has a lot of ideas about how to market a spa and attract clients to her business. She also has a good sum of money that she has been saving from a severance package from her 15-year corporate career, and she feels confident that between that and some family money she will have enough capital to back her business in the start-up phases.

Because Mirasol relocated for massage school, she doesn't have a very strong network and is still learning the lay of the land. She isn't as familiar with the demographics of the different markets in the area, though she has a few ideas for locations based on areas where she likes to spend her own time and money. She explores some of the more upscale areas where she thinks her spa could be successful, but is discouraged to see that they all already have several established spas. She wonders if there might be some up-and-coming retail areas that would suit her needs, but she hasn't found any yet.

Mirasol has traveled to many countries, and really wants to incorporate the aesthetic from some of her travels in Southeast Asian countries into the décor of her spa and the products she plans to sell. She has done a lot of research on private labeling, and wants to create a line of custom body products, as well as teas and spa snacks for her guests. However, she has never manufactured products or designed a spa before and is uncertain about the technical and logistical specifications spas might require. Having never worked in a spa before, she isn't entirely sure what equipment she will need or how she should staff her spa. Though she is anxious to get started, Mirasol wants to take the time to make sure she does things right.

You are a good friend of Mirasol's, and because you have experience with developing good locations for wellness businesses, she comes to you for advice.

Case Study Questions

1. How do you think Mirasol should approach her location situation? How would you do it if you were in her situation?
2. Would you recommend that Mirasol enlist the help of any professionals? If so, what kinds of professionals might be helpful to her in this stage of development?
3. What do you see as Mirasol's strengths? What are some ways in which she is at a disadvantage?
4. Mirasol wants to start her own private-label line, including teas and foods. Knowing what you know, what would you recommend she do first before investing any money in development or packaging?
5. What are some of the considerations that Mirasol should think about when shopping for space for her spa? What unique needs will she have that other massage therapists might not be concerned with in their location search?
6. Help Mirasol flesh out her location mix. Is there anything she is overlooking or hasn't considered?
7. Do you think Mirasol is ready to launch a spa business? Why or why not? As her business coach, are there any alternative approaches she might try?

CHAPTER

10 Organizing and Legal Structuring

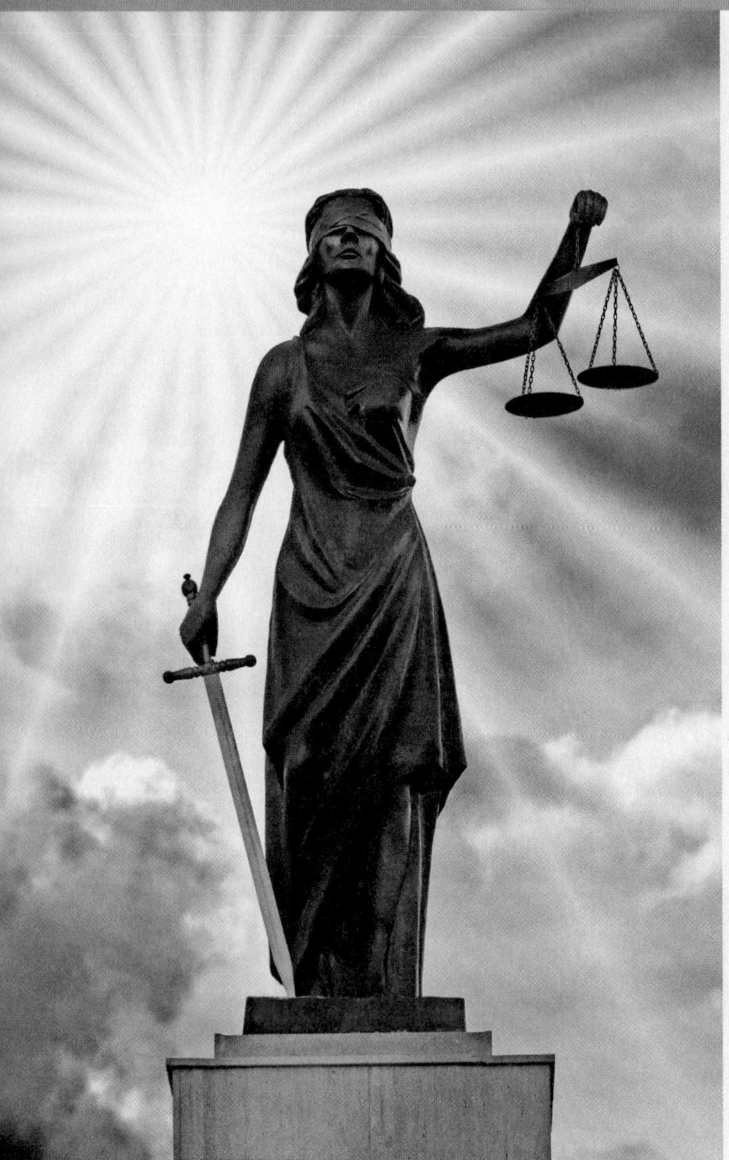

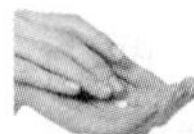

CHAPTER OUTLINE

LEARNING OBJECTIVES

1. Explain the importance of following legal protocols when starting a business
2. Identify different legal structures for your business
3. Demonstrate the value of a business name
4. Provide an overview of business taxes
5. Provide an overview of permits, licenses, and legal requirements for small businesses
6. Explain responsibilities as an employer
7. Investigate insurance coverage for your practice
8. Examine the elements of insurance billing for your clients
9. Analyze legal considerations of bringing your business online

KEY TERMS

anticybersquatting consumer protection act *166*
board of directors *159*
C corporation *159*
CAN-SPAM Act *166*
commercial property insurance *164*
corporation *159*
cybersquatting *166*
deduction *161*
disability insurance *165*
Employer ID Number (EIN) *161*
fictitious business name *160*
general liability insurance *164*
health insurance claim form *165*
home-based business insurance *164*
I-9 *163*
IRS tax audit *162*
legal structure *156*
limited liability company (LLC) *158*
partnership *158*
product liability insurance *164*
S corporation *159*
shareholders *159*
sole proprietorship *158*
tax avoidance *161*
tax evasion *161*
taxes *161*
trade name *160*
trademark *160*
unemployment insurance *165*
W-2 *163*
W-4 *163*
W-9 *165*
worker's compensation *165*

LEARNING LEGALESE: WHAT YOU NEED TO KNOW FOR YOUR MASSAGE BUSINESS

If you like laws and sausages, you should never watch either one being made.

—Otto von Bismark

As a business owner, you will be responsible for knowing and adhering to all of the local, county, state, and federal laws and regulations that govern not only massage, but small business in general. While it may not be necessary to get a legal degree or become a tax specialist, you should keep abreast of your responsibilities and ensure that you are conducting your business legally. As the common maxim observes, ignorance of the law is neither an excuse nor a protection from the law. The following "Put It in Writing" exercise will give you an overview of your familiarity with some of the requirements of starting and maintaining an above-board business.

The United States has a fairly litigious (quick to take legal action) culture and you want to take every measure possible to protect both yourself and your business. It is important to follow the rules and all of the established laws when setting up any business; this will not only help you avoid trouble down the line, but will help you and your business be viable parts of your community. This chapter will give you an overview of the five steps to registering your business, as well as ongoing requirements for keeping it running. The five steps to registering your business include:

1. Determining the legal structure of your business
2. Registering your business name
3. Establishing your tax obligations and obtaining your federal tax ID number
4. Registering with your state revenue agency
5. Acquiring all necessary licenses and permits

You'll also get some other important tips on issues such as intellectual property, registering trademarks, paying taxes, and special considerations for conducting any of your business online. However, nothing in this chapter is meant to be construed as legal counsel or a replacement for seeking legal advice from a legal professional. Remember that this book merely provides an overview, and is not intended to offer an exhaustive list of requirements at the federal, state, or local level; always be sure to check with local authorities on any current regulations that may affect you. Always consult an attorney, accountant, or government agency with specific questions, concerns, or confusions (after all, this wouldn't be a chapter on legal issues without a disclaimer!).

ORGANIZING? STRUCTURING? IT SOUNDS LIKE BUILDING A HOUSE

And in a way, it is! As you've seen in many other chapters of *The Business of Massage Therapy,* starting a business is very much like building a house. It all starts with a solid foundation. The first step in registering your business is choosing the appropriate foundation, or legal structure, for your business. A **legal structure** is the type of business entity in which you organize your business. Legal structures differ in terms of financial, tax, and legal responsibilities, and many factors go into selecting the appropriate structure for each business.[1] When you are getting started, make sure that the legal structure you select takes into account all of your unique and special needs. Seek input from your attorney and accountant to make sure the legal structure you choose is the best one for you.

LEGAL STRUCTURES AT A GLANCE

- *Sole proprietorship:* A business owned entirely by one individual, who is responsible for all obligations and debts of the business.
- *Limited liability company (LLC):* A business structure that provides limited personal liability for the debts and actions of the business, pass-through taxation, and relative flexibility.
- *Partnership:* A legal structure that involves two or more people who invest their time, money, efforts, labor, and talents to share ownership and responsibilities of a business.
- *Corporation:* Considered legally to be separate and distinct from its owners, a corporation can be sued, pay taxes, and enter into contracts. Corporations have shareholders and a board of directors.
- *C Corporation (C Corp.):* An organization that is taxed at both the business level and the individual level.
- *S Corporation (S Corp.):* Known as a "pass through" entity, similar to a partnership, because taxation happens only at the owner level. There are certain requirements for a company to qualify as an S Corp.

The most common types of legal structures for smaller massage businesses include sole proprietorships, limited liability companies, and partnerships. Businesses with larger-scale operations often incorporate into S corps. and C corps. A brief description of the legal structures you might consider for your business follows, along with each structure's relative advantages and disadvantages. You will also find lists of some of the federal tax forms you will need to create each type of legal structure. The lists given are not complete, and some forms may not apply; check with your local authorities, attorney, or Small Business Center to ensure you utilize the correct forms for your fabulous and unique business.

Sole proprietorships are among the most common and simple business entities in the United States at present.[2] In a

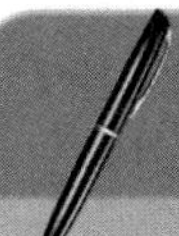

PUT IT IN WRITING

Legal Eagle or Legal Beagle?

1. A(n) _____ is a hybrid of a partnership and a corporation, and allows the owners to participate in management of the business without assuming unlimited liability.
   a. S corp.
   b. sole proprietorship
   c. C corp.
   d. Limited liability company
2. When someone writes original material, it is their _____. Copying material from someone else's website and placing it on your own without giving credit to the source is a violation of _____.
   a. property, common sense
   b. intellectual property, copyright
   c. work, implied contracts
   d. magnum opus, civil liberties
3. Legally structuring your massage business refers to _____.
   a. sending a check to the Secretary of State
   b. having a lawyer help you remodel your office
   c. filing the appropriate paperwork and following specific processes to become a sole proprietorship, LLC, S corp., C corp., or partnership
   d. having clients sign a waiver
4. Writing something untrue about another massage therapist in your online blog that damages his/her professional reputation is an example of _____.
   a. gossip
   b. slander
   c. a vendetta
   d. libel
5. Alisha's trade name is very similar to that of another company. She receives a letter telling her that her website intentionally confuses and baits their customers and that she may face legal action if she does not stop using her website immediately. This is an example of _____.
   1. a cease-and-desist letter
   2. really bad karma
   3. something to ignore
   4. a good reason to seek legal counsel
6. As a massage therapist and business owner, there may be practices that violate professional _____ but do not violate any laws.
   a. associations or memberships
   b. ethics or boundaries
   c. attire
   d. networks
7. Willfully and intentionally withholding a portion of or the entirety of all of your income and tips from your massage business is considered _____.
   a. a risky business practice
   b. an honest mistake
   c. tax law dismissal
   d. tax fraud/tax evasion
8. As a massage therapist working on your own, it's important to have _____ insurance.
   a. personal, malpractice, and product liability
   b. personal disability
   c. automobile and health
   d. all the above
9. As a massage business owner with employees, law requires that you have _____.
   a. uniforms
   b. workers' compensation insurance
   c. employee handbooks
   d. business contracts
10. You should contact government authorities at the _____ level to ensure that you are fulfilling all the license and permit requirements to operate a small business.
   a. city and county
   b. state and federal
   c. all of the above
   d. none of the above

Scoring Guide

1) a = 3 b = 1 c = 2 d = 4
2) a = 3 b = 4 c = 2 d = 1
3) a = 3 b = 1 c = 4 d = 2
4) a = 2 b = 3 c = 1 d = 4
5) a = 4 b = 2 c = 1 d = 3
6) a = 3 b = 4 c = 1 d = 2
7) a = 3 b = 1 c = 2 d = 4
8) a = 3 b = 3 c = 3 d = 4
9) a = 1 b = 4 c = 3 d = 2
10) a = 3 b = 3 c = 4 d = 1

Now tally up your score, and see where you are:

34–40: Legal Eagle: Perhaps you've been to law school, have a love affair with the IRS, or just can't get enough of *Law & Order,* because you certainly know your stuff! You are in a great position to run a sound and law-abiding business. You might even consider doing a little moonlighting to help your friends organize their businesses!

26–33: Legal Connoisseur: You know a great deal about the legal issues of running a business, and are in a strong position for your business. Since you have such a solid foundation, you're also in a prime position to learn more about legal areas where you might have less experience or familiarity.

18–25: Legal Aid: You know some of the main legal parameters of running a business, but take the time to brush up so you don't run afoul of the authorities unintentionally.

10–17: Legal Beagle: You've heard of the law, and you know that there are some of them out there that might be relevant to you. However, if you're going to run a successful and long-lasting business, you will want to read this chapter carefully. You might also check out some of the free classes provided by a local business development center to make sure that everything is in order.

sole proprietorship, the business is owned and managed by one individual who is responsible for all operations and owns all of the assets of the business. In essence, this means that the sole proprietor *is* the business, and is also liable for any business obligations or debts.

There are no formal requirements for forming a sole proprietorship, unless you choose to operate under a name other than your own (such as "New You Massage" or "Bliss by Becky"). This is considered a fictitious business name: you'll learn more about this in the next section. One of the advantages of a sole proprietorship is that it is the simplest, least involved, and most affordable of all the business organization options. It also grants complete control to you as the business owner. In addition, sole proprietorships pay only one level of income tax and the owner can collect all the profits generated by the business.[3] Also, a sole proprietorship is relatively easy to dissolve if you decide you don't want to be in business any longer.[4] Sole proprietorships are automatically dissolved should the owner die.

However, sole proprietorships have disadvantages as well. Sole proprietors often find it more difficult to raise money for their business, and are often limited to personal funds and personally borrowed money for start-up and operating capital. If the company loses money, the proprietor has all the liability for the losses. Sole proprietorships can have a great deal of risk as the owner assumes unlimited liability. If your business gets sued or involved in a lawsuit, your personal assets can be tapped (and zapped!) very quickly.

To form a sole proprietorship, you may need the following forms.[5] Check with your local business development center, as this information can change.

- Form 1040: Individual Income Tax Return
- Schedule C: Profit or Loss from Business (or Schedule C-EZ)
- Schedule SE: Self-Employment Tax
- Form 1040-ES: Estimated Tax for Individuals
- Form 4562: Depreciation and Amortization
- Form 8829: Expenses for Business Use of Your Home
- Employment Tax Forms

A **limited liability company (LLC)** is a business structure that provides limited personal liability for the debts and actions of the business. Often referred to as a hybrid of partnerships, sole proprietorships, and corporations, LLCs can provide the benefit of pass-through taxation while allowing relative flexibility in management.[6] In LLCs, profits flow through to the owners, similar to a partnership or a sole proprietorship. LLCs are formed by filing articles of organization with an individual state, and the rules governing LLCs varying from state to state. LLCs allow for multiple owners (owners are known as "members"), and they may be individuals, corporations, or other LLCs. Because most states allow "single member" LLCs, or entities with only one owner, many massage therapists chose this organizational structure for their business.

However, LLCs are not the magic bullet of business organization. Companies that hope to grow significantly over time and attain investors would be ill-advised to structure as an LLC. LLCs are typically simpler to set up than corporations, but more complicated and costly than sole proprietorships or partnerships. Some states do not allow certain kinds of businesses to form as LLCs (typically financial or insurance businesses). Since the status of LLCs varies from state to state, be sure to check out the applicable rules in your own state. Incidentally, the federal government does not recognize an LLC as a classification for federal tax purposes, and LLC business entities must file a corporation, partnership, or sole proprietorship tax return[7] (check with your tax advisor for more information).

The following forms are commonly associated with LLCs (remember to check for the most current requirements first).

- Schedule C (Form 1040): Profit or Loss from Business
- Schedule E (Form 1040): Supplemental Income and Loss
- Schedule SE (Form 1040): Self-Employment Tax
- W-2 and W-3: Wage and Tax Statement, and Transmittal of Wage and Tax Statement
- Form 940: Employer's Annual Federal Unemployment (FUTA) Tax Return
- Form 1040: U.S. Individual Income Tax Return
- Form 8832: Entity Classification Election

A **partnership** is a legal structure that involves two or more people who invest their time, money, efforts, labor, and talents to share ownership and responsibilities of a business. Types of partnerships include general partnerships, joint ventures, and limited liability partnerships. In partnerships, co-owners share in the profits and losses of a business. Typically, each partner has a level of control in the business. Because a partnership is a legally binding relationship, where all parties are entitled to gains and are liable for losses, it is important to be objective about crafting partnership agreements (see Chapter 13 for more information).

There are many benefits to starting a partnership for your massage business; it can be daunting, nerve-racking, and lonely to start a new business all by yourself, and partnerships can help ease the burden. Bringing in other talented practitioners with complementary skills can exponentially increase your service offerings to clients, and can give you the advantage of new ideas and perspectives. Your knowledge capital and financial resources are likely to be expanded as well. Partnerships can be formed fairly easily, and your ability to raise capital is increased. Like a sole proprietorship, partnerships are only subject to taxation at one level; the profits "pass through" to the individual partners who report income and losses on their individual tax returns.

Partnerships afford the owners slightly less control, as all decisions must be made jointly and the profits must be shared. Partnerships hold extensive liability—partners are held jointly and individually liable.[8] This means that you can be held responsible for anything that you do as well as for legal obligations and debts incurred by your business partner, even without your knowledge. Like a sole proprietorship, it also means that your personal assets can be vulnerable. If

PITFALLS

Many people go into professional partnerships fairly casually, without taking the time to create a legal agreement or plan the partnership strategically. A partnership is like a marriage—no one wants to think of a breakup, but many have been burned by not thinking ahead. Regardless of your initial relationship with your partner(s)—friends, family members, associates—enter into a business partnership with objectives spelled out. An exit strategy for each partner should be discussed, agreed upon, and included in the legal documents for the partnership. See Chapter 13 for more on pros and cons of partnership.

the business is unable to pay its debt obligations, creditors have claims against individual partners' assets.

The following are some common tax forms associated with a partnership (remember to check for the most current requirements first).

- Form 1065: Partnership Return of Income
- Form 1065 K-1: Partner's Share of Income, Credit, Deductions
- Form 4562: Depreciation
- Form 1040: Individual Income Tax Return
- Schedule E: Supplemental Income and Loss
- Schedule SE: Self-Employment Tax
- Form 1040-ES: Estimated Tax for Individuals
- Employment Tax Forms

Some massage businesses are formed as corporations. Authorized and chartered in the state in which it is formed, a **corporation** is a unique entity unto itself. A corporation is considered legally to be separate and distinct from its owners, and it can be sued, pay taxes and enter into contracts.

Corporations have shareholders and a board of directors. **Shareholders** are the owners of the corporation, and they typically purchase their ownership stakes in the company. Shareholders have limited liability in the business, because the assets and liabilities are owned by the business itself. The shareholders elect a **board of directors,** which has central decision-making authority and often employs managers to oversee operations of the business.[9]

There are different kinds of corporations, but the two most common are C corporations and S corporations (named for their relevant rules in the Internal Revenue Code).[10] A **C corporation** (C corp.) is an organization that is taxed at both the business level and the individual level—in other words, both the corporation pays taxes on business profits and the shareholders pay taxes on the same income when it is distributed. This "double taxation" is a main disadvantage of C corporations, and many attempt to avoid it by filing for S corporation status. A Subchapter **S corporation** (S corp.) is known as a "pass through" entity, similar to a partnership, because taxation happens only at the owner level. There are certain requirements for a company to qualify as an S corp., and any company not meeting or maintaining the requirements is automatically a C corporation.[11]

There are many benefits to operating as a corporation. Because only the corporation itself is responsible for liabilities, many entrepreneurs and investors find this structure to be advantageous in the protection of personal assets. Ownership equity can be sold to shareholders in the form of stocks, and therefore corporations also have a better ability to raise significant capital in the beginning and during the life of the company. And since the corporation is its own entity and separate from the owners, the business goes on in the event of ownership change or shareholder death.

You've already seen the disadvantage for C corps. when they are taxed at two levels, but corporations have other challenges to consider. They are often much more costly, complicated, and time-consuming than other forms of organization. Corporations are also monitored by federal, state, and some local agencies, resulting in much more paperwork and organization.[12]

The following are some of the forms typically used in C corporations (don't forget to check for current requirement information):

- Form 1120 or 1120-A: Corporation Income Tax Return
- Form 1120-W: Estimated Tax for Corporation
- Form 8109-B: Deposit Coupon
- Form 4625: Depreciation
- Employment Tax Forms
- Other forms as needed for capital gains, sale of assets, alternative minimum tax, etc.

Some of the forms required for an S corporation (is that the sound of you checking for current requirements?):

- Form 1120S: Income Tax Return for S Corporation
- 1120S K-1: Shareholder's Share of Income, Credit, Deductions
- Form 4625: Depreciation
- Employment Tax Forms

GETTING ORGANIZED
Paperwork

In the previous sections, you were given a list of potential paperwork you will need to file for each business structure (whether initially or for tax purposes). As you begin to decide which structure will work best for you and your business, you might find it very helpful to keep a list of these forms in your *Business of Massage Therapy* notebook to stay organized. Remember, however, that forms requirements can be changed or updated at any time, so be sure to keep your notebook updated as well!

- Form 1040: Individual Income Tax Return
- Schedule E: Supplemental Income and Loss
- Schedule SE: Self-Employment Tax
- Form 1040-ES: Estimated Tax for Individuals
- Other forms as needed for capital gains, sale of assets, alternative minimum tax, etc.

WHAT'S IN A NAME? HOW TO NAME YOUR BUSINESS

What's in a name? That which we call a rose By any other name would smell as sweet.

—William Shakespeare

The second step in getting your business going is choosing a business name. Naming your business can be an incredibly exciting process, but it is important to approach it strategically. The name you choose for your business is a very important decision and can impact your success going forward. Choosing a weak or overly complicated name can make it much harder for you in the long run. Ideally, a business name should be easy to use, memorable, and evoke a certain feel ing. It should be simple and easy to spell. A successful business name conveys the purpose of your business, and inspires clients to learn more about what you have to offer them. Your business name can affect how easily you are remembered, or how easily you are found online or in directories.

Of course, many holistic practitioners elect to use their own name and credentials rather than a unique name for the business (such as Basil Stephens, LMT or Carrie LaPre, L.Ac). This works best when you *are* your business, and don't intend to employ other practitioners or offer services beyond the scope of your own skills. Entwining your own name with your business allows you to build both a business and personal brand with the same efforts. If you would rather not use your own name, most states require that you register a **fictitious business name,** which allows you to do business without creating an entirely new formal identity. It also helps you to brand your business effectively with a unique and compelling name. If you choose to operate your business under a fictitious business name (also known as "assumed name" or "doing business as" [DBA]) you will have to file it with the state. The exact rules on fictitious names vary from state to state, so check your local regulations.[13]

Many therapists choose to use a geography-specific name (Big Sur Massage or Cameron Station Holistic Healing), which can help target customers to find them more easily. Others like to incorporate the specific type of work they do into their name (Javi's Sports Therapy, Radiance Reiki, or Lou's Swedish Massage), while others like to focus on the desired benefit for the client (Live Pain Free Massage, Therapy for Optimal Athletics, or Bliss Through Bodywork). Such names are good because they offer a "visual" element for clients, who can actually imagine living pain free or experiencing that bliss if they work with you. Such names evoke the mission of the business and suggest a compelling solution that might motivate clients to take action to give you their business. You might avoid names that try to be too clever or trendy. Business names always influence client opinions of you and your business, so choose wisely.

Before you fall in love with a name, you will want to make sure that it is available. You don't want to open up "Serenity by Sarah" if there is another "Serenity by Sarah" registered down the road or in a nearby town. Not only might this complicate your ability to expand your operations in the future, it can dilute your brand and confuse clients. It might also get you into some trouble with licensed trade names that are protected. A **trade name** is a company name that identifies and symbolizes a unique business and brand. This is not to be confused with a **trademark,** which is a distinctive word, symbol, or indicator used on goods and services to represent their origin and to distinguish them from the products or services of other businesses. An example of a trade name is Nike, and an example of a trademark is the Nike swoosh.

If you plan on expanding operations or getting involved with interstate transactions, you would be wise to run a preliminary search in the U.S. Patent and Trademark database. If your name is available, you can begin the process of applying for a national trademark. This can take a long time and a chunk of money, but it can be well worth it to protect your business and defend your brand in the long run.

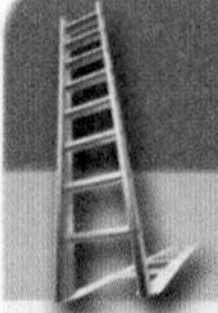

FIRST STEPS

If you don't yet have a business name in mind or selected, and you don't know where to start, begin with a little competitive research. Look at people or businesses in your area with similar service offerings and evaluate the names that they have chosen. What catches your attention? What makes you want to learn more? Are there some names that you find forgettable or even displeasing? Seeing what works for others can help you brainstorm your perfect moniker.

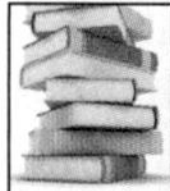

HELPFUL RESOURCES

You can check the availability of names and register a name for your business through the website of your Secretary of State. You can also conduct free trademark database searches and find more information on the patent and trademark registration process by visiting the U.S. Patent Office at www.uspto.com.

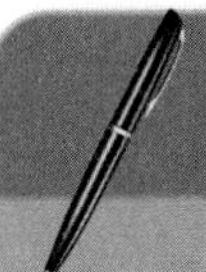

PUT IT IN WRITING

Naming Your Business

Perhaps you have a few names already in mind, or you have already homed in on a specific name. If you are struggling to narrow it down or aren't sure your chosen name is the right one, run it through the exercise below. See if it matches some of the common criteria for a successful business name.

If you feel truly attached to a particular name and it doesn't fare too well with the above criteria, don't despair or throw it out yet. These are just suggestions. While it may be more difficult, there are always ways to brand and grow your business with uncommon names (just think Xerox, Nike, or Kleenex—if they did it, so can you!).

Name	Memorable?	Evoke Feeling?	Easy to Remember/Spell?	Positive Connotation?	Informative?
________	________	________	________	________	________
________	________	________	________	________	________
________	________	________	________	________	________
________	________	________	________	________	________
________	________	________	________	________	________

ESSENTIAL INFORMATION ABOUT TAXES FOR YOUR BUSINESS

The next step in getting your business in operation is registering and organizing for your tax liability. **Taxes** represent the percentage of an individual's income or a business's gross profits that is imposed by the government in order to support public services. The type of taxes you will have to pay for your business will depend on many factors, such as what legal structure you choose, if you are employing people, and if you are selling tangible items. Tax law is the same for everyone—no one is immune from paying taxes. The thought of reading about taxes may seem as appealing as a root canal, and you may just elect to pay an accountant or professional adviser to handle all of the taxes for the business rather than handle them yourself. Even if you do this, you would be wise to gain a basic understanding of your tax obligations as a business owner. This can help you make more informed choices, as well as identify tax advantages that can save your business money. It will also make your relationship with your accountant or adviser much more productive.

Businesses are required to register with their state for one or more tax-related identification numbers, as well as licenses and permits. You learned of many of the tax forms needed for different business entities when deciding on a structure for your business. Many massage therapists supplement their service income by selling complementary products such as lotions, CDs, therapeutic tools, oils, ointments, and so forth. If you are going to be selling retail products, you will need to file with your State Revenue Department for a Sales and Use Tax account (also known as seller's permit or resale license in certain states).

If you plan on having employees, are operating your business as a partnership or corporation, have a Keogh plan, or are paying a non-resident alien, you will need to obtain an Employee Identification Number. An **Employer Identification Number (EIN)** is used to identify a business entity, and is also known as the Federal Tax Identification Number. You can apply for an EIN online through the Internal Revenue Service's website (www.irs.gov). You will probably also need to file a State Employer ID number.

You will most likely need to file your taxes quarterly (every three months), and you should do your best to stay abreast of changes to tax codes and applicable laws (which can happen often). Being aware of tax laws can help you take advantage of tax breaks and legally minimize your tax liabilities.[14] This is known as **tax avoidance,** the practice of using legal means to lower taxes owed. Tax avoidance is a very common practice among businesses and individuals. In contrast, **tax evasion** is the intentional deception of the government through means such as concealment, misreporting, or failure to file. While tax avoidance can be done legitimately, tax evasion is illegal. There are several tax-cutting strategies that individuals and businesses employ, such as deferring tax liability through investments and pension plan contributions and using all available deductions. A **deduction** is any expense that the government allows individuals and businesses to subtract from gross income, lessening the amount taxed. For example, the cost of laundering your linens or the mileage put on your car are deductions that massage businesses can take on gross income.

It is very important to keep impeccable financial records, and to track all expenses and income. This will not only make it easier for you and/or your accountant to file your taxes in a

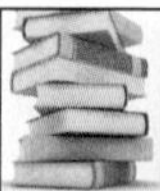

HELPFUL RESOURCES

To find out information on specific legal and tax regulations in your area as well as a wealth of other small business resources, visit www.business.gov.

timely fashion, but will make life much easier if you are ever subject to a tax audit from the Internal Revenue Service. An **IRS tax audit** is a thorough examination of a taxpayer (whether an individual or a business entity), tax returns, and supporting records and documents. The goal of an IRS tax audit is to ensure that you or your business have complied with the laws and requirements of fulfilling your tax obligations.

Whether you are a sole proprietor or employ many people, it is always a good idea to maintain a special savings account set up exclusively for taxes so that you are not caught unaware by your tax obligations. Also, as a massage therapist, remember that all of your tips are considered taxable income, and should be reported on your individual income tax. In addition, many massage therapists and holistic practitioners engage in barter for goods and services. This is also considered taxable by the government[15] (see Chapter 13 for more information on bartering services).

DEATH BY PAPERWORK: MORE LICENSES, PERMITS, AND LEGAL REQUIREMENTS FOR SMALL BUSINESSES

The next step in getting your business on board is making sure that you have obtained all local and state licenses and permits. In Chapter 4, "Professional Issues," you learned about the kinds of licenses, certificates, and permits you need to operate as a massage professional. There are also typically licenses and permits that you must obtain in order to carry out business, regardless of industry. As you saw in Chapter 9, "Location, Location, Location," you may need special permits to operate a massage business in your home, in certain zones, or at all. This is based on local and state laws. This section will cover a few of the common licenses, permits, and other legal requirements you may need for your business. As you should have ingrained into your mind by now, check with your secretary of state, small business administration, or other local authorities to learn the specifics of your area.

The following is a list of common licenses that you may need for your business:[16]

- *Occupational License:* This allows you to perform certain regulated occupations. If you live in a place that regulates massage therapy, you will likely have obtained this license before going into business for yourself. You can get this license through city and county building or planning development departments.

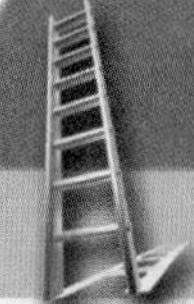

FIRST STEPS

Look at the list of licenses and permits to see which relate to the business you are planning. Are there any that aren't on the list? Take your business plan (or a good solid idea of what you want to create) and head down to your city and county building. They'll be happy to help you sort out exactly which permits you will need to get your business up and running (and happy to collect your money for those permits, too!).

- *Business Licenses:* This license basically allows you to conduct business in your city, and can be obtained from a county clerk.
- *Building Permit:* If you are planning on modifying, building, or massively reconstructing your business space, you will need to file with the city and county planning department.
- *Zoning Permit:* Slightly different from a building permit, a zoning permit looks at how a building project fits into the community. Check with city and county planning department.
- *Health Permit:* Many cities require that the local health department approve you and your operating space before you start carrying out business.
- *Alarm Permit:* If you have installed a fire or burglar alarm, some cities require that you have an alarm permit. You can get this from your city and county or fire department.
- *Signage Permit:* Many cities require permits for external signage (this can relate to sidewalk signs and sandwich boards as well). Check with your city and county or planning department.

WHO'S THE BOSS? REQUIREMENTS FOR EMPLOYERS

The employer generally gets the employees s/he deserves.

—J. Paul Getty

If your business model includes employing other therapists or staff, you will have a few unique legal requirements (see Figure 10-1 ■). If you don't already have one, you will need to start by obtaining a federal Employer Identification Number (EIN) from the IRS. You will want to establish a recordkeeping system up front, as the IRS requires that you keep all employment taxes on file for four years.

Insurance
Business licenses, permits
Local, state, and federal taxes
Workers' compensation, disability and unemployment insurance
Marketing
Providing a safe, clean environment and materials necessary for service delivery.
Organizational and administrative support
Responsibilities of Employers

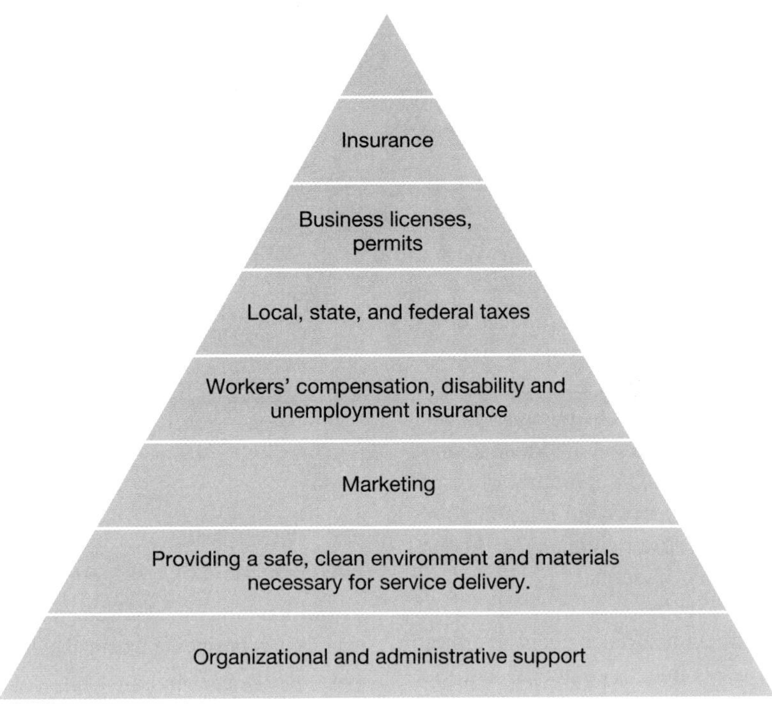

FIGURE 10-1

Employers are responsible for many things, including insurance, licenses, workers compensation and disability, taxes, and providing a safe work environment.

There are several forms you will need to be aware of as an employer. A **W-4** is an income tax withholding form, and must be filled out and signed by an employee on or before his or her date of hire. Employers in turn submit this signed form to the IRS. Employers are required to report all wages paid and all taxes withheld to the federal government each year. A **W-2** is a wage and tax statement that employers complete for each employee, sending forms to both the Social Security Administration and the employee (for his or her own income tax reporting).[17] Check with your state to see if you are responsible for withholding state income tax for your employees as well.

In addition to the W-2 and W-4, another important form for employers is the I-9. All employers are required to verify a candidates' legal right to work in the United States. The **I-9** is the federal government's form for verification of employee eligibility, and must be completed within three days of hire.[18] Employees must provide documents and identifications as specified on the I-9. Unlike the W-4, the I-9 is not submitted to the government, but rather kept on file with the employer and subject to scrutiny in the event of a workplace audit.[19]

If you are new to having employees, you will probably need to register with the New Hire Program in your state (as required by the Personal Responsibility and Work Opportunity Reconciliation Act of 1996).[20] As the employer, you will be responsible for reporting all newly hired or rehired employees within 20 days of date of hire. You will also need to have workers' compensation insurance, and some states require that you have disability insurance for all employees. Some businesses are required to register for and pay unemployment insurance tax. Check with your state's workforce agency to see if your business is responsible for unemployment insurance.

State and federal laws require all employers to prominently display various posters that inform employees of employer responsibilities and employee labor rights in full view in the workplace. And of course, you will be required to file your quarterly taxes for the business, and are responsible for reporting information on all wages subject to Medicare, Social Security, and income tax withholdings.

Because of all the myriad steps involved in employing other individuals, many business owners elect to forego employees altogether and work with independent contractors. You learned the distinction between employees and independent contractors in Chapter 2. Employers are typically not responsible for withholding income taxes, Social Security, or Medicare from independent contractors. If you plan on bringing other people into your business, but want to bring them on as contractors rather than employees, make certain you fully understand the difference in designations.

Incorrectly designating status to avoid dealing with additional hassles, tax liabilities, or additional expenses can result in penalties and consequences from the IRS.[21] Proceed cautiously in this area.

INSURANCE COVERAGE FOR YOUR BUSINESS

Return for a moment to the house metaphor introduced at the beginning of the chapter; if the structure of your business is a foundation, and all the steps to get licenses and registered are building blocks, then insurance is your business's roof, protecting it from all of the external elements. In Chapter 7, "Abundance from Within," you saw the importance of insurance for protecting your personal assets and learned about some different kinds of insurance. Your company will benefit from this same protection, and adequate coverage can literally make or break your business.

A short conversation with an insurance agent may help you understand your business's insurance needs, as those needs will vary depending on several factors including size, scope, location, legal requirements, mobility, and so forth. As you saw in the last section, local and federal laws may require you to have disability insurance, unemployment insurance, and workers' disability insurance if you have employees. Even if you are not required by law to have any kind of insurance, you will want to be sure that your business is protected from the unexpected. Failure to do so could devastate you and your business. The following is an overview of some of the types of insurance that savvy business owners have in addition to their personal coverage (Figure 10-2 ■).

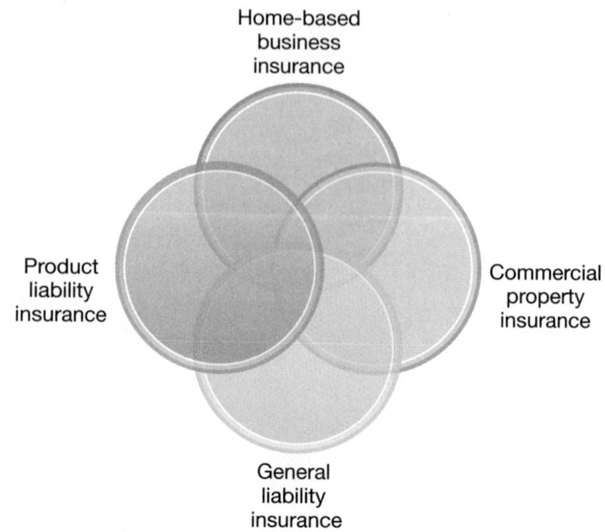

FIGURE 10-2

In addition to personal coverage and other required insurances, many smart business owners also invest in home-based business insurance, as well as commercial property, product liability, and general liability insurance.

General liability insurance: This covers expenses of bodily injury to clients, guests on your business property, or damage to property caused by business product or service. It can also cover costs of defending lawsuits. Injury done to you or your employees is typically not covered by liability insurance.[23] Many bodywork associations provide therapists with liability coverage specific to the massage industry.

Product liability insurance: This protects a business from injury claims related to the manufacture or sale of products, medicines, foods, or goods. Degree of product liability relates to where you are located, as well as your placement in the supply chain:[24] If you are creating products for resale or private use with your clients (such as scrubs, oils, or creams), you may want to invest in this type of insurance; if you are buying a mass-distributed product and using it according to specifications, you probably won't. Fortunately, many industry-specific insurance carriers include product liability.

Commercial property insurance: This covers loss and damage of company property due to events such as fire, smoke, wind, hail, vandalism, and civil disobedience. In addition to physical property (computers, building, etc.), this insurance helps recover lost income and damages due to business interruption.

Home-based business insurance: This covers home-based business losses (which are often not covered by homeowners' insurance policies). If you are operating your practice out of your home, you may need to purchase this additional coverage.

PITFALLS

According to a recent article in *Massage Today,* the vast majority of spa and wellness center owners are misclassifying their workers as independent contractors.[22] According to the article's author, most in the industry "would not pass an IRS audit." However, because the penalties for misclassification are so steep, and the IRS is getting stricter with wellness practitioners, do not make the mistake of misclassifying workers to save on tax expenses, especially when doing so could capsize your business down the road.

Fun is like life insurance; the older you get, the more it costs.

—Kin Hubbard

INSURANCE REQUIREMENTS FOR EMPLOYERS

In addition to the insurances above, you may have additional insurance needs if your business employs others.

Unemployment insurance: Unemployment insurance is a federal-state program that provides temporary income to workers who become unemployed through no fault of their own. It is jointly financed through federal and state employer payroll taxes.[25] Under certain conditions, businesses with employees are required to pay unemployment insurance tax. If your business is, you must register with your state's workforce agency.[26]

Workers' compensation: This covers the cost that the employer is responsible for in the event of injury to an employee that is hurt on the job. It also provides employee death benefits if someone is killed on the job. Workers' compensation is required by law for any business with employees.

Disability Insurance: Some states require employers to provide their eligible employees partial wage replacement coverage for sickness or injury that is not work related. At the time of writing, these states include California, Hawaii, New Jersey, New York, Rhode Island, and Puerto Rico.[27]

THE OTHER SIDE OF INSURANCE: BILLING FOR YOUR CLIENTS

With all of the scientific research behind it, massage therapy is increasingly covered by insurance companies as billable therapeutic service. Every state allows massage therapists to bill insurance companies for treatments of clients injured in automobile accidents or injured on the job (through workers' compensation insurance).[28] As with any regulation subject to change, be sure to keep tabs on the evolving insurance rules in your area.

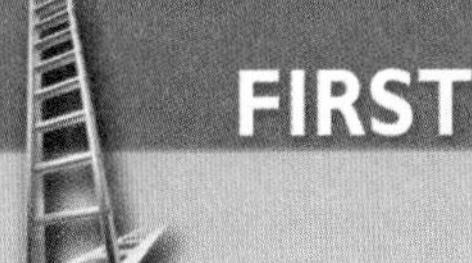

FIRST STEPS

Insurance billing can be very beneficial to some and very difficult for others. As you try and decide if this is an acceptable or appropriate payment method for your business, ask around about other therapists that bill insurance. Ask about their experiences, their successes, and their challenges with this option. If you decide to go this route, see if you can't benefit from the learning curve of others rather than recreating the insurance billing wheel.

Many therapists elect to accept insurance as an alternative payment option for services. This can be of great benefit to both client and practitioner, and can be a great advantage for a massage business. Some clients struggle to pay for massage out of pocket, and will only seek therapy from practitioners that offer the insurance billing payment option. Some practitioners report that accepting insurance has a snowball effect and has helped to grow their business into a profitable and successful venture very rapidly. However, you want to include this into your practice strategically, as there can be pitfalls and legal considerations to consider before adopting insurance billing as part of your business model.

Any massage therapist that bills for insurance will need to educate himself or herself thoroughly on state laws, insurance company policies, billing codes, and protocols. Many therapists erroneously think they can charge more for insurance clients than those paying out of pocket, but this is unethical (and in many places illegal).[29] Clients will need to obtain a diagnosis and prescription for massage therapy from a primary health care provider in order for therapists to bill their insurance. Massage therapists can not make this designation on their own, and any treatment that is billed to insurance must be associated with the stated condition.

Accepting insurance as a method of payment generally involves a good deal of paperwork. Most insurance companies will require a W-9 form from those practitioners submitting billing forms. A **W-9** is an IRS form that companies use to request a taxpayer identification number. It is typically sent to consultants, independent contractors and other self-employed workers, and provides your social security number or EIN for your business.[30] You will need to fill out the **Health Insurance Claim Form,** a standardized document for insurance billing in the United States. It is also very important to keep very good SOAP notes, both for your own records and to provide to the insurance company. As you remember from Chapter 4, SOAP notes are forms that document the work performed in therapeutic massage sessions, and allow therapists to track the subjective, objective, assessment, and plan components of each session. Insurance companies may also require that you use their specific coding, which may differ from what you have learned in school or in insurance billing seminars.

One thing to keep in mind when considering insurance billing for your business is that it can often take a very long time to be paid by insurance companies; practitioners or businesses that don't have enough additional cash flow to ride out the wait may be in trouble.[31] Make sure that you figure out a system that supports your business during times when accounts receivable may be high with insurance claims, but inflow is nonexistent for awhile. Here are a few other tips to ensure smoother sailing on the insurance sea:[32]

- *Document, document, document:* Write your SOAP notes to accurately reflect your treatment approach, and indicate client progress. Use the proper forms required by the company, and make sure to fill them out correctly.

- *Use the most current, proper codes:* The American Medical Association releases an annual manual with all known medical procedure codes. Make sure the codes you use are accepted by insurance companies.
- *Always follow doctor's prescription, and stay within your scope of practice:* Remember that it isn't your role to diagnose, and insurance will likely only cover treatments prescribed by a primary health care provider.
- *Do your homework:* Make sure that an insurance company will actually cover your treatments before providing therapy: as much as you want to help people, you don't want to end up not being paid for your valuable service.

CYBERLAW: PROTECTING YOURSELF AND YOUR BUSINESS ONLINE

Using the Internet to build and grow your business can be very rewarding and beneficial. As you will see in Chapter 15, "Leveraging the Internet," the Internet has become a valuable and powerful asset for massage businesses. Many of the steps and rules of the road for conducting business (such as truth in advertising) are the same in online businesses as they are in regular brick-and-mortar ones. However, doing business online can carry additional legal considerations, particularly in the area of privacy, security, copyright, and taxation. You will learn more about online security, privacy, copyright, and other legal considerations in Chapter 15. In the meantime, it is important to preview a few legal considerations with using the Internet to promote, build, and conduct your business. Even if you are not planning on selling anything online, e-commerce laws relating to copyright and online marketing still apply to you. A number of legislative initiatives regulate and affect all business conducted online, and the rules can be complicated and change quickly, just like the online world itself.

Earlier in the chapter you learned how to research name availability for your business. You will want to do the same thing to research your domain name availability, and will ideally be able to find a domain name that not only mirrors your business name but does not infringe on anyone else's trademark. As more and more businesses are moving online, cybersquatting has become an issue. **Cybersquatting** is the act of registering or using a domain in bad faith, with the sole intention of profiting from someone else's trademark or brand recognition. This can be with the intention of selling a domain for profit, or to generate business by piggy-backing off of another domain's popularity. The **Anticybersquatting Consumer Protection Act** of 1999 makes this activity illegal.[33] This is important to know in order to protect your own trademark from others, as well as to avoid unintentionally (or intentionally) cybersquatting on someone else's mark.

If you plan on doing any e-mail marketing, such as promotional notices or e-newsletters, you will want to be aware of the legal parameters. The **CAN-SPAM Act** of 2003 is a law that regulates commercial e-mail in the United States and aims to protect recipients from unwanted and unsolicited e-mail. An acronym for *Controlling the Assault of Non-Solicited Pornography and Marketing Act,* CAN-SPAM basically mandates that all e-mail messages must offer a method for recipients to unsubscribe (opt out of the mailing list) and contain the sender's valid physical postal address.[34] An important thing to remember is that you can only carry out unsolicited electronic marketing to a person who has given you their permission to be on your subscriber list, whether by opting in electronically or doing a "soft opt-in" (i.e., giving your business card or filling out a client intake form). Note that some autoresponder services will only allow you to send messages to individuals who have opted in to your list electronically.

The Internet can be a great way to boost your business, and an exciting way to help it grow. Always safeguard the privacy and information of your clients, follow the rules, and use common sense when conducting your business online.

Congratulations, you legal guru you! You have just worked through a lot of weighty and substantial legal information! You've learned how to structure your business optimally, how to protect it from the unexpected, and how to navigate the regulations and rules to ensure your business not only survives, but thrives. Continue to keep aware of laws and stay in line with what is expected of you as a business owner, and you will always be in a great position to build the best business possible!

PUT IT IN WRITING

Legal Trouble

Have you ever known anyone who has run into legal problems or challenges with their business? Maybe you know someone who received a cease and desist letter for using a trademarked domain name, or perhaps someone who got into trouble with the IRS? Write about some examples of others' challenges, and things you will do differently in your own business.

____

____

____

____

____

CHAPTER SUMMARY BY LEARNING OBJECTIVES

1. **Explain the importance of following legal protocols when starting a business** The United States has a fairly litigious (quick to take legal action) culture, and you want to protect both yourself and your business. It is important to follow the rules and established laws when setting up any business; this will not only help you avoid trouble down the line, but will help you and your business be viable parts of your community. Some of the basic steps to registering your business include: 1) Determining the legal structure of your business; 2) Registering your business name; 3) Establishing your tax obligations and obtaining your federal tax ID number; 4) Registering with your state revenue agency; and 5) Acquiring all necessary licenses and permits.
2. **Identify different legal structures for your business** Legal structures differ in terms of financial, tax, and legal responsibilities, and many factors go into selecting the appropriate structure for each business. The most common types include sole proprietorship and limited liability companies. Businesses with larger-scale operations often incorporate into S corporations and C corporations.
3. **Demonstrate the value of a business name** The name you choose for your business is a very important decision and can impact your success going forward. A successful business name conveys your business's purpose, and inspires clients to learn more about what you have to offer them. Your business name can affect how easily you are remembered, or how easily you are found online or in directories. When choosing a business name, make sure that it is available and not violating anyone else's registered trademark or trade name.
4. **Provide an overview of business taxes** The type of taxes you will have to pay for your business will depend on many factors, such as what legal structure you choose, whether you are employing people, and if you are selling tangible items. Tax law is the same for everyone—no one is immune from paying taxes. While some techniques legally allow you to avoid some taxes, tax evasion is illegal. Many small businesses must file taxes quarterly.
5. **Provide an overview of permits, licenses, and legal requirements for small businesses** After filing for taxes, the next step in getting your business on board is making sure that you have obtained all local and state licenses and permits. There are typically licenses and permits you must obtain in order to carry out any business, regardless of industry. Check with your local authorities to see what occupational and operational licenses and permits you will need for your business.
6. **Explain responsibilities as an employer** If your business model includes employing other therapists or staff, you will have a few special legal requirements. If you don't already have one, you will need to start by obtaining a federal Employer Identification Number (EIN) from the IRS. You will want to establish a recordkeeping system up front, as the IRS requires that you keep all employment taxes on file for four years. You will be responsible for completing and filing forms such as the I-9, W-2, and W-4. You will also have to be aware of regulations on workers' compensation, unemployment, work place safety, and so forth.
7. **Investigate insurance coverage for your practice** Insurance helps protect your business from the unexpected, and adequate coverage can literally make or break your business. Insurance needs vary depending on several factors including size, scope, location, city requirements, mobility, and so forth. Insurance products such as general liability, commercial property insurance, and employer-specific insurance can be essential for your business.
8. **Examine the elements of insurance billing for your clients** Any massage therapist billing for insurance will need to educate themselves thoroughly on state laws, company policies, billing codes, and protocols. Most insurance companies will require form W 9, Health Insurance Claim Forms, and session SOAP notes. Following certain steps can minimize hassles and expedite payment from insurance companies.
9. **Analyze legal considerations of bringing your business online** Many of the steps and rules of the road for conducting business online (such as truth in advertising) are the same in online businesses as they are in regular brick and mortar ones. However, doing business online can carry additional legal considerations, particularly in the area of privacy, security, copyright, and taxation.

ACTIVITIES

Quiz: Identifying Organizing and Legal Structuring Words and Concepts

1. Mary knows that she wants to organize her business as a corporation, but does not want to be subject to "double taxation." What other type of organization might she apply for?
   a. sole proprietorship
   b. S corporation
   c. C corporation
   d. 401c-3
2. Denali loves to create her own all-natural oils and body scrubs for client treatments. One day a new client calls to tell Denali that he broke out in hives after her treatment and had to go to a doctor. In the event that that client decides to sue, what kind of insurance coverage do we hope that Denali has?
   a. Product liability insurance
   b. Flood insurance
   c. Workers' compensation
   d. Malpractice
3. Petra is trying to decide on a name for her new business, and really admires one of her very popular competitors, Siren Spa. She decides to call her company "Siren's Spa." What might she be violating?
   a. ethics
   b. code of competition
   c. the speed limit
   d. trademark and trade name laws
4. Not only does Petra decide to name her business Siren's Spa, but she purchases the domain name "sirensspa." Not only does this direct more traffic to her site from people looking for her competitor and bring her more business, she also hopes that the original Siren Spa might offer her some money for the domain she has purchased. What is this an example of?
   a. good business conduct
   b. cyberstalking
   c. cybersquatting
   d. trademark violation
   e. both c and d
5. Which of the following is *NOT* one of the first steps of getting your business legally organized and operational?
   a. determining the legal structure of the business
   b. acquiring all necessary licenses and permits
   c. creating your succession plan and exit strategy
   d. registering your business name
   e. registering with the state revenue agency
6. Which act protects individuals from unwanted and unsolicited e-mails?
   a. Children's Online Privacy Protection Act (COPPA)
   b. Truth in Lending Act
   c. Controlling the Assault of Non-Solicited Pornography And Marketing Act (CAN-SPAM)
   d. Electronic Signatures in Global and National Commerce Act (ESGNC)
7. A/an _____ is used to identify a business entity, and is also known as the Federal Tax Identification Number.
   a. Employer Identification Number (EIN)
   b. Tracking device
   c. Employer pin
   d. Employer Identification Badge
8. The Internal Revenue Service requires that employers keep all employment taxes on file for _____ years.
   a. 2
   b. 10
   c. 4
   d. 25
9. As a massage business owner with employees, it is important (and often required) that you have
   a. workers' compensation insurance
   b. unemployment insurance
   c. disability coverage
   d. all of the above
10. A _____ is any expense that the government allows individuals and businesses to subtract from gross income, lessening the amount taxed.
    a. judgment
    b. deduction
    c. contribution
    d. payment

Discussion Questions

1. When you think about creating a name for your business, what factors are the most important to you? Creativity? Catchiness? Inherent meaning? Why do you think some names make a business successful, while others can be a liability? Can you think of examples on either side?
2. Many massage therapists report aversion to some of the concepts in this chapter, such as legal organization, taxes, and insurance. Why do you think this is? What sort of issues (if any) come up for you when you consider these aspects of running a business?

Case Study

Robert and Jackie

Robert and Jackie are both successful massage therapists who have known one another for several years. After a long conversation about their mutual goals, their complementary strengths and weaknesses, and their vision for a shared business, they decide to become partners in a new massage business venture. Unwilling to jeopardize their friendship and mutual respect, they draft a contract that clearly spells out one another's roles and responsibilities in the new endeavor. They also draft a contingency plan should either partner decide to leave the business or be unable to continue in the partnership for reasons such as illness and death.

While Robert is taking the lead on filing all the paperwork to organize their partnership, Jackie begins to do the research and to take the steps to file their business name. After a search in the U.S. Trademark Database, she finds that the name they have chosen, Wellspring Massage, does not have a trademark on it and they are free to use it. Robert and Jackie do not file their own trademark on the name, knowing that the process can be long and costly, and figuring that they will go down that road when their business takes off. Instead, they just register their name with their Secretary of State, where it is also available. Jackie purchases an available domain name that works with their business name.

With all the pieces in place, Robert and Jackie start looking at their tax structuring. They know that they want to bring other people in to provide massages for the business's clients, and will need to bring in people who will wear the Wellspring uniform and comply with the structured work schedule. They are also planning on offering new hires training, in part to regulate operations and in part to intentionally craft a culture within the company. Feeling a little overwhelmed at all that is required to hire employees, they decide to classify their workers as independent contractors for tax purposes. They both feel relieved to be passing on a lot of the expense and hassle to the contractors.

They register with their state revenue agency and begin to acquire their necessary licenses and permits. They are disappointed when the city tells them they will need to petition for a special-use permit due to zoning laws, a process that will take much longer and cost much more than they anticipated. As a result, their grand opening will be delayed. To recover the expenses, they have to restructure their pricing model slightly. They also decide to forego some of the insurance that their agent recommends they get, deciding that it is just too costly to do it all and that they probably won't need it anyway.

Finally, after all their permits are in place and all their organizing, structuring, and paperwork are in line, Jackie and Robert excitedly begin preparing for their grand opening. They buy a list of geographically targeted e-mail contacts and start sending out massive blasts to everyone in the area, announcing their arrival in the neighborhood and offering promotional specials. They store all of these contacts in their database, planning to send regular e-mails in the future. They do not include any information about opting out in their e-mails.

It is around this time that Jackie and Robert hear about you, a holistic business consultant, and ask you for your input on their process. You listen patiently to their story.

Case Study Questions

1. What do you think about the way Jackie and Robert came to form their partnership? Do you think they made good choices? Was there anything you might have done differently?
2. How likely do you think it is that a company name would be available with the Secretary of State, the Federal Trademark database, and still have an available domain name? Do you think many companies have so much luck, or do you think they have to go through several names before finding a match? What has been your experience?
3. Do you think Robert and Jackie should wait to file their own trademark application for their business? Do a little research for them and find out the requirements for a suitable trademark, as well as the steps to go through the process with the U.S. Patent and Trademark Office.
4. What do you think of Robert and Jackie's decision on worker classification? Do you foresee any problems that you should share with them? Can you offer them alternative solutions?
5. Robert and Jackie hit some snags with permits that ended up costing them time and money and delayed their grand opening. Do you think this is common when opening a business? Do you think there is anything they might have done instead that would have saved them time and money?
6. What can you tell Robert and Jackie about their decision to purchase an e-mail list for their e-mail marketing campaign? What is your advice for their future campaigns?

CHAPTER 11

Marketing Fundamentals

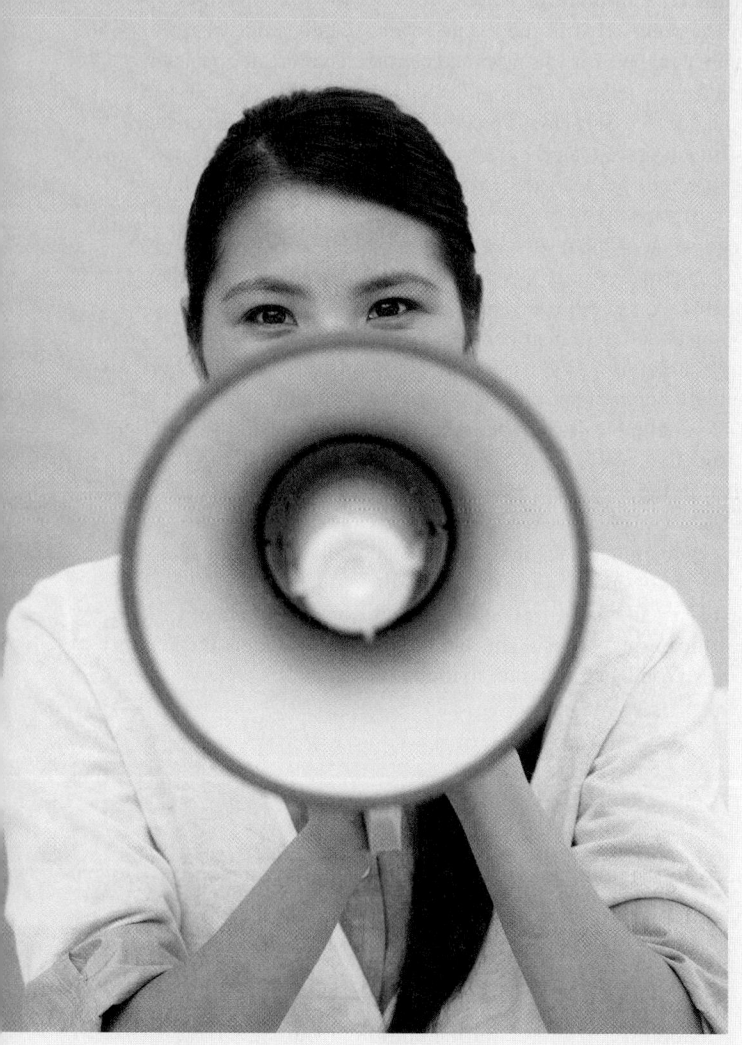

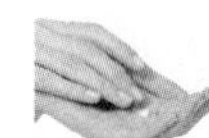

CHAPTER OUTLINE

LEARNING OBJECTIVES

1. Define marketing
2. Explain the marketing mix and define the "four Ps" of marketing
3. Define product and placement, and explain how to structure price
4. Explore the various components of promotion, and learn how to leverage customer service as a marketing strategy
5. Explain the purpose and makeup of a marketing plan
6. Write a mission statement
7. Examine trends in the massage industry
8. Identify a target market
9. Describe a company analysis and identify and assess competition
10. Define and explore a SWOT analysis
11. Introduce implementation tactics to help achieve marketing goals

KEY TERMS

advertising *178*
budget *183*
community relations *180*
company analysis *183*
company culture *184*
competitive analysis *185*
competitive edge *185*
consistency *172*
customer service *178*
differential pricing *175*
discounting *175*
executive summary *181*
implementation tactics *185*
industry analysis *182*
marketing *172*
marketing mix (the four Ps of marketing) *173*
marketing plan *180*
mission statement *181*
placement *173*
premium pricing *175*
price *173*
product *173*
promotion *175*
public relations *178*
publicity *180*
SWOT analysis *185*
target market *183*
value-added *175*
word of mouth *178*

MARKETING

Marketing is not only much broader than selling; it is not a specialized activity at all. It encompasses the entire business.

—Peter Drucker

The word "marketing" is used a lot in business, but it is not necessarily understood by those using it. **Marketing** refers to any activity that serves to let your market know about you, attract customers to your product or service, and keep them coming back for more. Marketing is how you match your capabilities to the needs of your potential and actual customers. Virtually everything you do to endorse your massage practice can be construed as a part of marketing—how you design your practice space, the business card you hand to people, the way you communicate, your website—anything and everything that promotes an image. In day-to-day interactions, people are constantly leaving an impression upon one another. Thus, it is important that you are consistent with all of your interactions. **Consistency** is the foundation of successful marketing. With your marketing materials, you will want to keep things looking the same. With your actions, you will want to do what you say you are going to every time.[1]

Although marketing encapsulates all that you do for your practice, there are specific marketing techniques that will help you and your practice stand out. The best massage skills in the world will not help you if people do not know about you, and marketing bridges that gap.

In this fast-paced, media-rich society, everyone is constantly bombarded with marketing messages. Consumers are exposed to endless commercial messages, which come in many forms: radio ads, TV ads, newspaper ads, billboard ads, ads in the mail, ads at sporting events, product placement in movies, and so forth. Advertising in the United States is a multi-billion dollar industry;[2] getting consumer attention is big business. Expert estimates vary, but general wisdom holds that the average North American is exposed to between 1500 and 16,000 marketing messages *daily*.[3] So how are you going to get the message about you and your wonderful massage business out there amidst all that noise? Let's start by looking at how others are getting their message about their products and services through to you; complete the "Put it in Writing" exercise below to see what has worked on you.

PITFALLS

Marketing is an ongoing part of any successful practice. Many people put a great deal of energy into marketing up front, and get discouraged when they don't see immediate results from their efforts. Client response is not an exact science—one massage therapist reported that some clients have called him *three years* after receiving his business card. It can take time to build a clientele, and steady efforts to keep it flourishing. Do not get discouraged if results are not always immediate.

You are a skilled professional with superlative hands-on skills. You care about your clients and trust in your ability to make a difference in the lives of those you work with. But before any of that happens, you need to develop and hone your massage marketing skills so that the community can benefit from your work. Putting together an effective marketing blueprint and program is one of the most important components in a strong and successful practice.

Before you start to worry that you will have to sell out your beliefs to become a master manipulator or perfect every sophisticated marketing technique, relax. The great thing about marketing your own massage business is that you get to be 100 percent yourself. You get to pick and choose the methods

PUT IT IN WRITING

Memorable Marketing

If the average person receives so many messages, how many does she remember in particular? Take a moment to think about what marketing messages you have seen or heard today: do any logos, brand names, or brand slogans pop into your mind? Write five of them down.

1. ______________________
2. ______________________
3. ______________________
4. ______________________
5. ______________________

Of all the messages to which you were likely exposed, why did those five stand out for you? Was it the use of humor? The quality you associate with the product or service? The fact that you've seen that ad so many times? Write down some of the reasons you think you remembered those five.

1. ______________________
2. ______________________
3. ______________________
4. ______________________
5. ______________________

PITFALLS

One of the attractions of a career in massage therapy is its seeming divergence from the "corporate" or "standard" business world. Though you are first and foremost a therapist, many practitioners fail to consider the sales involved in a successful career and ignore marketing altogether. Keep in mind that while it may be a wonderful holistic business, it is still a business!

and messages you send out to convey your personality, your integrity, your values, and what you truly have to offer. At its essence, marketing strives to create an experience for customers, one that you consistently convey through every point of contact individuals have with you—your business card, your voice mail message, your brochure, your website, your consistent professionalism, and of course, your massage service itself. Think of marketing as a creative way to tell the story of you and the glory of massage to the public.

THE MARKETING MIX

Marketing is not one single thing, but rather an umbrella term that combines four marketing activities known as the **marketing mix.** The marketing mix includes product, placement, price, and promotion, and is also known as the *four Ps of marketing* (Figure 11-1 ■). The **product** refers to the good or service being marketed, which of course is massage in this case. It can also specify any classes, additional services, or retail products you may sell in your business; examples of retail include aromatherapy oils, vitamin supplements, bath and body products, and so forth.

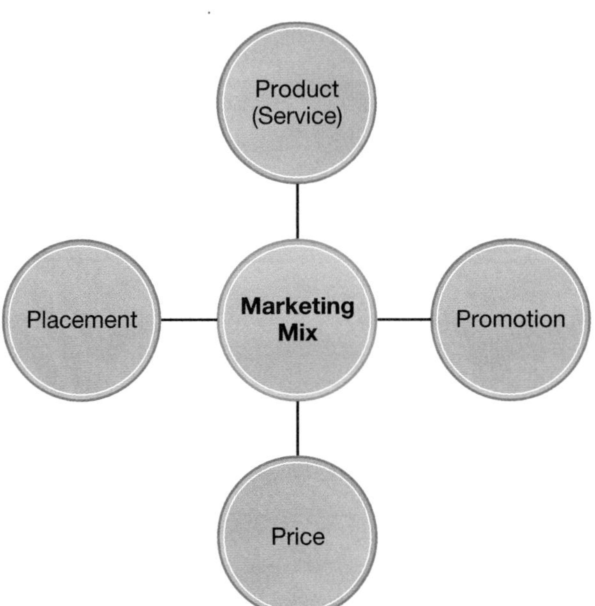

FIGURE 11-1

Your marketing mix includes your product (service), price, promotion, and placement.

Placement refers to the location where a product or service can be purchased, and is often referred to as a "distribution channel" in marketing parlance. As a massage therapist, your placement will be wherever you perform your massages: in your office, at a client's home, at a clinic, at a resort, and so forth.

> *Most folks are motivated a lot more by a pressing problem or fear of loss than by the chance for gain. Make your marketing explore the customer's frustration and pain. Have your product or service be the cure.*
>
> —Kevin Nunley

Price is the amount a customer pays for a product or service. It is another important ingredient in your marketing mix, and one that should not be arbitrarily chosen. As a massage therapist, it can be very difficult to put a price on your service. It can be an emotional issue to claim that the time and energy you put forth during a massage is quantifiable. It can also be hard to put a number on the consistent value you are creating for clients, as their needs and response to treatment may change. However, to be fair to your clients and yourself, prices should be consistent. A number of factors go into properly determining your price structure:

- material costs
- rent expense
- staying competitive within your market
- how much your clients can and will pay (clients' perceived value)
- how much you think your work is worth (your perceived value)
- length of session
- work location (office, home, corporate setting)
- ethical considerations
- your financial goals
- value added for client
- therapist education and experience

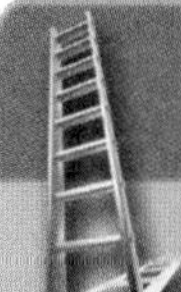

FIRST STEPS

One of the best ways to create a reasonable price structure is to look at what other therapists are charging in your area. Call around or go into the offices of your competition. What is the range of prices being charged by others doing comparable work to your own? If you were to charge a similar price, could you cover your expenses and meet your financial goals?

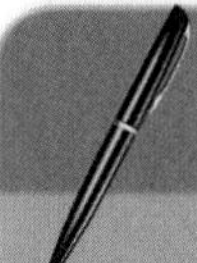

PUT IT IN WRITING

What's It Worth to You?

What am I willing to pay for massage? While there are many factors that go into structuring price, as listed above, you can't expect clients to value your services more than you yourself do. Figure 11-2 ■ can help you get an idea of your own price points when receiving a massage, and can help you identify appropriate ranges for your own price structure. Fill in the boxes with the different amounts that you would pay for each of the listed services in different contexts. This may be based on your experience paying for massage in the past or solely upon your financial expectations and limitations. When you finish, look back on your answers. Based on what you would pay, what do you think others would be willing to pay you?

	Therapist's Office	**Home Visit**	**Medical Clinic**	**Day Spa Setting**	**Discount Massage Chain**
The therapist just graduated from massage school					
You received a referral for the therapist from a close friend					
Therapist has been practicing for seven years; you got his name from phone book					
Read article about therapist in favorite magazine					
You just lost your job but really need a massage					

FIGURE 11-2

As you set your price structure, it can be helpful to evaluate how you value different services in different locations, while many factors effect effective pricing, it is helpful to explore your own perceptions and relationship to value and price.

PITFALLS

A word of caution on differential pricing; it is not always wise to charge different customers different prices for the same service. In order for this kind of selective pricing to work, different customer groups (i.e., students, retirees, military personnel) must be selected on justifiable criteria (i.e., fixed incomes). In addition, customers paying the full price might feel slighted or unfairly charged if they find out from someone else that others are getting a better deal. In order to avoid sticky situations and to be fair to all your clients, you might make mention of your discounts in your marketing literature.[4]

TABLE 11-1 Sample Service Menu

Service	Price
60-minute massage	$65
90-minute massage	$80
Ayurvedic herbs included in massage oil	$+10
Hot stones included in massage	$+20
Aromatherapy add-on	$+15
30-minute Reiki session	$+25
Exclusive package (includes 60-minute massage, hot stones)	$80
Royal package (includes 60-minute massage, Ayurvedic herbs, hot stones, aromatherapy)	$100
Luxury package (includes 90-minute massage, hot stones, aromatherapy, Reiki session)	$125

Even with a standard price in place, it is standard business practice to offer occasional discounts or differential pricing on your services. **Discounting** refers to temporarily reducing the set price for a good or service as an incentive for purchase. For example, you may offer all your clients a 10 percent discount if they buy a package of five massages at once. Or you may send out a flier or e-mail campaign advertising a $20 discount for all Valentine's Day gift certificates. **Differential pricing,** or discriminatory pricing, occurs when different classes of customers are charged different rates. This sounds much more unethical than it actually is; senior and student discounts at the movie theaters are examples of differential pricing.

On the other side of the pricing decision spectrum is premium pricing. Also known as prestige pricing, **premium pricing** occurs when prices are set above those of the competitors to enhance the perceived value of the service and attract luxury-seeking clients.[5] This is often the case when one pays for a massage on a cruise or an elite day spa. Some clients believe that higher prices indicate better quality. You may also find that temporary premiums are necessary for practical reasons; for example, you may have different prices for a massage in your office during your set hours and for an outcall massage at a client's home after normal business hours.

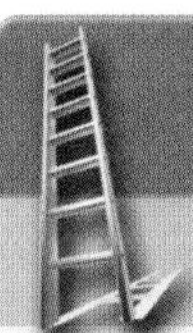

FIRST STEPS

Type "massage discount (your city)" or "massage specials (your city)" into your favorite search engine. What comes up? Take a look at what discounts are being offered by other therapists in the area. Why are they being offered? First time clients? Holiday specials? Package deals?

Many therapists include **value-added** services into their service menu to substantiate their premium pricing. Offering a client a free product sample or an add-on of a service such as hot stones generates a perceived value for the customers that may be more valuable to them than a discount.[6] And often, the initial investment for value-added services such as paraffin wax or aromatherapy treatment is quickly returned by the revenue they generate.[7] Customers are often more likely to pay for such perceived value at a premium. Incorporating lymphatic drainage, reflexology, energy work, Raindrop therapy®, or craniosacral treatments into your repertoire are all examples of value-added services (see Table 11-1 ■).

Take a moment to observe the price effect with package deals. Clients enjoy a greater discount the more expensive the package becomes. As a client adds on more services, notice how the premium pricing is happening even while the illusion of discounting occurs. A client may be saving money by bundling services, but a therapist is making more than they would by just offering 60- or 90-minute massages, without expending much more energy. The benefit of value-added services is that they can generate more revenue without doing much more work. They can also boost your competitive edge by offering clients choices and added benefits.[8] Just make certain that you choose value-added services that resonate with you and are aligned with your overarching practice.

GOT PROMOTION?

The final P in your marketing mix refers to **promotion,** or the communication you put into the market about your goods and/or service. Essentially, promotion is how you get the word out about you, your service, and the other three Ps in the marketing mix. Elements of promotion include customer service, word of mouth, advertising, public relations, and publicity.

PITFALLS

In many major cities, online discounters such as Groupon and LivingSocial have gained a huge following by featuring large discounts of 50% at various local businesses. Often marketed to business owners as a great marketing opportunity, these sites will often target massage therapy businesses. While it's true that you may get a lot of people in the door this way, be aware of the limitations of this business model. First of all, you will only be paid a percentage of the sale price, which means you could make as little as 20% of your regular price. If you are a solo practitioner, this could burn you out very quickly if a lot of discounts are sold. In addition, many people who purchase these coupons are out for deals only, and will not be back for another service at regular prices. If you participate, do so knowingly!

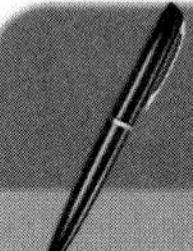

PUT IT IN WRITING

What's Your Price Point?

While many factors will go into setting your price point (such as the going rate in your area and the quality of service), it is very important that you set a rate that you are comfortable with and that reflects your values and goals. In order to do this, it is important to understand your own relationship to cost, value, and charging others. As a consumer, do you gravitate towards discounts or premiums? Take this quiz to uncover some of your thoughts.

1. When I go shopping:
   a. I splurge on the highest fashion, the most gourmet foods, and the most posh things. I'm worth every penny.
   b. I always look for sales. I won't buy anything that's not on a discount.
   c. If I need something, the cost really doesn't matter.
   d. I'd prefer to buy things on sale, but I'll spend more if I think I'm getting a good value.
2. When I spend a lot of money on something:
   a. I feel guilty and like I wasted my money.
   b. I feel like the product or service is more valuable. I only spend my money on high-ticket items.
   c. I know it was a rare event, but worth it.
   d. Who cares? It's just money.
3. When I am considering buying something:
   a. I don't waste time shopping around. I buy the first thing I see, regardless of the cost.
   b. I spend hours doing consumer research. I'm looking for a good price, but if I believe I'm getting the best value, I'll spend more for it.
   c. I shop only on price—whatever store is selling it for the lowest price, that's where I'm buying.
   d. I buy the most expensive thing. That way I know I'm getting the best value.
4. When someone gives me a discount on a service:
   a. I'm delighted, and will definitely be back as long as they keep giving me the deal.
   b. I obviously don't think they value their service very much.
   c. I'm pretty happy to save money, though I'll be back when the price returns to normal.
   d. I just tip them the difference. It's all the same to me.
5. If I'm getting a massage, I will likely go to:
   a. Whomever I like. The price doesn't matter.
   b. Normally I would go to someone I can afford, but every now and then I might splurge and go to a luxury spa or buy myself a more luxurious service than usual.
   c. The most exclusive spa in town. Hey, if they're charging that much, it must be worth it, right?
   d. The cheapest place I can find. A massage is a massage is a massage, but price is most important to me.

Scoring Guide

Now that you've completed the quiz, go back and score it.

1) a = 4 b = 1 c = 3 d = 2 4) a = 1 b = 4 c = 2 d = 3
2) a = 1 b = 4 c = 2 d = 3 5) a = 3 b = 2 c = 4 d = 1
3) a = 3 b = 2 c = 1 d = 4

Now add up your scores:

17–20: The Epicure. You always want the finest, and believe that price is the best indicator of the worth of a good or service. You expect to pay more for value, and you will probably feel comfortable charging higher prices for your services.

13–16: The Fiscally Abstracted. You do not spend much time evaluating the relationship between money and value. This will help you be flexible and adaptive with your pricing structure. Just make sure the lackadaisical attitude is not a way of avoiding underlying issues.

8–12: The Financial Libra. You are constantly measuring the monetary scales. Though you appreciate a low price, you often equate value with higher prices. You may feel comfortable charging less than some competitors, but will up-sell your value-added services (see below).

5–7: Pleasantly Parsimonious. Value and price are aligned for you; the lower the price, the more the value you perceive as a consumer. As a therapist, you may be more comfortable pricing your services lower along the accepted range. In addition, you may offer discounts or discriminatory pricing to entice price-sensitive clients like yourself.

Regardless of where you score, go back through the quiz and examine your answers. Are there any areas that concern you about your relationship to price and value? Can you foresee how your answers might be a benefit or a challenge to your practice? Keep in mind that you will have to balance internal feelings with external conditions, such as going rate in your market, skill level, and competition.

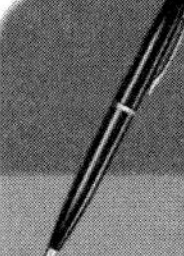

PUT IT IN WRITING

Show Me the Value for My Money!

In the space that follows, brainstorm some ideas for value-added services that you might like to incorporate into your massage practice. Maybe you have experienced something nice in a treatment you have received. Maybe there is something you have always wanted to try. After you think of some ideas, jot down what you would pay for each service. Then write what you think someone else might be willing to pay. Do not worry if the numbers are different; look at the difference, then ask yourself what you would be comfortable charging.

Service	What I would pay	What clients might pay
______	______________	______________
______	______________	______________
______	______________	______________
______	______________	______________
______	______________	______________
______	______________	______________
______	______________	______________
______	______________	______________
______	______________	______________
______	______________	______________

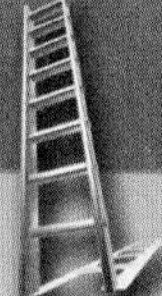

FIRST STEPS

Developing Your Own Customer Service Strategy

Regardless of the form your career takes (employee, contractor, private practitioner, business owner), it is very important that you develop and hone a great customer service strategy. Complete the following statements, then look at some common customer service tips that follow. It might prove useful to store your responses in your *Business of Massage Therapy* notebook so you can brush up on your customer service plan from time to time.

1. To me, great customer service is ____________________.
2. When I think of an instance where someone went above and beyond for me as a customer, I think of ____.
3. When I had that positive experience, I felt ______________________________ about the company.
4. When I think of an instance where someone treated me very rudely as a customer, I think of ________________.
5. When I had that negative experience, I felt ______________________________. about the company.
6. My approach to customer service has typically been ____.
7. In the past when I have had to deal with a difficult customer, I have handled the situation by ____.
8. When I think of great customer service as a massage therapist, the three most important things are ____.

Common Tips for Great Customer Service

While your approach to customer service will reflect your unique personality and values, the following are common tips for great customer service. Read through the list, and then brainstorm a few of your own ideas.

- Always employ the Golden Rule, treating clients the way you want to be treated as a consumer.
- If you have employees, hire people who can deliver great customer service naturally and provide training on your specific brand of customer service. Make expectations clear.
- If you have employees, empower them to make customer service decisions. This could mean encouraging your people to develop strong therapeutic relationships with your client base, or allowing them to provide discounts, refunds, or free products.
- Solicit feedback from your clients and be prepared to take action or make changes based on the responses.
- Have a clear idea of the wants and needs of your target market, and seek to solve their problems.
- Sharpen your listening skills so you can custom-tailor each experience to the clients' needs and wants.
- Be prompt in communication with clients. Even if you can't answer every incoming phone call, stay on top of voice mails, e-mails, and other forms of contact. Don't make clients wait for a response from you.

Brainstorm a few more ideas about great customer service and write them out here.

____
____
____
____
____
____

Do what you do so well that they will want to see it again and again—and bring their friends.

—Walt Disney

Due to the hands-on and personal nature of the business, customer service is one of the most important elements of marketing for massage. **Customer service** refers to the client care activities, both material and intangible, that support the delivery of a business's core product or service. Customer service also helps to build loyalty by meeting and exceeding client expectations. At its root, business is really about the management of relationships, and just about nothing helps foster client relationships better than exceptional customer service. This can include providing consistently excellent massage, as well as anticipating client needs and delivering above them. Even following up with helpful information, sending birthday discounts, and providing confirmation calls are part of a good customer service strategy (see Chapters 3 and 14 for more information on minimizing no-shows through cancellation policies and confirmation calls).

If you do build a great experience, customers tell each other about that. Word of mouth is very powerful.

—Jeff Bezos, founder of Amazon.com

The better and more polished your customer service, the faster you can benefit from word of mouth. **Word of mouth** refers to informal communications by those who have experienced your massage, including recommendations and referrals that clients make on your behalf. Word of mouth marketing is also known by its other aliases: viral marketing, grassroots, buzz marketing, product seeding, and referral programs.[9] Estimates show that a satisfied customer will tell three people about a product or service that he likes,[10] leading to the old adage that your best salesperson is a satisfied customer. With enough contented clients, your business can quickly grow exponentially and lead to a lucrative practice. Word of mouth marketing can be incredibly effective and a cornerstone of any good business. But be careful! While a happy customer will tell three people, the flip side of word of mouth is that a dissatisfied customer will tell *eleven* people about a product or service that he does not like.[11] And since people can be dissatisfied for any number of reasons (no matter how wonderful you are), and there is very little control you can exercise about what others say,[12] it will be important for you to take proactive measures to promote yourself as well. Word of mouth can definitely be a great marketing mechanism, but make sure you have other tools in your toolbox! And ultimately, the best mouth out there to promote your practice and get your business booming is your own.

There are several other promotion techniques to choose from. Advertising, public relations, and publicity are all facets of promotion. Advertising is often one of the most prominent components of promotion for small companies. Often erroneously confused with or used interchangeably with marketing, **advertising** is the way in which you get your marketing message out into the world. Remember, *marketing* refers to the collection of activities that you systematically perform in order to promote your business; *advertising* is just one ingredient in the four Ps of the marketing mix. Advertising is the public paid promotion of your good or service, and there are several different advertising media available from which to choose. Advertisements for massage can be found in magazines, online, in newspapers, on radio, and even on television. Look for them in phone books, at bus stops, on grocery carts, and in your mail box.

PITFALLS

Many people starting out in business often believe that the only way to get clients in the door is to spend a lot of money on advertising. This is not necessarily the case. Expensive ads do not guarantee a larger volume of clients or huge profits. Many new therapists go broke trying to place glossy ads in high-end magazines, and are very discouraged when the phone never rings.

The average consumer needs to hear or see an ad *seven* times before a buying decision is influenced.[13] It will be very difficult, if not impossible, to reach your target customers that many times with high-cost advertisements, particularly when you are just starting your practice. Do not make the mistake of believing that spending more will earn you more. For low-cost/no-cost tips, see the end of this chapter.

Creating effective marketing materials can be somewhat time consuming, but remember that your promotional pieces can be your first point of contact with potential customers. They will establish your image, and it is important that they be professional, somewhat sophisticated, and aligned with the image you want to project to the world. Unless you have a background in marketing or graphic design, you may want to consider getting some help preparing your marketing materials or use prepared promotional pieces. If you feel very confident in your ability to make an affordable and eye-catching advertisement, by all means do so, but don't feel bad if you need a little help.

Public relations refers to how you as a practitioner project yourself and interact with the community around you. Anything you do to promote interest in your products/services and promote a favorable impression of yourself and your business is public relations. Public relations are aimed less at directly boosting sales, and more at promoting your overall image within your community.

For massage therapists, community relations can be an effective and fruitful aspect of public relations.

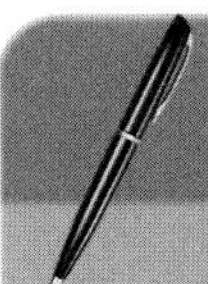

PUT IT IN WRITING

Different Ads, Different Markets

To help you brainstorm about creating an ad for your massage business, try this exercise. See if you can come up with an ad for the products and services in Table 11-2 ■, none of which are massage related. The idea is just to get your creativity flowing. Imagine you have been chosen as the advertising executive for these products' accounts. Pick *two*, and read their product/service description. Start by thinking of your target market (see the description of target markets later in this chapter). In the space provided, write out any descriptive words that you think could or should be included with a magazine advertisement to help sell your product or service. Next, with words or images, include the kinds of visuals that would be useful for an ad to compel readers to purchase your product or service.

Product/Service 1 descriptive words:

____

____

____

____

Product/Service 1 images:

Product/Service 2 descriptive words:

____

____

____

____

Product/Service 2 images:

Bonus: See if you can find some actual ads for product/services similar to those you chose. What were the similarities and differences from your ad?

TABLE 11-2 Different Ads for Different Markets

Pet Drinks Flavored Water. Delicious flavors specially designed for your dog or cat, with the added vitamins and nutrients they need.	**Evergreen Resort.** With 140 trails and 8 months of fresh powder, we've been entertaining winter sports enthusiasts for over 50 years.	**The Habit Breaking Pen.** This pen has no discernable smell, but releases a terrible taste whenever one puts it in the mouth.	**Travel Buddy.** I speak over 10 languages and have traveled with people who don't want to trek alone for over 15 years.
Beer with a Cause. 30% of the proceeds of this new beer line, which includes both lager and ale, go to a local charity.	**Art to Your Door.** Not everyone can afford to own art, so why not rent it like a movie? Go online now to start your subscription to some of the best original art around.	**Salad Gum.** This gum has all the vitamins and nutrients of a full salad, without actually having to eat one.	**Dance Lessons.** Specializing in tango, salsa, and merengue, we are a married couple who have been teaching dance for over 20 years.
Green Wedding Planner. With over 100 green weddings planned, I can help you create that special day and do something good for the planet.	**Bad Breath Detector.** When you want to be sure, measure the state of your breath with this halitosis detector. Has experienced 95% accuracy in trial tests.	**Concrete Furniture.** The latest in upscale home furnishing, our coveted concrete furniture is long lasting and made to order. We specialize in interior tables and countertops.	**Hypnotherapist.** Founder of the local hypnotherapy association, I specialize in smoking cessation, weight loss, and anxiety reduction.

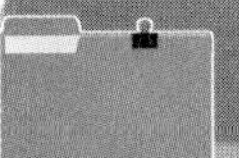

GETTING ORGANIZED

Guess what comes next! Do the same thing for your own massage service, and create a sample first ad. You may not choose to use it for the public just yet, but put your ideas and your sample ad into your *Business of Massage Therapy* notebook for the time when you are ready to start the advertising component of your marketing.

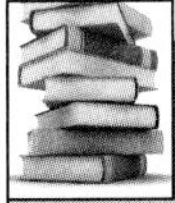

HELPFUL RESOURCES

There are many online resources that offer inexpensive ways to create your ads. Office Depot Online, Vistaprint, and FedEx Kinko's can help you with design and layout for postcards, fliers, or sample print ads. Also, check out books on creating great low-cost advertisements, like *Marketing Without Money for Small and Midsize Business: 300 Free and Cheap Ways to Increase Your Sales* by Nicholas Bade (2005, Halle House) or *How to Get Big Results from a Small Advertising Budget* by Cynthia Smith (1995, Carol Publishing).

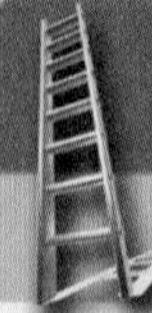

FIRST STEPS

Volunteering massage is a great way of engaging in community relations, especially when you are just starting out. Are there any upcoming events in your neighborhood where you could volunteer your services? It is great for building relationships, and a wonderful way to give back to your community. And who knows? You may even get some new clients due to your generosity (and exposure).

Community relations refers to activities that develop and strengthen relationships with the community, often through philanthropic activities. Volunteering to give massages to participants at a local fundraising walk for cancer, donating a massage to a local school's charity auction, or teaching free massage classes at a community school are all great examples. Engaging in community relationships helps connect you to your neighbors and positions you and your massage business as part of a vibrant community.

Publicity is another component of promotion, and, unlike advertising, is typically free. **Publicity** is any attention that is garnered for you (or that you garner for yourself) and your massage practice. Publicity can take the form of feature articles, online mentions, radio or television appearances, giving a speech or talk, press releases, sponsorship deals, seminars, trade fairs, and so forth. If you open your practice in a new area, or expand your business, send a press release to the local media announcing your arrival or new changes. Local news is there to report what is going on in the local community, and you are a part of that! Press releases will be explored more in Chapter 12, and you can find a template and sample press release in Appendix B.

Some advantages of publicity are that it is typically free or low cost, and can lend an air of credibility to you and your service. Think how much credence you give to a product or service that is positively spotlighted on the news; it *earned* exposure, it didn't *pay* for it. The downside, just as we discussed with word of mouth (a variation of publicity), is that you have little to no control on what others say about you. The old adage "any publicity is good publicity" may be true for celebrities, but not necessarily for massage therapists.

THE MARKETING PLAN

Now that you understand the importance of marketing and some of the prime ingredients in its mix, it is time to look at the important role of a marketing plan. A **marketing plan** is a document that details your marketing goals and the detailed steps you will take to achieve them. It is a blueprint for action and, done properly, a roadmap to success. With clear objectives and realistic steps, your marketing plan should be a reference to use as the basis for all marketing endeavors.

Many start-up companies use their marketing plan as a key component to acquire funding from banks, venture capitalists, or outside investors.[14] However, even if you have no intention of seeking outside money and would not dream of showing your marketing plan to anyone else, it can still be an invaluable tool for your successful practice. A well thought out marketing plan will help you understand:

- Who you are
- Where you are
- Where you want to go
- How you are going to get there
- What you value
- What is going on in your market
- Which customers you want to target, and how to reach them
- What you are up against in terms of competition
- What your four Ps mean for your company
- Your strengths, weaknesses, opportunities, and threats (SWOT)
- The steps you will take to achieve your marketing goals

HELPFUL RESOURCES

There are many resources to help you leverage publicity to give your practice a boost. Check out *Power Publicity for Massage Therapists* by Paul Hartunian (2006, Clifford Publishing) and *Guerrilla Publicity* by Jay Conrad Levison (2002, Adams Media Corp.). Also, take a look at www.publicity101.com or Elizabeth Yarnell's www.denverpublicity101.com.

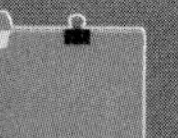

GETTING ORGANIZED

A marketing plan template and sample are included in Appendix B. Make a copy, and fill out the sections to create a marketing plan of your own. Put it into your *Business of Massage Therapy* notebook, and look back over it periodically to help you execute your marketing strategies.

Although marketing plans can differ in their components and intricacy, a common approach is the 10-point plan. The 10-point plan includes:

I. Executive Summary	A short overview of your company that highlights the main points of your marketing plan.
II. Mission Statement	Why are you in the massage business? What are you setting out to do? What values drive your business?
III. Industry Analysis	What is happening in the local massage industry? At the national level? What current trends are important to your company?
IV. Target Market	Who are your potential customers? How many of them are there? What are their needs, and how do they make purchasing decisions?
V. Company Analysis	An overview of your business, including goals, culture, and experience.
VI. Competitor Analysis	Who are my competitors? Why are they my competition? What do I have that they don't?
VII. Four Ps	How will I define my product/service and placement? How will I structure price? And what promotional tactics will I use?
VIII. SWOT Analysis	Strengths, Weaknesses, Opportunities, and Threats.
IX. Implementation Tactics	Step-by-step actions to accomplish your marketing goals, with specific target dates.
X. Conclusion	Sum it up!

An **executive summary** is a lavish name for an introduction. It is a miniature version of what the rest of your marketing plan contains. It helps give readers a clear overview of your business, and is a useful and concise reminder that you can access quickly. Some therapists choose to write their executive summary before the rest of the marketing plan, and then use it as an outline. Others choose to write the plan first and then go back and write the executive summary. Do whatever works best for you.

MISSION ACCOMPLISHED: WRITING A MISSION STATEMENT

A **mission statement** is an important part of your marketing plan and a fundamental tool for any massage practice. A mission statement is informed by what you value and what drives you forward. A mission statement reflects your company's raison d'etre, and should help guide and influence your daily decisions.[15] It encapsulates you and your company's goals and purpose in a concise and straightforward way.

HELPFUL RESOURCES

Examples of Mission Statements

- Establish Starbucks as the premier purveyor of the finest coffee in the world while maintaining our uncompromising principles while we grow. (Starbucks Corporation)[16]
- Our reason for being is: To serve our customers' health needs with imaginative science from plants and minerals; To Inspire all those we serve with a mission of responsibility and goodness; To empower others by sharing our knowledge, time, talents, and profits; and To help create a better world by exchanging our faith, experience and hope. (Tom's of Maine)[17]
- The mission of Southwest Airlines is dedication to the highest quality of customer service delivered with a sense of warmth, friendliness, individual pride, and company spirit. (Southwest Airlines)[18]

Here are some mission statements relevant to massage therapy:

- The mission of Serenity Bodyworks is to provide consistently superlative therapeutic massage so that clients can achieve and maintain optimal physical and emotional health. (Serenity Bodyworks, Denver, CO)
- To provide exceptional care to every client, every day with a spirit of warmth, friendliness, and personal pride. (Earthling Day Spa, Charleston, SC)
- To provide massage and facial services and products that are of the highest quality, offering value for your money, and use of the latest and most effective practices in the spa industry. (Creations of Clarity Spa, Round Rock, TX)
- To promote relaxation of mind and body to better cope with stresses of today's hectic pace and environment.
- To provide nurturing care for men and women through physical manipulation of muscles, tendons, and joints and increasing awareness of potential causes of physical stress. (Sheng Chi Massage, Fairview Park, OH)

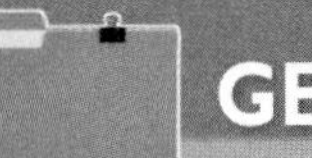

GETTING ORGANIZED

Do some research to find the mission statements of companies that you admire. They do not all have to be from massage therapists or holistic practitioners; try and find a broad range. When you find some, whether online or from printed materials, compile them and use these in your *Business of Massage Therapy* notebook to help you write your own.

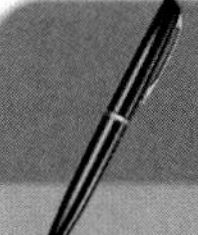

PUT IT IN WRITING

Mission Possible: Building Your Mission Statement on Your Core Values

A mission statement is built upon the foundation of your core values. To help you identify your core values, complete the following exercise. Write the first thing that comes to mind, without thinking about your answer.

1. The one word I would use to describe myself is ____________________.
2. One word that others use to describe me is ____________________.
3. The two qualities I look for in a partner are ____________ and ____________.
4. The person I most admire is ____________. I admire him/her because he/she represents ____________ to me.
5. I don't imagine I could live without ____________.
6. The two most important people in my life are ____________ and ____________.
7. One thing that I am the most proud of is ____________.
8. If I could create anything, I would want it to be ____________________.

Now copy the words you chose to complete the sentences above in the spaces below:

________ ________ ________
________ ________ ________
________ ________ ________

This should give you a good idea of what you truly value. Now put your values into action and included them in your mission statement. (If you need help thinking of core value words, go to Appendix B for another values exercise.)

EXAMINING CURRENT TRENDS IN THE INDUSTRY

> *It takes as much energy to wish as it does to plan.*
>
> —Eleanor Roosevelt

The next part of the marketing plan is current trends, or **industry analysis.** In order for your marketing endeavors to be successful, it helps significantly to understand what is happening in the world of massage in your area. Industry analysis facilitates your understanding of your position in the local market. Take an objective look at the trends of massage in your area. Perhaps you have noticed an abundance of new day spas nearby, or seen more advertisements for individual therapists in your favorite community paper. Perhaps a low cost, high volume franchise has moved into town. Maybe you have heard that enrollment is up at the local massage schools, or that a number of massage schools are closing down.

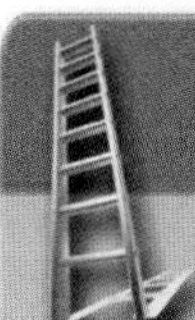

FIRST STEPS

Call around to different schools and see what trends they are observing locally. Contact your secretary of state's office or other regulating authorities and see if the number of registered and licensed therapists has increased or decreased in the last few years. Go online and type "(your city) massage trends)" and see what you find.

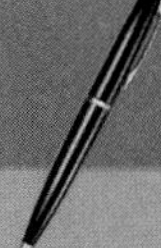

PUT IT IN WRITING

Characteristics of Success

Doing an industry analysis also helps you to determine what the key success factors are in the massage industry. What does it take to make it in this market? For example, if one of the trends in your area was an economic downturn, a successful practitioner might be resourceful and financially flexible. Write out four characteristics that would make someone successful in the current market situation.

1. ____________________
2. ____________________
3. ____________________
4. ____________________

Once you've identified those four things, you can honestly assess which of them you have and which you do not. This will also help you in subsequent sections of your plan.

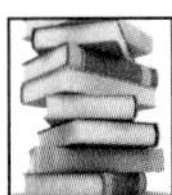

HELPFUL RESOURCES

There are several resources out there to give you a better understanding of trends in your industry. Most public libraries have a business resource department, and access to many national and regional business databases. These resources will also help you as you research your target market and your competitors. If you get confused or are not sure how to find what you are looking for, the business librarians are there to help you out. If you want to see national trends, look at online sources such as the U.S. Department of Labor's Bureau of Labor Statistics (www.bls.gov) or www.hoovers.com.

Many small business owners and executives consider themselves at worst victims, and at best observers of what goes on in their industry. They sometimes fail to perceive that understanding your industry directly impacts your ability to succeed.

—Kenneth J. Cook, author of *The AMA Complete Guide to Strategic Planning for Small Business.*

HITTING THE TARGET

Your **target market** consists of those that you identify as your potential customers. Therapists cannot (and probably should not) try to be all things to all clients,[19] and targeting your market based on what you have to offer will help narrow your marketing focus. As an entrepreneurial therapist, it is important to have a clear picture of whom you are trying to reach with your marketing endeavors; you will also want to understand as accurately as possible what it is they want. Who are they? What needs do they want met? What are the characteristics of your target market? Try to be as specific as possible. Consider elements such as age, income level, physical activity, gender, geography, education, and so forth (see Figure 11-3 ■).

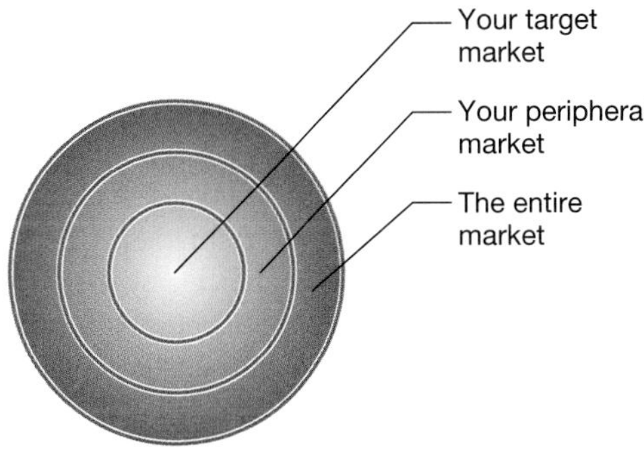

FIGURE 11-3

Identifying and understanding your target market can help narrow your marketing focus.

US AND THEM: ASSESSING YOURSELF AND THE COMPETITION

In the **company analysis,** you get to talk all about you and your business. Whether you are getting started or looking to improve your existing business, this is the time to talk about all the great things about your company. All the work you did on goal setting in Chapter 8 can be included in this section. This is also the place to talk about your **budget** for marketing.

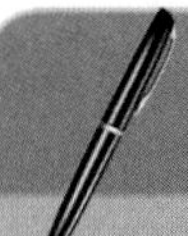

PUT IT IN WRITING

Hitting the Target

Write out a description of who you want to reach with your marketing message. Who will find your services most helpful? Try and be as detailed as possible. The following description of the target market for a crafts store might be helpful:

> Alpaca's is targeting women in the 24–55 age range, because all consumer research has shown that women in this range are the most likely to spend money on crafts. There are 540,000 women between the ages of 24 and 55 in the Denver Metropolitan area.[20] The median household income is $39,500. We are targeting our product to all women who make $45,000 or more, as we believe that is the level where individuals begin to have more disposable income for craft supplies. Our customers are educated, having completed at least a bachelor's degree. They are looking for a sense of community and connection that they will find at our fusion coffeeshop/craftstore, where classes, presentations, and group meetings will take place.

Now you try:

1. My target market is:

____

____

____

2. The need that my target customers want solved is:

____

____

____

3. I can solve it because:

____

____

____

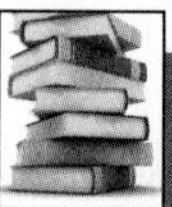

HELPFUL RESOURCES

There are many resources to help you identify and describe the demographics of your target market. Check out the *Country and City Data Book* published by the U.S. Department of Commerce and *Survey of Buying Power Data Service* published by Sales and Marketing Management. Also look at the demographics in your immediate area by going to www.yourstate.gov and finding "demographics."

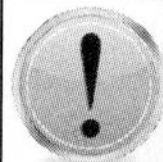

PITFALLS

Many therapists go into business without taking stock of themselves or assessing the market around them. Perhaps they don't think it is important to know with whom they are competing, or don't see how the changing trends can affect their practice. Knowledge is power, and the more you know about the conditions of the massage market around you, the better prepared you will be.

A budget estimates how much you will be able to spend for each activity. Many marketing experts recommend that companies aim to spend 20 percent of their resources on marketing. However marketing budgets are relative to the unique goals and capacity of each business, and you will be responsible for determining and committing to your own budget. What is a realistic amount to spend on each activity in order to sell your practice to your target market?

You can also explore the company culture that you have or would like to create. **Company culture** refers to the shared values, practices, and behaviors in a company.[21] Even if you're the only person in your massage business, you still have a company culture, usually defined by your personality and the experience you create for your clients. Some entrepreneurs might want a culture marked by fun and humor. Others might want a culture that is rooted in peacefulness and calm. What do you want your culture to be? The company analysis is also a good opportunity to explore your past professional experiences, whether in massage or elsewhere. How have these experiences prepared you to

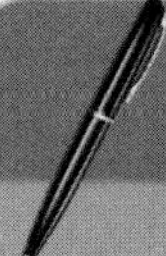

PUT IT IN WRITING

Assessing the Competition

Remember those four key success factors you identified in the industry analysis section? You have already applied them to yourself; now look at the competition. The chart below is a tool often used in decision management, and can also be used to assess your competition.[23] Look at the key success factors that you identified in the industry analysis section. Do your competitors have them?

Say the four characteristics you identified were: technique, consistency, good location, customer service. Now give each one of those criteria a weight of importance. If you think customer service is the most important, give it a 4. If you think consistency is least important, give it a 1. Now chose five of the competitors you listed and plug them into your chart, and rate each one from 1 to 10 on your four different criteria. Multiply the score times the weight given, and sum up your competitors. Table 11-3 ■ gives an example assessment.

The objective of this exercise is threefold: it helps you assign value to success characteristics, it helps you gauge your competitors, and it helps you to quantify what you like and dislike about another's service. From here you can learn from your competitors with gratitude and respect.

Now you try it: use Table 11-4 ■ to do your own assessment.

TABLE 11-4 Factors for Success

	Weight
Weighted Score	

TABLE 11-3 Factors for Success

	Weight	All About You Day Spa	True Touch	Greg Great, LMT	Happy Hands	Sara Smee, CMT
Technique	2	7	5	8	2	6
Customer Service	4	6	6	6	9	7
Good location	3	5	8	3	7	5
Consistency	1	5	8	3	6	5
Weighted Score		**58**	**64**	**52**	**67**	**60**

do well in your practice? Do you possess any of the four key success factors you designated in your industry analysis section?

It is also very important to perform an impartial **competitive analysis** to see what you are up against. Knowing who your competitors are and what they are doing will help you navigate a successful marketing plan. It will also help you define and sharpen your own competitive edge in relation to other therapists. A **competitive edge,** or competitive advantage, is what sets you apart. A competitive advantage can be due to your technical massage expertise, specialized modalities, lower prices, a high marketing budget, your location, or anything that gives you an advantage over the competition. Ideally, your competitive edge should be sustainable and continue over time.[22] Your competitive analysis should do the following:

- Determine who your competitors are. You can identify as many as you like.
- Where are they located? Are their offices close to your office?
- Why have you defined them as a competitor? Similar massage techniques? Similar price structure? Geographic proximity?
- How do your competitors reach their clients (website, mailings, street visibility, etc.)?
- What do you like about what they are doing?
- What do you dislike about what they are doing?
- What do you see as your competitive edge?

You have already learned the four Ps of marketing (product, placement, price, promotion), and now you can put them into your plan. Here you can define your product and/or service. Where will you perform your service or sell your products? You can set your initial price structure, exploring any discounts or premiums you would like to include. Here is also the place to state the types of promotional activities you think would be most beneficial to reach your target market. Come up with a promotional mix (advertising, public relations, word of mouth, etc.) that will advance your practice.

SWOT ANALYSIS

Throughout the chapter you have been exploring the characteristics about your mission, your industry, your target market, your business, and your competitors. All these activities have primed you for the SWOT analysis, one of the most powerful tools in your marketing plan. A **SWOT analysis** is an examination of your Strengths, Weaknesses, Opportunities, and Threats.[24] SWOT is merely a description of the internal and external business conditions for your massage practice. A SWOT analysis can be applied on a micro- or macro-level of the business; in other words, you can use it as a strategic tool when making decisions both small (selling a new kind of aromatherapy oil to clients) and large (starting your own company). Performing a SWOT analysis (see Figure 11-4 ■) can help you look at yourself and your business in a comprehensive, objective way; it can help identify aspects and prospects you might otherwise not have considered.

	Helpful (supports goals)	*Harmful* (can hurt goals)
Internal (personal or professional aspects)	**Strengths** Examples: -good reputation in community -financial reserves -ongoing education -marketing expertise	**Weaknesses** Examples: -high rent costs -working in poor location -lack of business experience -disorganization
External (environmental conditions)	**Opportunities** Examples: -unmet need among customers -new market trend -can expand retail -competitors leaving area	**Threats** Examples: -increase in competition -massage demand is seasonal -price battles -faltering economy

FIGURE 11-4

A sample SWOT analysis from a massage business, assessing its strengths, weaknesses, opportunities, and threats.

- *Strengths:* These include personal or professional aspects that are helpful to achieving your objectives and goals for your massage practice. These are "internal," meaning they relate only to you or your business.
- *Weaknesses:* These include personal or professional aspects that are harmful to achieving your objectives and goals for your massage practice. Like strengths, weaknesses are internal.
- *Opportunities:* These are environmental conditions that are helpful to achieving your objectives and goals for your massage practice. These are "external," meaning they exist outside of your immediate sphere of control.
- *Threats:* These are environmental conditions that are harmful to achieving your objectives and goals for your massage practice. These are external.

As you go through your SWOT, ask yourself how you can use each strength in your practice. Once you have recognized weaknesses, think of ways you can grow or work with those areas. How can you take advantage of the opportunities around you and at the same time defend against possible threats?

MAKING IT HAPPEN: IMPLEMENTATION TACTICS

Implementation tactics will be the next part of your plan. Implementation tactics are the way in which you break your goals down into small, manageable, pieces. You mentioned your goals for your massage practice in the "Company Analysis" part of your marketing plan. This is the part where you put forth tangible and actionable steps towards accomplishing those goals. Recall from Chapter 8 that effective goals are SMART (Specific, Measurable, Attainable, Realistic, and Timely). The implementation tactics will help you achieve your SMART goals by breaking them down into manageable pieces. Having a plan of action that is clear and specific will make your goals all the more achievable.

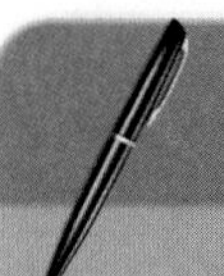

PUT IT IN WRITING

Got SWOT?

Take the time to fill out a SWOT of your own (use Figure 11-5 ■). Take an honest assessment of yourself and your environment for all the categories. Maybe there are some things you had not considered before. There is no judgment in a SWOT analysis, so just write down whatever comes to mind.

	Helpful (supports goals)	*Harmful* (can hurt goals)
Internal (personal or professional aspects)	**Strengths**	**Weaknesses**
External (environmental conditions)	**Opportunities**	**Threats**

FIGURE 11-5

Fill out your own SWOT analysis to assess your own Strengths, Weaknesses, Opportunities, and Threats.

Giving yourself a date to accomplish your tactic will help you carry out your plan. This section is often just a timeline of your goals, and the tactics and deadlines you have assigned to each one.

Imagine that you chose the following three primary goals: creating a business card and a brochure, setting up a website, and finding and engaging in three creative low- or no-cost marketing activities. Your plan might look like the one shown in Table 11-5 ■.

The final section of your Marketing Plan is your conclusion. Here is the place to sum up all that you have explored in your plan. It might also be a good place to decide how you will measure the success of the plan in the future. How

TABLE 11-5 SMART Goals

Goal	Tactic	Description	Completion Date
Goal 1: Create business card and brochure	1a.	Gather cards and brochures from other massage therapists whose designs I admire	1/15 Completed_______
	1b.	Decide what information I want in my brochure. Make a rough draft of the card and brochure	1/20 Completed_______
	1c.	Go online to price designing my own card through a discount printer such as VistaPrint or FedEx Kinko's	1/22 Completed_______
	1d.	Design my card and brochure within my budget, buying as many as I think I will need	1/25 Completed_______
Goal 2: Set up a website	2a.	Look at websites of other holistic practitioners, deciding what I like and dislike	2/1 Completed_______
	2b.	Decide what I can afford for website design and maintenance	2/4 Completed_______
	2c.	Register a domain name	2/10 Completed_______
	2d.	Choose a service provider and a package I can afford	2/15 Completed_______
	2e.	Help design my site the way I want it	2/16 Completed_______
	2f.	Take a course on web design and maintenance at the local community school to continue improving site	2/25 Completed_______

TABLE 11-5 SMART Goals

Goal	Tactic	Description	Completion Date
Goal 3: Find three low- or no-cost marketing techniques	3a.	Go through *The Business of Massage Therapy* for ideas and resources	3/2 Completed______
	3b.	Ask four other therapists what free/inexpensive marketing has worked for them	3/9 Completed______
	3c.	Search online sources for marketing tips	3/12 Completed______
	3d.	Chose the three that are best for me	3/14 Completed______
	3e.	Implement the first	3/15 Completed______
	3f.	Implement the second	3/20 Completed______
	3g.	Implement the third	3/25 Completed______

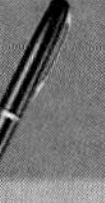

PUT IT IN WRITING

Implementation

Now you! Return to the work you did on goals in Chapters 2 and 3, and select three of your top goals. Now fill out Table 11-6 ■ based upon those goals. There is space provided for four tactics per goal, but you may find that you need fewer or more than that to accomplish your goal. Be creative, and try and think of as many detailed steps as necessary to help you achieve your desired outcome.

TABLE 11-6 SMART Goals

Goal	Tactic	Description	Completion Date
Goal 1:	1a.		Completed______
	1b.		Completed______
	1c.		Completed______
	1d.		Completed______
Goal 2:	2a.		Completed______
	2b.		Completed______
	2c.		Completed______
	2d.		Completed______
Goal 3:	3a.		Completed______
	3b.		Completed______
	3c.		Completed______
	3d.		Completed______

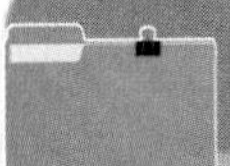

GETTING ORGANIZED

Now gather all the sections that you have completed in this chapter and compile them together. Congratulations, you marketing guru you! You have completed your marketing plan! Not only are you a skilled therapist, but you have also proven yourself to be an astute and wise entrepreneur as well. Well done!

will you know when your goals have been met? Just as with any conclusion, it can be short and succinct and should merely be a summary of what you have already said.

Keep in mind that a marketing plan is not a one-time undertaking. As was explored before, marketing is a dynamic and ongoing activity. Economic factors, changing customer needs, increased competition, and a host of other dynamics can shift your market conditions at any point. A successful massage therapist is always receptive and proactive when responding to such changes. You can always go back to your initial marketing plan to make any necessary adjustments or strategic changes as conditions dictate. The great part about marketing is that nothing is ever set in stone. You are always free to adjust your strategy.

CHAPTER SUMMARY BY LEARNING OBJECTIVES

1. **Define marketing** Marketing refers to any activity that serves to let your market know about you, attract customers to your product or service, and keep them coming back for more. Marketing is how you match your capabilities to the needs of your potential and actual customers.
2. **Explain the marketing mix and define the "four Ps" of marketing** The marketing mix includes product, placement, price, and promotion, also known as the four Ps of marketing.
3. **Define product and placement, and explain how to structure price** The product refers to the good or service being marketed. Placement refers to the location where said good or service can be purchased by the consumer. Price is the amount a customer pays for a product or service. Prices in a massage business are based on many factors, including the therapist's costs and financial goals and the ranges set by other therapists in the area. Discounting and premium pricing are different pricing strategies.
4. **Explore the various components of promotion, and learn how to leverage customer service as a marketing strategy** Promotion is the communication you put into the market about your goods and/or services. Elements of promotion include word of mouth, advertising, public relations, and publicity. Customer service is a very important part of good marketing, and relates to the client care activities, both material and intangible, that support the delivery of a business's core product or service.
5. **Explain the purpose and makeup of a marketing plan** A marketing plan is a document that details your marketing goals and the detailed steps you will take to achieve them. It is a blueprint for action and, done properly, a roadmap to success. With clear objectives and realistic steps, your marketing plan should be a reference to use as the basis for all marketing endeavors.
6. **Write a mission statement** A mission statement is informed by what you value and what drives you forward. It is based on your core values.
7. **Examine trends in the massage industry** Industry analysis helps to understand the current trends in the local and national massage markets, thus helping guide marketing strategies accordingly.
8. **Identify a target market** A target market consists of those that are identified as potential customers. Targeting customers helps to narrow the focus for marketing activities by defining who the target customer is, what problem he or she needs solved, and how the company is going to solve that for him or her.
9. **Describe a company analysis and identify and assess competition** The company analysis is an exploration of the goals, experience, and culture within a company. It is also an exploration of the financial budget for the company. Competitive analysis helps to understand the who, what, why, and where of the competition. It also helps to define the company's competitive advantage in relation to the market.
10. **Define and explore a SWOT analysis** A SWOT analysis is an exploration of a company's strengths, opportunities, and threats. It helps the company understand internal and external conditions.
11. **Introduce implementation tactics to help achieve marketing goals** Implementation tactics help achieve the goals set forth in the marketing plan by developing a time line for completion.

ACTIVITIES

Quiz: Identifying Marketing Words

1. Jenna is interviewed for a local newspaper that is interested in her volunteer massage for cancer survivors. This is an example of:
   a. targeting
   b. publicity
   c. branding
   d. advertising
2. A marketing mix consists of:
   a. target market, company analysis, current trends, competitor analysis
   b. product, place, price, promotion
   c. advertising, publicity, press release, word of mouth
   d. flour, butter, milk, eggs
3. In a SWOT analysis, strengths and weaknesses refer to _____ conditions.
   a. internal
   b. external
   c. market
   d. uncontrollable
4. A step-by-step action to accomplish a goal is known as a _____.
   a. map
   b. tactic
   c. plan
   d. deadline

5. A client receives a great massage and tells all his friends about you. This is best known as _____.
   a. discovery
   b. advertising
   c. placement
   d. word of mouth
6. Goals should be:
   a. EASY (early, accessible, simple, yearly)
   b. TRUE (timely, relevant, useful, evident)
   c. SMART (specific, measurable, attainable, realistic, timely)
   d. BEST (believable, effortless, stress-free, easy)
7. You have been approached by an acupuncturist, another massage therapist, a reflexologist, and a chiropractor who are interested in putting together a marketing campaign with your practice. They feel that marketing together will help propel everyone's businesses, while sharing the cost and responsibility. This is an example of _____.
   a. direct competition
   b. accommodating
   c. cooperative marketing
   d. a wellness center
8. You are a prenatal massage therapist. You have just read an article in the paper that reports a huge surge in birthrates in your area due to many factors; the article also predicts that this trend should continue. This is an example of a/n _____ for your business.
   a. threat
   b. community relation
   c. opportunity
   d. disaster
9. You have a client who is finishing her bachelor's degree and is not currently working. You have told her that you will reduce the price of her massage until she graduates. This is an example of _____.
   a. premium pricing
   b. price gouging
   c. client privilege
   d. differential pricing
10. As a therapist who specializes in temporomandibular joint therapy (TMJ), Pusma's _____ includes men and women who are burdened with the localized TMJ disorder.
   a. target market
   b. friends
   c. market conditions
   d. key customers

Case Study

Steve's SWOT

Steve is a massage therapist who specializes in sports massage. He has been practicing massage for nine years. During that time, Steve has devoted a lot of energy into mastering his craft and positioning himself as an expert. He teaches sports massage at the same massage school where he graduated, and volunteers massage at local sporting events and races. He also gives lectures to the sports groups he participates in about the importance of massage in an athletic routine. In addition, he sells supplementary products such as vitamins, sports creams, and self-massaging accoutrements. Steve lives in a town that prides itself on its athleticism and healthy activity. When Steve started his massage career, there were few sports massage therapists in his area; however, in the last five years his competition has tripled, and seems to only be increasing. Steve's goal is to grow his business by 30 percent, while still being able to have time to teach, lecture, and volunteer. He is developing a marketing plan to help him meet his goals. Do a SWOT analysis for Steve. What are his strengths, weaknesses, opportunities, and threats? Write them in Figure 11-6 ■.

	Helpful (supports goals)	*Harmful* (can hurt goals)
Internal (personal or professional aspects)	**Strengths**	**Weaknesses**
External (environmental conditions)	**Opportunities**	**Threats**

FIGURE 11-6
SWOT analysis.

CHAPTER 12

More Marketing for Massage

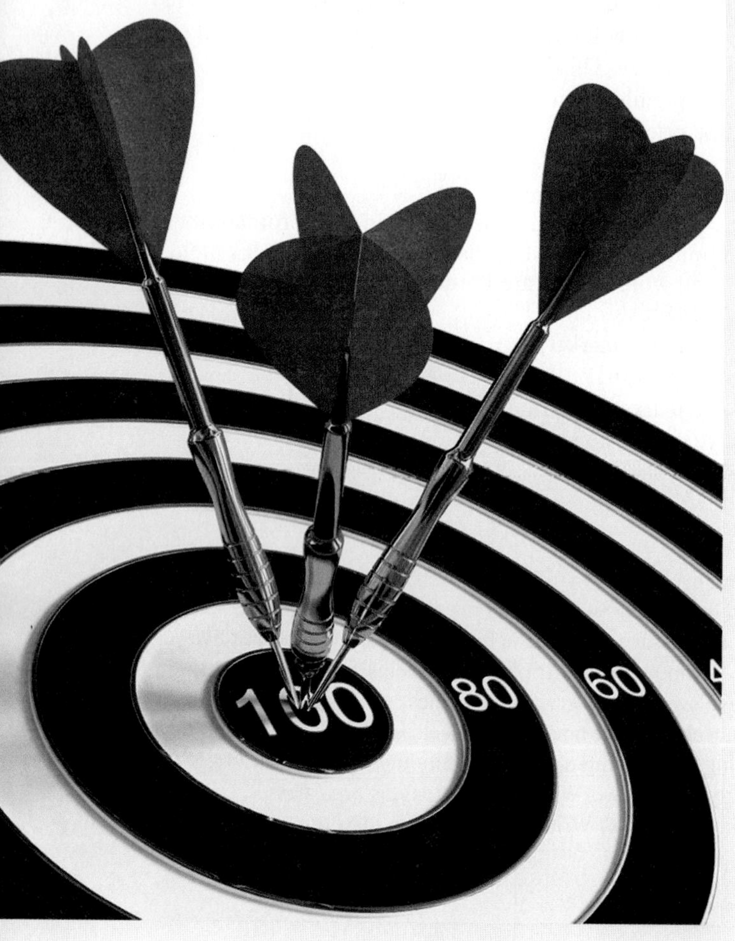

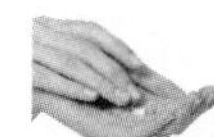

CHAPTER OUTLINE

LEARNING OBJECTIVES

1. Discuss why marketing is important for the massage professional
2. Evaluate marketing considerations and challenges unique to the massage industry
3. Identify essential marketing materials for massage therapists
4. Examine the anatomy of a business card
5. Introduce cooperative marketing, low-cost and no-cost marketing techniques and tools
6. Illustrate how to craft and deliver an elevator pitch for the massage therapist
7. Explore niche marketing for different massage modalities and different target markets
8. Examine the role of communications in marketing massage
9. Learn ways to "recession-proof" your practice through marketing
10. Identify ways to manage marketing information overload and exhaustion

KEY TERMS

auto responder *202*
brochure *195*
business card *196*
call to action *197*
communications *202*
conversion process *200*
cooperative marketing *198*
demand *193*
discretionary spending *203*
flyer *195*
information overload *206*
logo *196*
low-cost/no-cost marketing *198*
market saturation *193*
marketing collateral *193*
marketing skills *193*
marketing systems *193*
marketing tools *193*
Maslow's hierarchy of needs *204*
newsletter *202*
niche marketing *200*
press kit *196*
press release *195*
price ladder *204*
qualified prospect *201*
recession *204*
referral *198*
supply *193*
supply and demand theory *193*
technology fatigue *206*
unique promise *200*
viral marketing *203*

MORE MARKETING? REALLY?

> *Next to doing the right thing, the most important thing is to let people know you are doing the right thing.*
>
> —John D. Rockefeller

Wait a second—wasn't the last chapter all about marketing? Is this deja vu? Not quite. Because marketing is such an essential component for any successful business, because marketing a massage therapy business brings with it its own unique set of challenges, and because many massage therapists get overwhelmed and opt for the "head in the sand" approach to marketing, *The Business of Massage Therapy* has two full chapters devoted to this important topic. The last chapter introduced the fundamental marketing concepts, such as marketing plans, the four Ps of marketing, and the SWOT analysis. These concepts are applicable across industries, and give you a good high-level understanding of the role of marketing for your business. In this chapter, you will expand on how to apply those concepts within the unique framework of a massage therapy practice through more targeted action steps. The necessary marketing skills to be a successful small business owner are very different from those required by a successful large company. And the necessary marketing skills to be a successful *holistic* business owner can be quite distinct from those of other small business owners. Even if you don't care for the idea of selling, there are lots of fun ways to market and grow your own business!

Ask yourself a question: What is the one thing that all successful massage businesses have in common? Perhaps you might think it is skilled therapists that make a business thrive. Or maybe you think it is great customer service that keeps people coming back. What about that genuine and passionate mission to help other people? While those are all essential components, there is only one thing that all successful businesses—across industries—have that separate them from the pack. That one thing? *Customers.* The best products and services in the world will not keep a business running if there are not customers coming through the pipeline on a consistent basis. And that is where marketing comes in.

It is with heartbreaking regularity that the same pattern occurs in the massage industry: talented, intelligent, passionate, and big-hearted individuals come into the profession with the belief that skills and intention alone will substantiate their healing career. They believe that their talented repertoire and great customer service will have them beating clients off with a stick. They believe that their authentic mission and skill will ensure client referrals, fill their calendars, and have them meet their financial goals.

But if practioners fail to market themselves and their businesses, all those skills could be for naught. Many give up on their business and go work for far less money and control, or leave the industry altogether, dispirited and disillusioned that all of their talents and best intentions did not bring them the success they sought. It doesn't have to be this way! As important as skills and mission are, and as wonderful as the laws of attraction and the power of positive thinking may be, none of these are sound marketing strategies in themselves. This chapter will help provide you with more tools for growing and sustaining a thriving holistic business.

This chapter will help you tap into your powerful potential to market your massage business and create great success for you, your employees, and your company. Successful

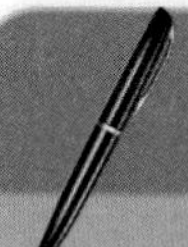

PUT IT IN WRITING

Me? A Marketer?

While it's true that anyone who works in this world is inevitably selling something, many therapists face personal roadblocks when it comes to marketing their business (and, in turn, themselves). Others find the process incredibly exciting and full of possibilities. It helps to identify where you are on the continuum before you move forward. Answer these explorative questions to uncover your feelings about marketing. And remember, there are no "right" answers; just pay attention to your responses.

1. When I read Chapter 11 on marketing, I felt ____________ and found the concepts ____________.
2. When I think about selling the service of massage therapy, I feel ____________.
3. When I think about selling myself as a massage therapist, I feel ____________.
4. For me, a description of a successful marketing campaign is ____________.
5. In order for me to be successful marketing my business, I would have to ____________.
6. My biggest opportunity to marketing my unique business is ____________.
7. My biggest challenge to marketing my unique business is ____________.
8. My competitive advantage in the market is ____________.
9. The three words I would use to describe my ideal client are ____________.
10. The three words I would use to describe the benefits of working with me are ____________.

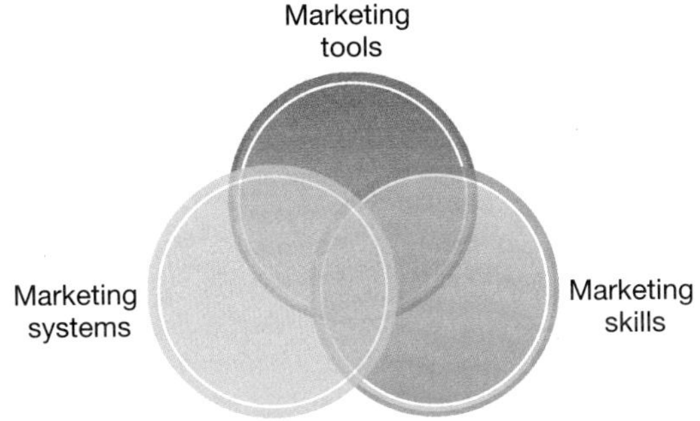

FIGURE 12-1

The three keys of successful marketing: marketing tools, marketing systems, and marketing skills.

marketing of any business is the culmination of three critical areas: marketing systems, marketing skills, and marketing tools. **Marketing systems** are the processes you have in place to identify leads, bait potential clients, convert them into actual clients, and retain them in your business. **Marketing tools** are the materials and technologies you will leverage to get optimal exposure and client conversion for your business. **Marketing skills** relate to your overall know-how and ability to leverage your systems and tools to optimize your success. Although each one is important, having strength in just one area won't get you nearly as far as fortifying all three pillars of marketing. Each one is interdependent with the others, and together they create a trifecta of marketing (Figure 12-1 ■).

EVALUATE MARKETING CONSIDERATIONS AND CHALLENGES UNIQUE TO THE MASSAGE INDUSTRY

As you have seen in earlier chapters, the massage industry is a dynamic one that has seen myriad changes over the last few decades. In fact, many would argue that the industry has changed substantially over the last few years, with great fluctuations both in the supply and demand side of the market. **Supply** is the total amount of products or services available for purchase in any given market, while **demand** is the market's desire and willingness to pay for a product or service. Supply and demand are closely interrelated forces: as demand for massage therapy has grown in recent years, the supply of therapists has grown with it. However, this is both an opportunity and a challenge for massage businesses. **Supply and demand theory,** an economic model that explains market forces, concludes that in a free and competitive market, increases in supply often result in a decrease in price (i.e., lower wages for therapists).[1] As consumers come to expect lower prices, many quality therapists are driven out of the market, driving down the supply.

In recent years, many of the corporate spas and franchise massage chains have helped satisfy the demand by increasing the supply of therapists while at the same time driving down consumer price points. Many in the industry maintain that massage therapy is reaching or has reached market saturation. **Market saturation** occurs when the amount of product or service has peaked due to increased supply, diminished demand, or other factors. When a market becomes saturated, growth typically becomes possible only through product or service improvements or increased consumer demand.[2]

So why is all of this important to you and your business's marketing? Certainly you don't need a degree in economics to market your business, but it does help to understand the changes in the landscape. Supply and demand definitely affects price points, and alter the competitive environment substantially. Although many would argue that these points are moot because there are always enough aching bodies to go around, it is naïve to think that heavy supply and stiff competition won't affect the way you will need to market yourself and your business. In addition, it is important to understand the increasing sophistication of the consumers themselves. Many of the old rules of marketing a holistic business (i.e., handing out a business card and hoping for the best) no longer apply in the way that they did 10 years ago. Increased competition in a technology-dependent and marketing-savvy world necessitates increased sophistication of your approach and an intentional strategy for getting people in the door (and keeping them coming back through that door).

FROM BUSINESS CARDS TO PRESS KITS: ESSENTIAL MARKETING MATERIALS FOR MASSAGE THERAPISTS

Not too long ago, a massage therapist reflected upon what she learned about marketing in massage school. She was told by her fabulous professors that all she would really need to promote her new practice was a business card, a brochure, and occasional promotional mail postcards announcing specials. If she felt adventurous, she might send out a newsletter from time to time. In spite of the amazing technical education she was given in massage, her business education left her actual practice flat and gasping for air. After a lot of lengthy research, classes, and working with a massage marketing expert extraordinaire, she learned that there are a lot more ingredients that could potentially (and successfully) go into her marketing mix, as shown in Figure 12-2 ■.

As you begin to bring your business into the light of day, it helps to have a lot of great marketing collateral on hand. **Marketing collateral** is a collection of any type of media that supports the promotion of your services and/or products. Collateral helps support your company's sales efforts; most marketing collateral typically hinges on your unique brand and ideally should have a cohesive look and feel to it. As you learned in the last chapter, the name of the game in marketing is *consistency*. Common examples of marketing collateral for any business include business cards, brochures,

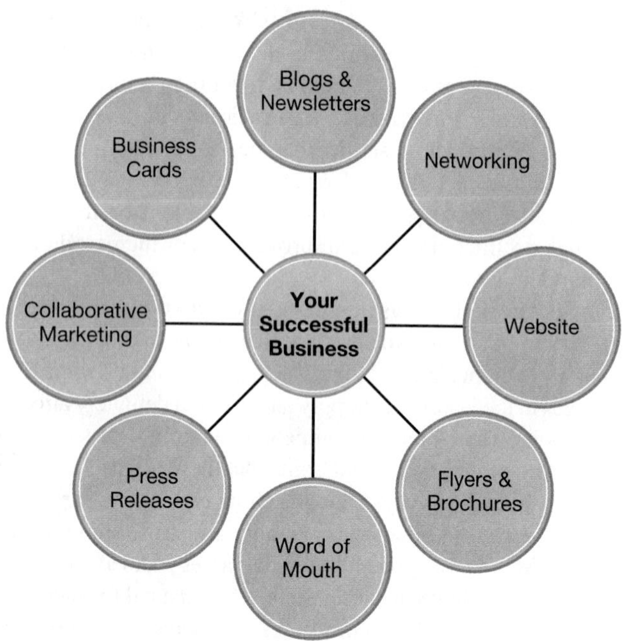

FIGURE 12-2

There are many tools for marketing success available to massage therapists, including websites, business cards, flyers and brochures, newsletters, press releases, networking, blogs, and much more.

press kits, sales packets, printed materials, signs and posters, websites, and paper and e-newsletters. Marketing collateral can also include the fun SWAG ("stuff we all get") like pens, keychains, hats, sticky notes, or other things that you yourself may have picked up from other companies over the years.

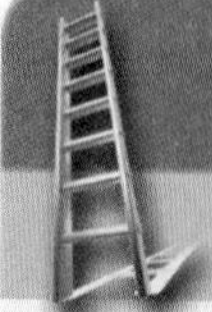

FIRST STEPS

Think of a time when you have been presented with someone else's marketing collateral. Perhaps someone trying to solicit your business left you with slick catalogue. Maybe a salesman gave you a sales kit filled with all of the company information. Or perhaps you went to a trade show and filled your bag with brochures, pencils, flashlights, and mugs from the various vendors there. Have any of these things ever helped to convert you into a customer? Did you ever feel compelled to do more research? Do you recall anything so compelling that you knew you wanted to work with a particular company? Reflect back, and jot down some notes in your *Business of Massage Therapy* notebook on marketing collateral that has worked for you as a consumer in the past.

In addition to consistency, one very important thing to keep in mind is the aesthetic of your collateral. Whether conscious or not, visual impact is essential to savvy consumers—remember what you learned in the last chapter about the sheer volume of images an individual sees every single day! Even with budget as a consideration, it is imperative to design your collateral with visual impact that compliments the image of your business, whether in printed or virtual form (see Chapter 11 for resources for inexpensive professional printing options). Distributing less-than-professional looking materials can have a negative effect on your business image, as people can be quick to write off homemade materials as

GETTING ORGANIZED

Useful Tools for Marketing Your Massage Practice

There are so many useful tools for a massage therapists to help them market their business successfully. Many of the concepts listed below will be explained throughout this and other chapters, but it can be very useful to have a handy list compiled when you get stuck with marketing ideas. Copy the list below and file it into your *Business of Massage Therapy* notebook. You might even add a few of your own tools that are not on the list below.

Business card
Brochure
Flyer
Press releases
Press kit
Sales packets
Signs
Posters
Word of mouth
Calls to action
Referrals
Newsletters
Blogs
E-zines
Elevator pitch
Auto responders
Networking
Collaborative promotion

Can you think of any additional tools not listed above that you could use to market your business? Write them here.

________________ ________________
________________ ________________
________________ ________________

being amateurish and reflecting lower quality of service. This can quickly erode consumer confidence and cost you clients (even if the opinion is wrong, client perception is all that counts in marketing). This is particularly true if you are planning on placing your price points at a premium, because more and more polished materials are becoming the minimum standards in the industry at every price point. Just take a look at the glossy campaigns put out by the budget massage chains.

You can distribute marketing collateral at trade shows, networking events, through e-mail, and of course on your website. One of the most basic and abundant forms of marketing collateral is the business card, which will be described in detail in the next section. Brochures are also very common. A **brochure** is a multifold pamphlet that succinctly explains the benefits of working with your business, while enticing potential clients to learn more. A well-written and well-designed brochure gets people's attention, sets you apart from the crowd, and engages people to actively pursue working with you. Brochures can be distributed personally, through direct mail, at trade shows, or on the exterior of your business location. Many therapists have had success leaving their brochure on information racks in hotels, tourist centers, or other friendly businesses.

Another useful piece of marketing collateral for massage therapists is a flyer. A postcard or **flyer** is a single-page pamphlet meant for distribution that is often used to advertise special events or promotions. Because they are typically less costly to produce and more likely to be read in a stack of junk mail than a brochure, flyers and postcards are often a good choice for direct mail campaigns.

In the last chapter you learned about publicity (part of promotion, one of the four Ps of marketing). Not all therapists are on par in skill level, and many consumers know this. In the land of massage, a lot of your business credibility comes from publicity in the form of word of mouth advertising, endorsements, and testimonials. Since publicity is the deliberate (but unpaid) attempt to persuade public opinion, you don't have to sit and wait for someone to say something nice about your wonderful massage or your fantastic business—you can always expedite the process. A good way to do this is through press releases. A **press release** includes information that is written by an individual or company representative and sent to media outlets with the intention of announcing something about a company, product, or service that is newsworthy and potentially of interest to the public. Press releases are not advertisements; rather they should include information that readers or viewers might want to know about. Press releases can be sent to newspapers, magazines, radio stations, television stations, or any other outlet that might reach your target market.

A well-written release can help increase your visibility and boost your traffic. The objective of a press release should be to provide information, not just to sell something. Press releases should be newsworthy and written with the media in mind. In other words, a good press release should answer the question "Why should anyone care about this?" There is a certain accepted protocol when writing a press release, so do a little research if you decide to send one out. Being outside of accepted norms can keep your press release from

FIRST STEPS

When creating your marketing collateral, you will want to focus not only on enticing prospective clients, but also on subtly differentiating yourself from the competition. Don't fall into the same rut of just describing you and your technique—focus on the problems you will solve and the benefits clients will get from working with YOU and your business. Make your copy pop and sizzle, and include calls to action over simply information (i.e., visit our website for a free gift, call today to schedule a free consultation).

PITFALLS

Many business owners believe that, because they are very excited about their business, everyone else will be, too. However, not everything is news, and your press release can be tossed without a glance if done improperly. Press releases can be great marketing tools when used properly, but you want to make sure you are following protocol and providing valuable news to media outlets. Follow these tips for a more effective release:

- Follow formatting guidelines. Samples of press release guidelines are available in Appendix B and online.
- Write in the third person. Don't use words like "I" or "we."
- Be newsworthy. Make sure that you are sharing news, not just selling something.
- Start strong, with headline and first paragraph telling the story and packing a punch.
- Illustrate impact. Has your business already solved a problem or filled a need? Share a success story, a quote or a testimonial from a happy client to show the benefit of your goods or services.
- Be timely to create a hook. Perhaps you can tie your press release to other current events or social issues.
- Avoid jargon. Remember that you are writing for a large audience that may not know industry lingo. If you use acronyms (like NCBTMB or TMJ), explain them first.
- Get permission. If you are quoting or referencing other sources, be sure that it is okay to do so.
- Be economical with wording. Try and avoid long-winded sentences and flowery or unnecessary language. Keep wording concise and to the point.

being read, and that is not what you want (see the Appendix B for a sample press release). A **press kit** is a compilation of print materials and marketing collateral that highlights key aspects of a company. While press kits are typically assembled for members of the media to provide background information about the business, more and more small businesses are redefining these kits into *informational packets* or *sales packets* for press and potential clients alike.[3] These kits typically include such information as publicity materials; brochures; fact sheets about history, mission, and key people; a copy of a recent newsletter; and a recent press release. No business is too small for a press kit. Think of a press kit as the spelled-out version of your business card—while a business card is a sampler of the "who, what, where, when, why, how," your press kit is the fleshed-out answers to all those questions.[4] And speaking of that old business card:

ANATOMY OF A BUSINESS CARD

Ah, the business card. That wonderful, ubiquitous, fantastic little worker bee of the business kingdom. Business cards are an indispensable part of your marketing campaign. A **business card** is a small card that identifies a person in relationship to a business and professional role. They are given out to people who might be potential clients, collaborative partners, or anyone else you encounter, and ideally convey the overall image of your business. They can be one of the most useful pieces of your marketing collateral, and reflect a lot about who you are as a massage therapist, as a professional, and as a business owner. For such tiny little billboards, business cards can pack quite a punch in a small amount of space.

So what should you include on your business card? A good business card offers all the essential information a potential client will need to follow up with you, either to schedule an appointment or to obtain more information (see Figure 12-3 ■). It should include company name (if you have one), your name, business address, phone number, e-mail address, and website. (A sidenote: many therapists who work from home or are not comfortable giving out their business address can write "Call for more information" or "By appointment only" in lieu of a physical address. Go with your instinct on that one.) If your business has a slogan or a logo, it should go on your card. A **logo** is a symbol or design that acts as a means of identification for a company or brand. Logos are important aspects of

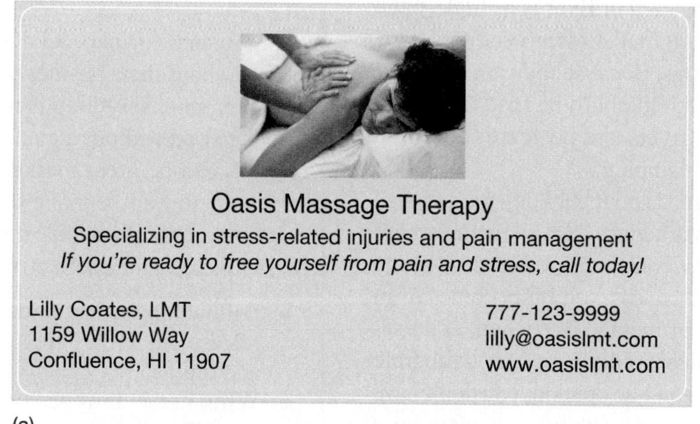

Oasis Massage Therapy
Specializing in stress-related injuries and pain management
If you're ready to free yourself from pain and stress, call today!
Lilly Coates, LMT
1159 Willow Way
Confluence, HI 11907
777-123-9999
lilly@oasislmt.com
www.oasislmt.com

(a)

Oasis Massage Therapy
Pain Retreat Reward Program
Buy 9 sessions, get your 10th massage free!
1 2 3 4 5 6 7 8 9

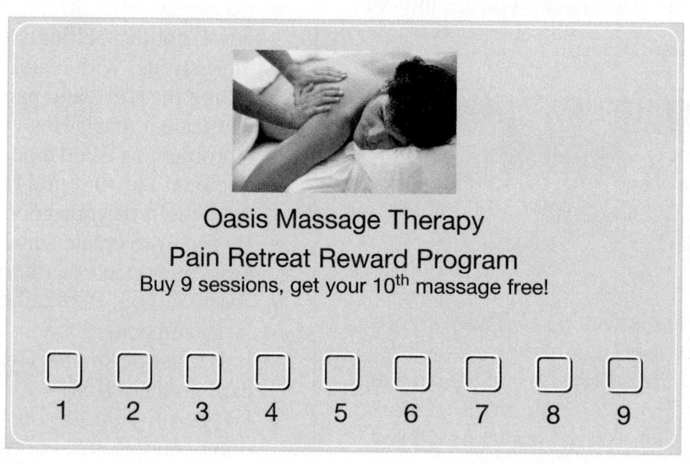

(b)

FIGURE 12-3

Business cards are tiny little billboards that can provide a lot of information about you and your business.

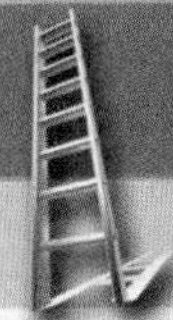

FIRST STEPS

Personal Branding

Remember all the discussion of personal brand in Chapter 2? Your business collateral and all your marketing materials can reflect and continue the personal brand you are working to cultivate. Remember to stay professional while incorporating the very unique aspects of the brand that is you!

branding your business, and should reflect the image you are trying to portray.

When you begin to design your business cards, remember that it is very important in marketing and branding to be consistent and cohesive with your design. Be intentional about your choices of color, content, style, font, card quality, and logo. Some massage therapists have been able to barter with graphic design professionals or graphic arts students to come up with some unique cards (see Chapter 13 for more information on bartering your services).

You might also want to add to your card information about the style of massage in which you specialize, such as neuromuscular or Feldenkrais, or the benefits of working with you, such as pain relief, reduced scar tissue, or increased proprioceptive awareness. Your card should also visually match all your other marketing materials, and provide visual incentives to read and retain the information. A good business card also features a **call to action,** words on marketing materials that urge the reader to take an immediate step closer to doing business with you. Examples of calls to action for a business card include: "Call today to reserve a session," "Visit our website for a free massage technique you can do anywhere," or "go to www.mycompany.com to learn the five things your doctor doesn't want you to know about massage." This call to action can be anywhere on your card, but due to limited space you might consider putting it on the back. Many professionals also use the back of their card for things such as appointment times, referral incentive programs, punch card promos to incentivize frequent visits or even reflexology charts (see Figure 12-3b for an example of maximizing the back of your business card).

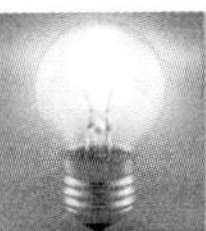

BRIGHT IDEAS

Kisha Lytle-Coffey, owner of A Beautiful U Massage, attaches small bags of bath salts to her business cards when she is promoting her spa parties at trade shows and events. People love this and always hang onto her card and remember her for parties and special occasions—long after they use the salts!

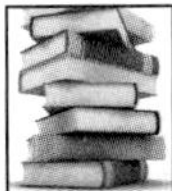

HELPFUL RESOURCES

There are many helpful resources out there to help you design your business card, create a logo, and create a marketing brand. Keep in mind that the more unique you want your marketing to be, the more expensive it can become. Graphic designers can charge multiple thousands of dollars to create custom logos. However, there are many companies out there that help small businesses economically create marketing campaigns. Check out companies like Vistaprint, Office Depot Online, and FedEx Kinko's.

Creating your cards is only one half of the equation; you will also want to get strategic about circulating them. Your business cards provide people the bridge from meeting you to working with you. You might even say so when you hand out a card with a phrase like "if you know someone who suffers from chronic pain, hang onto this card." Make sure to have an ample supply of business cards on you at all times—you never know when you might need them, or when someone might ask for a handful to distribute to friends or coworkers. Nothing looks less professional than scrawling your name on a ripped off piece of paper, so always be prepared to market your business!

When designing your business card, you can be creative while still maintaining a professional image. As with all of your marketing materials, you will want your business card to reflect the professional image you are aiming to convey. You will want to keep it simple. If it is too complicated, no one will read it. However, you want to make your business card stand out from the crowd. Some therapists have had success with unique business cards, such as making zig-zag edges, oversized cards, magnetic cards, or attaching a free gift to each card. Play with some different ideas, and choose what feels best for you and your business.

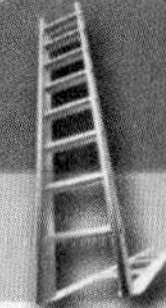

FIRST STEPS

Before you create your business card, go on a card hunt! Make it a goal to grab as many business cards as you can in the next week. Get some from the competition, but also track some down from other types of businesses and other industries as well. Notice what catches your eye, and also pay attention to cards that you do not care for.

THRIFTY MARKETING: LOW-COST MARKETING TECHNIQUES AND TOOLS

Even if you grasp the importance of marketing for your business, you may still have hang-ups about the expenses. Many new or struggling businesses let marketing fall by the wayside because they agonize over the expense. Never fear! Some of the most successful, high-earning wellness businesses were started on a shoestring, and today there are abundant cost-effective techniques that can complement your holistic practice. There are also many ways you can propel your business in a collaborative way. In your marketing plan, you did an analysis of your competition. Remember that your competition can also be your support. **Cooperative marketing** is the practice of jointly promoting distinctive businesses, and is something you can undertake with other massage therapists, other holistic practitioners, or other businesses in general. Marketing alliances can be undertaken with chiropractors, aromatherapists, acupuncturists, counselors, physical therapists, doulas, nutritionists, and so forth. Anyone in your circle of influence can become a cooperative marketing partner.

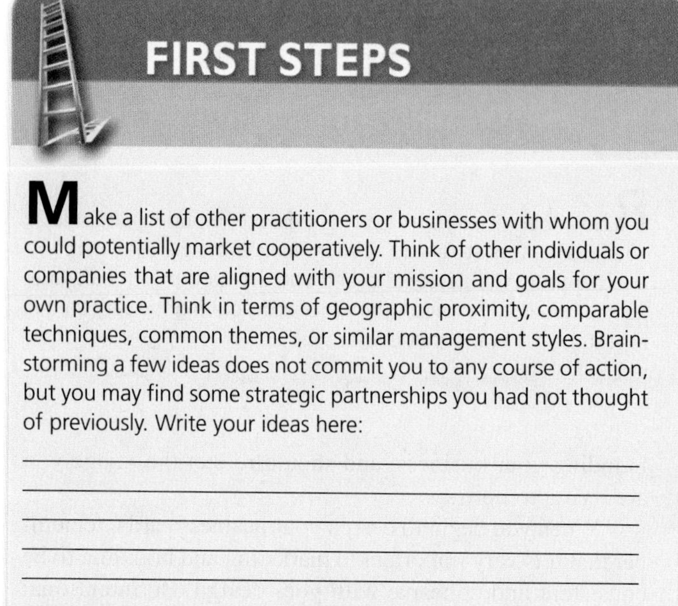

FIRST STEPS

Make a list of other practitioners or businesses with whom you could potentially market cooperatively. Think of other individuals or companies that are aligned with your mission and goals for your own practice. Think in terms of geographic proximity, comparable techniques, common themes, or similar management styles. Brainstorming a few ideas does not commit you to any course of action, but you may find some strategic partnerships you had not thought of previously. Write your ideas here:

____

____

____

____

____

____

> *Great discoveries and improvements invariably involve the cooperation of many minds.*
>
> —Alexander Graham Bell

Partnering with others to promote your business has many advantages: it can reduce the financial outlay for advertisements or websites, alleviate some of the time and responsibilities involved in marketing, help you network with other professionals in a supportive way, and also help you psychologically ease into the world of marketing as part of a collaborating team rather than a lone wolf.[5]

Depending upon the scope of your practice, the size of your business, and your level of experience, you may be very attracted to **low-cost/no-cost marketing** techniques. You don't need to spend excessively to have effective exposure. One great low-cost/no-cost technique is to leverage the already potent power of word of mouth advertising, which you learned about in the last chapter. Give your clients a reason (aside from your inherent talent, of course) to promote you by asking for and rewarding referrals. A **referral** is an endorsement of a good or service, typically by someone who has experienced it and was pleased. Talk to your satisfied clients and invite them to tell friends and family about you, and even to distribute your marketing collateral on your behalf. To give clients an extra incentive to talk you up, offer discounts on massage for each client they send your way. Many therapists not only give a discount to the person doing the referring, but also mark down the initial session for the new client who comes in through an existing client. This way, everyone wins and word of mouth can work rapidly. Because it costs so much more to attract a client than to keep a client,[6] the short-term cost of offering referral discounts are often recovered quickly.

PITFALLS

Many therapists feel conflicted over the issues of both competition and collaboration. As healers, we tend to be resistant to cutthroat rivalry with our competitors. Yet many often have a hard time collaborating with other businesses for fear of losing clients or potential income. Often, a balance between the two is necessary. Examine your levels of comfort with both competition and collaboration.

A strong word of caution, however. Some therapists have taken to implementing this same system with other holistic practitioners, offering money or discounts for each referral. While professional referrals are very common, and can be an important part of your collaborative marketing efforts, be certain that your motivations are in the right place. Be cautious of employing an incentive or money-based referral program with other practitioners. Doing so could cause a conflict of interest and be a breach of ethics. The NCBTMB even states that massage therapists should "refuse any gifts or benefits which are intended to influence a referral, decision or treatment that are purely for personal gain and not for the good of the client."[7] When it comes to building practitioner referral networks, make sure that the best interests and needs of the client are the basis of all referrals.

The following are a few more suggestions for low-cost/no-cost marketing in addition to those already mentioned throughout the chapter:

- *Chair massage:* Chair massage is a great, portable way of marketing your practice. What better way to inform people of your talents than to let them experience a "hands-on" sample of your skill? Many therapists do chair massage in venues with high concentrations of their target market—hospitals, sporting events, wellness fairs, and so forth. Some charge, some volunteer their time; either way, they get a lot of exposure and hand out a lot of business cards.

- *Educate your clients:* Remember, marketing relates to your existing clients as well as to potential ones. In order to get clients coming back, it may help to educate them on the value of your service and the benefits provided. Let them know what regular massage can do for them and their well-being. You have spent time and money studying massage; they have not. You can informally educate your market in conversation, in your brochures, on your website, in newsletters, with flyers, and in e-mails. Be careful not to overload people with information, but hit on the educational highlights and focus on the benefits.
- *Teach a class:* You will also want to think about formally educating your target market. If your location allows, you can teach a lunchtime class in your space, or sign up to teach in your area. Teaching a class on massage at the local community school or a local sports group is a great way to get your name circulated. It also helps position you as an expert in your field. And, as they say, the best way to learn is to teach. (As a bonus, this free marketing might actually *pay you!*)
- *Community boards:* There are many tangible and virtual community boards upon which therapists advertise their services for free. Grocery stores and coffee shops often have a board for community members to post upon. Kijiji, Craigslist, Froogle, and Fremont are all online boards. www.craigslist.com is a popular site for anyone who wants to post ads for free, and 30 million visitors go there every month to buy, sell, and trade. (Because anyone can use these sites, you may have a harder time reaching your target market and you must be conscientious of security concerns. See Chapter 15, "Leveraging the Internet," for more information.)
- *Newsletters:* Many therapists find regular newsletters to be a wonderful and inexpensive marketing tool. Contributing to the educational theme, newsletters are a great way of informing current and potential clients of massage trends, benefits, and, of course, you! Done professionally and consistently, they can build client loyalty, keep you fresh in clients' minds, and announce your services to your target market. Newsletters can also enhance your credibility by establishing you as an expert. Using your database and subscriber lists, these can be delivered through traditional mail or e-mail (which is increasingly more common). Along with your business card and brochure, you can also hand out your newsletters in person at health fairs, sporting events, or workshops.
- *Give sample massages to possible referrers:* Referrals can be a cornerstone of a marketing strategy. Offer to give a free massage to another professional who also serves your target market: doctors, chiropractors, TMJ dentists, personal trainers, midwives, yoga teachers, and so forth.
- *Create a referral program for clients:* Many therapists offer discounts, retail gifts, or special prizes as part of their referral programs. Referral programs reward clients for their endorsement of your services. This entices existing customers to "sell you" to their friends and families.
- *Volunteer at community events:* Break out your massage chair and volunteer your services at local fundraisers, sporting events, or any other community event. This is a great way to enhance your community relations and get your name (and hands!) out there. You can also donate gift certificates to local charities or school auctions. Remember, volunteering and donations can also be tax deductible for your business (see Chapter 10).
- *Send birthday, holiday, or special occasion cards to your clients:* The time and expense it takes to send a card to a client celebrating a special occasion is nothing compared to the meaning it can have. Such a gesture can go a long way towards building client loyalty. You can also include a special discount to entice clients to schedule their next appointment.
- *Build a referral network of other massage therapists and holistic healers:* There will be times when the needs of your clients extend beyond the scope of your practice. Establish a good network of skilled practitioners to whom you can refer your clients. Doing so demonstrates your openness and integrated philosophy to clients, and can help build loyalty. Other therapists and holistic healers will be more likely to refer back to you as well.

PUT IT IN WRITING

Parsimonious Marketing

There are loads of free or inexpensive ways to promote your business. What other low-cost/no-cost marketing ideas can you come up with? Brainstorm some ideas in the space provided below. Then circle your top three choices and put them into action!

____

____

____

____

____

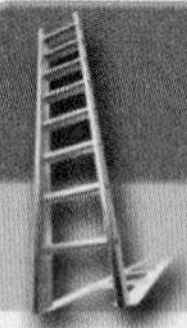

FIRST STEPS

Most small business development centers and local community schools offer inexpensive classes on marketing that are targeted towards small business owners. Check out the ones in your area, and find out what they have to offer. Not only will you learn additional ways to make your practice even more successful, classes are a great way to continue your education while you network with other professionals and members of your target market.

HOW TO CRAFT AND DELIVER YOUR ELEVATOR PITCH

In Chapters 1 and 2, you heard about elevator pitches, those quick 10- to 30-second summaries of who you are, what you do, and why people would want to work with you. These are fabulous little marketing and career advancing gems. An elevator speech encapsulates your **unique promise,** the exceptional and inimitable qualities that you possess as well as the benefit those qualities consistently bring to others. Your unique promise is the compelling solution that you provide in response to the pressing problem of your niche market.[8]

An elevator pitch is a prime player in your **conversion process,** the systematic way in which you turn prospects into customers. In other words, the conversion process is the way in which you build relationships with others to turn possible customers into happy clients. You want to give people a compelling reason to not only take your marketing materials, but to read and hold on to them, follow up with you, and become regular clients.

An elevator pitch is not only a marketing and sales tool, but a communications and teaching tool as well. It gives you a chance to shine in the subject that you love the most as you inform people who probably do not know as much as you do about massage. Your pitch should be designed with clients' needs in mind, be solutions-focused, and should provide just enough information to keep people engaged but not overwhelmed. Providing too much information on what you have to offer can make people tune out (tip: do not include an in-depth analysis of proprioceptive neuromuscular facilitation or the deleterious effects of stagnant hyluronic acid in the muscles when crafting your elevator pitch!!). As pitch experts advise, "think drinking fountain, not fire hose."[9] Potential clients are interested in the big-picture solutions that you can provide for them, not the intricate details of the inner workings of the body that you have spent so many long hours learning. At the same time, you don't want to be overly vague or general, or simply say "I'm a massage therapist", which does not paint much of a picture.

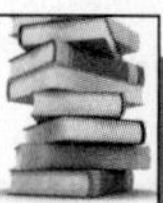

HELPFUL RESOURCES

For more information on inexpensive ways to market your massage practice, check out the Spalutions! and Bodywork Biz, websites or www.thebodyworker.com. They all offer tips and advice on how to market yourself and your practice.

So how do you create an elevator pitch? Focus on your ideal clients. What is their goal? What is their vision? Can you think what inspires them to action? Now think of some of your actual client success stories. If your ideal client were telling someone else about you, what might they say? Incorporate all those ideas into your pitch—but remember your Cs. According to pitch expert Chris O'Leary, there are nine Cs of writing a pitch. A good pitch should be:

- Concise
- Clear
- Compelling
- Credible
- Conceptual
- Concrete
- Consistent
- Customized
- Conversational

Great job! By having a compelling pitch you are head and shoulders ahead of the competition. Once you get it down—practice, practice, practice. And then practice some more. Be ready to give your pitch at any time, anywhere, and to anyone. The idea isn't to have a canned presentation, but to be fluent in your own fabulousness so you won't get tongue tied or miss great opportunities. And remember, your goal is not only to promote your business, it is to earnestly educate and be of service in the world. Authenticity has everything to do with elevator pitches, and they can create beneficial learning experiences for others!

NICHE MARKETING: ENSURING YOUR MARKETING MESSAGE GETS TO THE RIGHT PEOPLE

It can be difficult to break through all the competing messages out there in order to ensure that your marketing message is reaching the right people. Do you remember in the last chapter where you learned that the average person can be exposed to thousands of marketing messages *a day?* With the near-constant bombardment that nearly everyone experiences, your marketing message can easily get tuned out or lost altogether. One way to counter this is to get laser sharp on your target market, your compelling promise, and your niche.

Niche marketing is a style of promotion that identifies and targets a specific client demographic. Niche marketing focuses on solving the specific needs of that group, which is

PUT IT IN WRITING

The Pitch

Jot down some notes for the following questions, and see if you can parse your brainstorm into a cohesive pitch, When you finish, keep it on file in your *Business of Massage Therapy* notebook for future reference.

1. Who is your ideal client?

 ____

 ____

2. What are her goals in life?

 ____

 ____

3. What are her struggles?

 ____

 ____

4. How can you help? What solutions have you already provided to others?

 ____

 ____

5. If your ideal client were to write a testimonial for you, what would it say?

 ____

 ____

 ____

6. Now try to sum it all up into a succinct pitch:

 ____

 ____

 ____

a subset of a larger market. For example, "working mothers" are a market, but "Latina working mothers in their 30s with family incomes over $120,000" is a niche market. A niche can be based on factors such as stage of life, professional interests, unique problems, or a collection of common characteristics, such as age or geographic location.[10] As a massage therapist, your niche is often going to relate to the problems they struggle with (such as postsurgical pain) and the solution you provide (decreased scarring, improved recovery time; see Figure 12-4 ■).

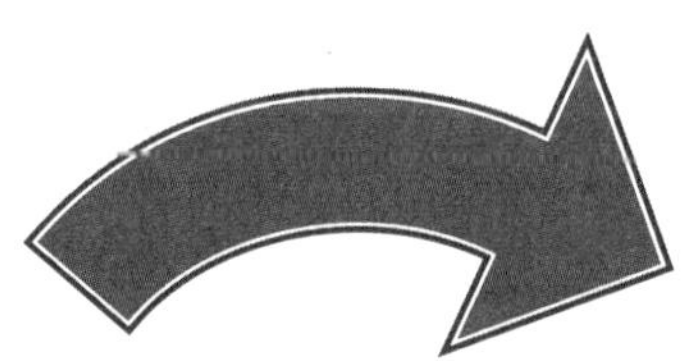

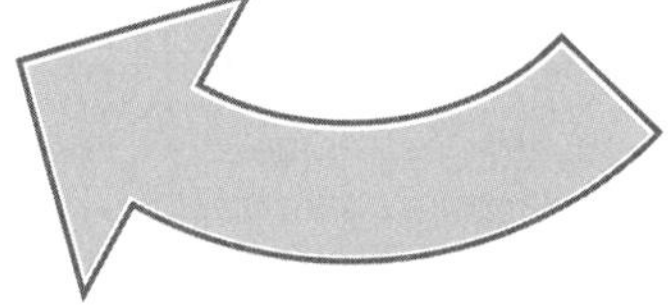

FIGURE 12-4

Niche marketing is a style of promotion that identifies and targets a specific client demographic.

Not all massages modalities are created equal, of course. Marketing that works for a day spa will not be as affective for an NMT therapist specializing in thoracic outlet syndrome, and vice versa. The TOS specialist might not fare so well at the bridal expo. And the spa might find few prospects sending their marketing materials to a local physical therapists' association. The spa would likely find more qualified prospects at that bridal fair. A **qualified prospect** is a potential buyer who has the necessary need, financial resources, motivation, and authority to make a buying decision on a good or service.

With a clear vision of your target and a succinct and well-honed message, you become a magnet for your ideal customers. You want to draw clients who "get it," rather than chasing those that don't. This will not only save you loads of energy, but will help make you more effective in your business by working with people who want what you have to offer and will keep coming back for more (and referring friends along the way)!

Some holistic practitioners balk at the idea of narrowing their niche, afraid that doing so will lose potential clients and won't be able to support a business. Another common concern is that narrowing a target market will exclude people in need. They go for the "spray-and-pray approach," hoping if they just cast their nets wide and throw marketing out into the ether, clients of all stripes are bound to beat down the door. However, most people find that the opposite happens—clients barely trickle and the phone doesn't ring. In fact, seasoned experts maintain that the more specific you can be about your target, the better your chances for success. Additionally, trying to cater to everyone will likely dilute your message

PITFALLS

Many therapists balk at the concept of a niche market for fear that they are excluding potential customers and getting trapped in one specialty only. While narrowing your focus has been proved again and again to simplify and enhance marketing efforts, don't think that making a niche market of pregnant mothers in their late 30s in Cleveland means you will never work with a nonpregnant client again in your life. You may find that you have an overlap in niches, or that people gravitate towards your work from different demographics. You can always work with whomever you want. This may be something to experiment with over time. Remember that targeting your markets is meant to simplify and strengthen your marketing message, not trap you into a corner.

and even your expertise. Drawing out a laundry list of all the styles of massage you learned in school and having a vague client profile can actually confuse clients. And as holistic business coach Marilyn O'Leary maintains, "confused people don't buy."

THE GREAT COMMUNICATOR: WHAT COMMUNICATIONS CAN DO FOR YOUR MARKETING

In this day of constant connection, viral marketing, Facebook, and Twitter, communication has become more important than ever. **Communications** is the practice of transmitting information or exchanging ideas with others, and is increasingly done through virtual and electronic means. Many small businesses are identifying the benefit of frequent contact with their target market. While massage is a historically "high-touch, low-tech" field, if you feel comfortable or have any interest in incorporating current technologies into your business, you may gain a substantial edge over the competition. You are going to learn more about using the Internet strategically, including information about blogs, newsletters, and e-zines in Chapter 15, "Leveraging the Internet," but this section will give you some information on incorporating social networking and other communication tools into your business.

Holistic practitioners have long incorporated newsletters into their business practices. A **newsletter** is a periodically distributed communiqué that addresses topics of interest and business-related information to a target market or subscribers. In the environmentally conscious electronic age, very few newsletters are printed on paper and snail-mailed (although this is a perfectly acceptable option). Newsletters are a great opportunity to educate your niche market on particular aspects of the work that you do. They can also include information on current specials, upcoming events, community occasions, health tips, or recent trends in the massage industry. Regular newsletters are multipurpose marketing tools—they can attract new clients, expose your other services to existing clients, bring back a client who hasn't thought to come in for awhile, educate, and strengthen your position as an expert in your field.[11]

Many small businesses are building their subscriber lists and sending out regular newsletters and communications via an auto responder service. An **auto responder** is a program that automatically responds to an incoming e-mail or delivers information via e-mail on behalf of a person or company. Certain paid services, such as Aweber Communications or Constant Contact, help you build a subscriber list while following legal guidelines to avoid spamming (see Chapter 10, "Organizing and Legal Structure"). They can also help you send out regular promotions, newsletters, surveys, or other communications tools via e-mail. They also help you track the statistics of your communications, so you can see who is actually reading the e-mail you sent or clicking on links to your website.

In recent years, the Internet has become an instant celebrity maker, as people are able to broadcast and share just about anything with just about anyone, who then pass that anything along to just about everyone else. Because of this "exponential potential," viral marketing has become a very

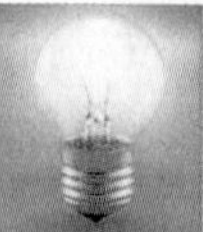

BRIGHT IDEAS

Targeting and Websites

As consumers are gravitating more and more towards identifying and acquiring goods and services online, websites are invaluable marketing tools for businesses of all kinds. They can also help you with your niche marketing, as people will be entering specific keywords to find a business just like yours. A well-designed and well-optimized website can be a mighty magnet for individuals in your niche market. You will learn about designing and managing websites in Chapter 15, and as you do, keep in mind ways that you can use this powerful tool to attract your niche market and catapult your business.

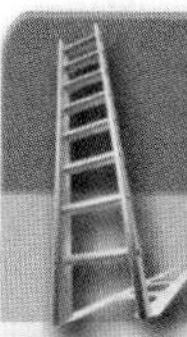

FIRST STEPS

Take It to the Life Lab

Go through your own e-mail messages and see how many of them have been sent from an auto responder such as those listed above. What do you notice about this kind of e-mail marketing? What do you like or dislike about it? What do you think of the aesthetic? How did you get on the mailing lists? Do the e-mails follow the anti-spamming rules?

powerful marketing technique. **Viral marketing** is a strategy that replicates word of mouth advertising, encouraging people to pass along a marketing message to others until it spreads exponentially (hence the name). While viral marketing may not be the answer for all holistic businesses, it may be a good option for you depending on your scale, scope, and company positioning.

You may not want to (and probably shouldn't) paste your personal exploits all over YouTube or Twitter yourself into oblivion, but fortunately you do not need to become a flash in the Internet celebrity pan in order to benefit from viral marketing. You can invite clients to share your newsletters, or include a referral incentive in your marketing materials that entices people to pass along your marketing. You could also create something valuable that gets forwarded—an e-book on stress management, or an article of five pressure points you can work at the office. Perhaps you specialize in a certain modality, such as pre-natal massage or reflexology; you could record and post a video of five basic techniques that could be done by a friend or partner, then suggest people share them with others. Think of creative ways you can use technology to propel word of mouth about you and your business.

Learning how to minimize your efforts while maximizing your impact is one of the key lessons for successful business owners. Because you just can't be everywhere at once, many therapists have incorporated video and audio messages into their websites and e-mail messages. Some even host their own e-radio shows. Many businesses put a welcome video on their website, or videorecord information about an exciting new service in one of their mass e-mails. This lends an extra air of familiarity and personalization to your message, while you only have to make one recording.

Some holistic practitioners who are really serious about growing their businesses exponentially have created teleclasses and webinars to communicate with large groups of their target market clients. Doing this drastically increases your income potential without changing your energy output. Naturally, as a massage therapist, you can't easily give a massage to more than one person at a time, or even attempt to give one through a teleclass. However, think about creative ways that you could turn your skills and knowledge into valuable information for a larger audience. Perhaps you could offer clients a stress-reduction workshop, or demonstrate stretches to avoid injury through a webinar. Think of ways to creatively apply your natural talents and interests in new ways.

Not ready for prime time? Relax—you don't have to be a cyberjunkie with a master's degree in Web 2.0 to apply the technologies discussed here! Although it is typically associated with the Internet, viral marketing can take place on a smaller scale offline. Techniques like incentivized referral programs operate under the same premise. One clever approach is to create a "same day" list, an exclusive list of clients who are willing to be called and offered discounted sessions when last-minute appointments become available. Not only does this give your clients something of perceived value through a discount, it also helps you build loyalty, grow your subscriber list, and keep your appointment calendar full when you have last-minute cancellations. Such an offsite technique can also be a part of word of mouth marketing.

Whether you are the sole therapist or are overseeing 20 others, it helps to tap into the power of the celebrity expert with your marketing and communications campaign. Every time you present yourself as an expert in your trade, whether offline or through videos, teleconferences, newsletters, blogs, and other means, you are building credibility and positioning yourself as a go-to resource in the minds of your target or niche market. To further develop credibility, it is a great idea to add an "In the News" tab on your website, and include any articles, profiles, or press releases that feature your business (even if you wrote them yourself). The more people see you this way, the better your business will thrive. And after all, that's what every business owner wants, right?

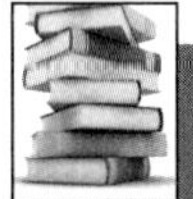

HELPFUL RESOURCES

These days, when it comes to communication and marketing, the sky isn't even the limit anymore. Many companies have sprung up around viral marketing and social networking (which often overlap). Many businesses use Ning, YouTube, Facebook, Squidoo, MySpace, Digg, Flickr, Photobucket, and Twitter to surreptitiously promote themselves or their business (always remember: don't be too pushy!). Sites such as www.gotomeeting.com or www.goconference.com can help you put on a teleclass. Use your PDF publisher to create an e-book, or check out such sites as www.lulu.com that can help you publish your own book. Wanna be a radio star? Sign up for your own show at www.blogtalkradio.com. Opportunities abound!

RECESSION DEPRESSION: PROTECTING YOUR BUSINESS THROUGH ECONOMIC STORMS

When everyone seems to be going against you, remember that the airplane takes off against the wind, not with it.

—Henry Ford

You know for a fact that massage is a viable and valuable service. However, when it comes to public perception and massage's place on the consumer survival pyramid, the reality is that many perceive massage as a discretionary spending item. **Discretionary spending** is the portion of an individual or group's outflow of money that is nonessential.

As wonderful as massage is, it is often one of the first line items to be cut when the economy turns or one's finances go sour. Because of this, massage therapy can often be an ebb-and-flow, feast-or-famine kind of industry.

Massage therapists and holistic businesses are often particularly hard hit in a recession. A **recession** is a period of time when the gross domestic product growth is negative for two or more consecutive quarters. Other indicators such as investment spending, employment, household income and expenditures, and business profits all tend to decline in a recession.[12] Unless you have been without any media outlets or have been seeing clients from under a rock somewhere, you have probably heard a lot about recessions in recent times, and have seen the near panic brought about by its mere mention. You have also probably experienced the effects of a recession directly; perhaps you or someone you know has been laid off from a job, or maybe your clients have cut back on sessions or ceased coming altogether.

When going through tough economic times, many companies have a knee-jerk reaction to cut marketing efforts and expenditures to save money. At a time when budgets are being cut across the board, this can seem to make sense in the short term. However it is important to understand that contracting your marketing efforts and budgets can actually hinder you during tough financial times and continue to stunt you when the economy recovers. Businesses that cut their marketing budgets also tend to see a subsequent decrease in sales. Bad economic times can actually be a blessing in disguise and great for businesses with disciplined marketing efforts. After all, someone is always making money out there and it might as well be you! Remember, there are all those low-cost and no-cost marketing techniques you can continue to employ even in lean times.

However, marketing in tough economic times is not just about continuing volume or carrying on as usual, especially for massage therapy. Part of successful marketing in this time is to be strategic about your positioning. It is important to be mindful and sensitive to the fears people are having in tough economic times, and to appeal to their basic needs. While a luxurious pampering session at a day spa might not be a need, being free of debilitating pain might be. (To be fair, a day of luxurious pampering may well *be* a need for some; it all depends on the target market.) Marketing activities should take into account the difference between needs and wants.

It might help to take a quick stroll through the needs pyramid presented by humanistic psychologist Abraham Maslow, and to look at ways to incorporate massage therapy and its benefits into the needs hierarchy.[13] **Maslow's hierarchy of needs** (Figure 12-5 ■) is a theory and model that evaluates human motivation from the most fundamental to the most advanced, often graphically depicted as a triangle. At the bottom of the needs pyramid are the basic physiological needs for an individual's survival: food, water, oxygen, and homeostasis. On the next level are the comfort and security needs: employment, productivity, family security. The third level involves love and belonging, and relates to how a person fits into his community, the friendships he is a part of, and his family harmony. The next level up is esteem: feelings of achievement, self-respect, respect from others, and confidence. Finally, the top level of the pyramid is self-actualization, and addresses the more transcendental needs such as morality, spirituality, meaning, and creativity.

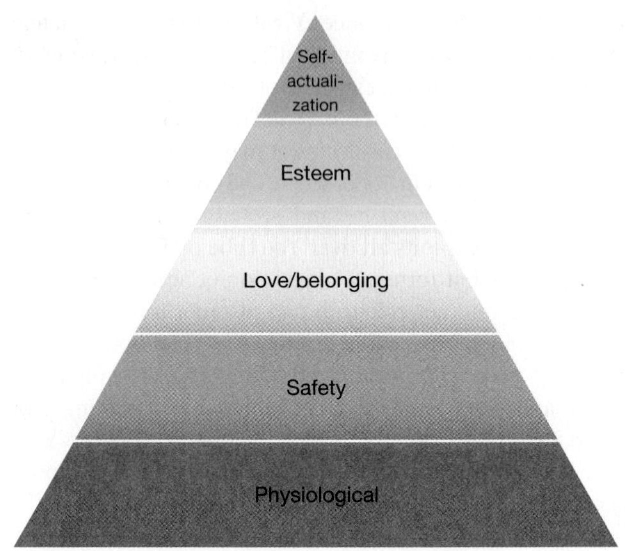

FIGURE 12-5

Maslow's hierarchy of needs.

Source: Maslow, A. (1954). *Motivation and Personality.* New York: Harper.

Even if your business model involves pampering over survival necessity, or if your prior marketing efforts have emphasized luxury, it is okay to change gears to attract and retain newly budget-sensitive clients. In fact, the smaller your business, the easier it can be to be agile with your marketing message. Another thing you may want to consider is expanding your services along a price ladder. A **price ladder** provides a variety of products and services at graduated prices in order to accommodate different clients' price sensitivity and commitment levels. For example, at the low end of the ladder you might have a free or very inexpensive class on pre-natal massage techniques for pregnant women and their partners. At the high end you might offer a massage retreat to a select number of VIP clients. Price ladders are always a good idea, but a comprehensive and adaptable one can be essential in challenging financial times.

You may also need to be more assertive during a recession, and it may become necessary to stretch outside of your comfort zone. Get out there and network, network, network! Pick up the phone and call old clients or potential leads

PUT IT IN WRITING

Hierarchy of Needs

Looking at the pyramid in Figure 12-5, how can you position your business and its services in a way that addresses the hierarchy of needs for your clients? For example, at the physiological level, regular massage helps maintain homeostasis and delivers nutrients and oxygen to ischemic muscles. At the love and belonging level, perhaps you have holiday gift certificates discounted for coworkers or family members. Brainstorm a few ideas for each level here:

Physiological:

____

____

Comfort and security:

____

____

Esteem:

____

____

Love and belonging:

____

____

Self-actualization:

____

____

During tough economic times, it may be more useful to focus your positioning on solutions to the more basic needs rather than the more esoteric ones. However, it is always helpful to have a firm handle and empirical examples of how massage can benefit a client's needs at every level.

directly, informing them of specials, new services, or upcoming events. Here are a few other ideas for holding it strong during a recession:

- Review all of the low-cost/no-cost marketing techniques you learned earlier in this chapter and put them to use. Then do some research and brainstorming to come up with even more. This will help you cut costs but stay visible.
- Give clients a discount for prepayment, or for buying in bulk through packages.
- Reward consistent clients with free gifts or discounts.
- Check out what the competition is doing to weather the storm.
- Continue to build that network of cross-collaborators and referring practitioners.
- Regularly assess your expenditures and evaluate if there are ways to cut money without cutting value (for example, a less expensive linen service or purified water distributor).
- Diversify your portfolio: add complimentary services to your repertoire, such as chair massage or in-room visits for hotels. Or you might start offering self-massage or couples' massage classes. Remember, you don't want to try to be all things to all people, but think outside of the box with the services you can offer that stay aligned to your overarching mission.
- Take the rescheduling lead: it's simple, but simply asking clients if they would like to reschedule after a massage can bolster your business. Many clients simply do not think to ask for a follow-up appointment, so taking the initiative can impact your bottom line.

Keep in mind that businesses of every size and industry can still grow and flourish in a recession. Bill Gates started Microsoft in the middle of a recession, after all. Also keep in mind that financial conditions are always in a state of flux, and you and your business can't afford to succumb to fear during down times. Keep positive and get creative about solutions—your perseverance and hard work will pay off, both in the short and long run.

IDENTIFYING WAYS TO MANAGE MARKETING OVERLOAD

You have absorbed a lot of information in this chapter and throughout the book. It can be a little overwhelming to process it all, especially if a lot of the information is new for you. As you already know, it can easily be all-consuming and stressful just to manage the business operations themselves, let alone all the ever-changing technologies and techniques of promotion. Understand that this is completely normal for anyone running a business. However the overwhelming feeling that can come with marketing a massage business and managing the supporting technologies deserves special mention.

PITFALLS

E-mail campaigns? Twitter? Webinars? A press kit? Social networking? A radio show!? Many people get overwhelmed with all the possibilities in marketing and therefore elect to do nothing at all. Don't let yourself get bogged down by all the choices, but rather experiment with what feels right for you, your personality, and your business goals. And remember, no one expects a perfect 10 the first time on the mat. If something doesn't work, try something else. Keep trying things out until you achieve your optimal marketing mix—and have fun!

The technological advances of the last century have been phenomenal: anecdotal evidence suggests that a person living a century ago might, if fortunate, accrue enough information in a lifetime to fill one single edition of today's Sunday *New York Times*.[14] That certainly makes for an interesting cocktail party factoid, but what does that mean for you? It goes without saying that processing more information in a day than your great grandparents amassed in a lifetime can overload the mind from time to time. **Information overload** results from the tremendous quantity of information that is presented almost constantly and that typically tends to be more than can be effectively processed by an individual. In our global world of 24-hour newscycles, overflowing e-mail inboxes and Twitter tweets, it often feels as though there is a constant information tsunami. The reality is that information overload and even fear of information overload can be a big barrier to your marketing efforts and your business.

What's more, as a business owner trying to keep up with all the rapidly evolving gadgets, gizmos, applications, software, sites, and "must–have" tools of a hyperconnected world, it is not uncommon to experience bouts of technology fatigue. **Technology fatigue** is the overwhelmed feeling that comes with the bewildering amount of rapidly evolving communications and information tools, such as social networking, e-mail marketing, online communities, and other "hands on" technological applications.

Chances are good that you entered the massage field because you are interested in a different kind of "hands-on technology." Maybe you don't like to labor over learning something new only to have that knowledge become obsolete in the blink of an eye. However, rather than declaring yourself a Luddite and shunning all technology in the name of self-preservation whenever information overload or technology fatigue set in, take a deep breath. Remember that not only is the livelihood of many small businesses entwined with these advances, they can offer amazing opportunities for you to not only survive, but seriously thrive. And in any market!

You have already learned many tips on self-care, but here are a few tips specifically intended to fend off (or at least manage) information overload and technology exhaustion while running your business:

- *Step back.* If you are feeling beholden to your mounting tweets or the rolling responsibility of updating your blog, go drink a cup or tea or step outside and go for a walk. The world won't end if no one knows how many sit-ups you just did.
- *Give yourself a "news fast" for a week.* Turn off the television and filter out the news on your computer. Sometimes you have to trust that the world will go on without you knowing about it.
- *Get organized.* Separate your e-mails into priority folders, and only devote so much time to responding. You might even make a Twitter or Facebook plan, so they don't begin to drain your time and productivity.
- *Evaluate benefits.* Don't apply technologies that don't really make sense or benefit your business model. Take time to really assess what, if any, advantage something will bring you and your business.
- *Outsource.* While it's good to have a cursory understanding of the technologies representing your business, you do not have to master every single detail. There are a lot of talented people and services out there who can do the work for you. Many savvy holistic practitioners even outsource their blogs, newsletters, and social networking tasks to free up time to focus on "hands-on" technologies. Hire people that play at the things you have to work at.
- *Unplug.* Close the e-mail and turn off the phone/BlackBerry/iPhone. As hard as this one can be for a 24/7 business owner, it is imperative to disconnect sometimes.

Incredible job! After two full chapters on marketing, you are now a promotion professional, a communications crackerjack, and a hands down marketing maestro! In addition to the fundamentals of marketing from the previous chapter, you have now learned how to craft strategic and impactful marketing materials and business cards, how to succinctly communicate the benefits of your business to anyone you meet, how to reach your niche market, how to keep your holistic business afloat in economic downturns, and how to manage the very real threats to marketing endeavors: information overload and technology fatigue. Armed with all of this information, you are now a marketing maven and poised to take your business to unlimited heights!

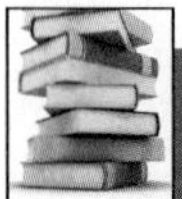

HELPFUL RESOURCES

If information overload becomes a real issue for you, check out *Surviving Information Overload: The Clear, Practical Guide to Help You Stay on Top of What You Need to Know* by Kevin Miller (2004, Zondervan).

CHAPTER SUMMARY BY LEARNING OBJECTIVES

1. **Discuss why marketing is important for the massage professional** Nearly all businesses rely on marketing to attract customers. However, many massage therapists shy away from marketing themselves and their business. Even with the best technical skills, a massage business cannot survive if it doesn't have clients.
2. **Evaluate marketing considerations and challenges unique to the massage industry** The massage industry requires practitioners and business owners to develop unique and adaptive marketing skills to stand out from the competition and survive economic changes. Because massage is such a personalized service, it carries a unique set of marketing considerations.
3. **Identify essential marketing materials for massage therapists** Marketing collateral is a collection of any type of media that supports the promotion of your services and/or products. It includes materials such as business cards, fliers, press kits, sales packets, printed materials, signs and posters, websites, paper and e-newsletters, and so forth.
4. **Examine the anatomy of a business card** A good business card offers all the essential information a potential client will need to follow up with you, either to schedule an appointment or to obtain more information. It should include company name (if you have one), your name, business address, phone number, e-mail address, and website. It should also match all of your other collateral, and include a call to action that prompts someone to learn more or follow up.
5. **Introduce cooperative marketing, low-cost and no-cost marketing techniques and tools** Cooperative marketing is the practice of jointly promoting distinctive businesses, and is something you can undertake with other massage therapists, other holistic practitioners, or other businesses in general. There are myriad low-cost and no-cost marketing techniques and tools available to massage professionals.
6. **Illustrate how to craft and deliver an elevator pitch for the massage therapist** An elevator speech encapsulates your unique promise, the exceptional and inimitable qualities that you possess as well as the benefit those qualities consistently bring to others. It is the compelling solution that you provide in response to the pressing problem of your niche market. An elevator pitch is a great way to express concisely what you have to offer and why people should work with you.
7. **Explore niche marketing for different massage modalities and different target markets** With the near-constant bombardment that nearly everyone experiences, your marketing message can easily get tuned out or lost altogether. One way to counter this is to get laser sharp on your target market, your compelling promise, and your niche. Niche marketing is a style of promotion that identifies and targets a specific client demographic. Niche marketing focuses on solving the specific needs of that group, which is a subset of a larger market.
8. **Examine the role of communications in marketing massage** Communications is the practice of transmitting information or exchanging ideas with others, and is increasingly done through virtual and electronic means. Many small businesses are identifying the benefit of frequent contact with their target market, using tools such as newsletters, auto responders, blogs, or e-mail. Some holistic practitioners use video on their websites, or host webinars and teleseminars as a way of communicating with a broad audience.
9. **Learn ways to "recession-proof" your practice through marketing** Although many companies cut marketing expenditures during tough economic times, it is more important than ever to continue marketing and to position your business strategically. Consider client needs versus wants in marketing endeavors, and implement low-cost and no-cost marketing techniques to ensure that you and your business remain visible and viable.
10. **Identify ways to manage marketing information overload and exhaustion** As an individual and as a business owner, it is very common to experience information overload and technology exhaustion when managing marketing tasks. Counter this by being strategic about technologies, and setting clear boundaries for use.

ACTIVITIES

Quiz: Identifying Massage Marketing Words and Concepts

1. A/n _____ is a potential buyer who has the necessary need, financial resources, motivation, and authority to make a buying decision on a good or service.
   a. sure thing
   b. qualified prospect
   c. client
   d. referral
2. Successful marketing of any business is the culmination of three critical areas: marketing _____, marketing _____, and marketing _____.
   a. skills, systems, tools
   b. systems, technologies, collateral
   c. tools, passion, esthetics
   d. skills, education, budget
3. The psychological theory that evaluates human motivation from the most fundamental to the most advanced needs is called _____.
   a. the All About Me Model
   b. the Pythagorean Theorem
   c. Cognitive Behavioral Theory
   d. Maslow's Hierarchy of Needs
4. What are essential components that a business card could have?
   a. name and phone number
   b. e-mail and website
   c. company logo, solutions provided, and a call to action
   d. all the above
5. A/n _____ is a compilation of print materials and marketing collateral that highlights key aspects of a company, and that is often sent to press or potential clients to market the business.
   a. sales kit
   b. press kit
   c. ad campaign
   d. both a and b
6. A/n ______ can be defined as a period of time when gross domestic product growth is negative for two or more consecutive quarters and can result in a decrease in spending on _____.
   a. depression, anything
   b. stagflation, necessary items
   c. recession, discretionary goods and services
   d. time of economic growth, education
7. According to Maslow, human beings cannot focus on any of their other needs when their _____ are not met.
   a. need for love and belonging
   b. basic physiological needs
   c. self-actualization needs
   d. vacation needs
8. _____ is a strategy that replicates word of mouth advertising, encouraging people to pass along a marketing message to others until it spreads exponentially. This is usually done online.
   a. Viral marketing
   b. Contagious targeting
   c. Marketing epidemic
   d. Outbreak networking
9. _____ is/are the processes you have in place to identify leads, bait potential clients, convert them into actual clients, and retain them in your business.
   a. Marketing tools
   b. Legal organization
   c. Social networking
   d. Marketing systems
10. True or False: When identifying a target audience, it is important to be as broad as possible to include as many potential clients as you can.
11. True or False: According to supply and demand theory, whenever the supply of a good or service increases, the demand and price for it automatically increase as well.
12. True or False: Cooperative marketing not only can be done with other complementary holistic practitioners or across other industries, it can be done with other massage therapists as well.
13. True or False: In the public's perception, massage therapy is often considered to be part of discretionary spending.
14. True or False: Bad economic times spell certain death for holistic businesses.
15. True or False: Although marketing is very important to a business, owners or managers do not have to do everything themselves. Many aspects can actually be outsourced to others.

Discussion Questions

1. What are your thoughts about collaborative marketing? Have you ever done if before? Have you seen it work for others? Discuss your experiences and beliefs about the ability to collaboratively work with others for everyone's mutual benefit.
2. Have you ever experienced information overload? What do you think of technology fatigue? Do you believe these are serious problems, or just an excuse? Discuss your thoughts or experiences around this topic, and brainstorm a few additional solutions to avoid information overload.

Beyond the Classroom: The Great Communicator Exercise

As you learned in this chapter, a lot of marketing involves communication. This can be in the form of newsletters, e-mails, blogs, articles, and other direct transmissions.

A. You may not feel that you have great writing skill, but business owners should be able to express the fundamentals of their business and their industry, both verbally and in writing. Come up with a few potential headlines for a blog post or an article. Write three zingers here:

1. ______________________________
2. ______________________________
3. ______________________________

Now take the one that resonates the most for you and write about it! Try and write at least a paragraph, but aim for three or four. Think about your niche market, incorporating its unique challenges and the solutions you or your information can provide. Check out other blogs that you might follow or articles that you have read in trade magazines for inspiration.

B. Earlier in the chapter you started working on your elevator pitch by brainstorming some ideas about your ideal client, his or her goals and struggles, and ways that you can help. If you didn't get a chance to flesh out your answers, take the time to do it now. Also take the time to thoroughly familiarize yourself with your pitch. If it helps, practice saying your pitch in front of a mirror. You might even record yourself saying your pitch and play it back so you can hear how you sound to others. Keep practicing and polishing that pitch until it shines!

CHAPTER 13

External Abundance: Financial Management for Your Business

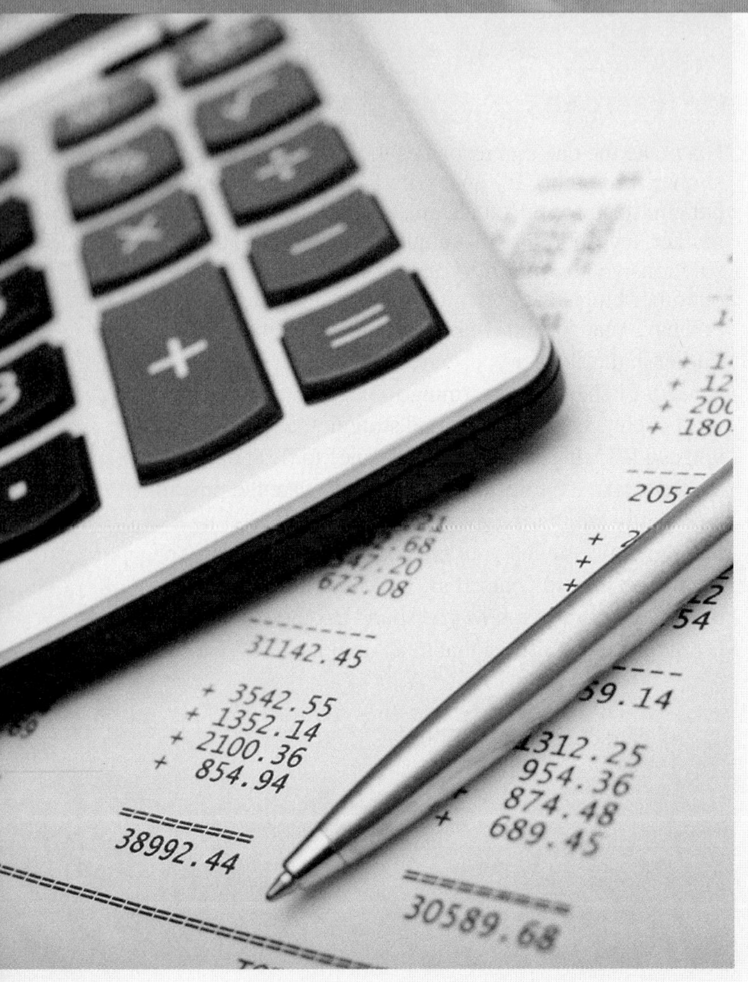

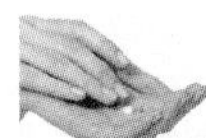

CHAPTER OUTLINE

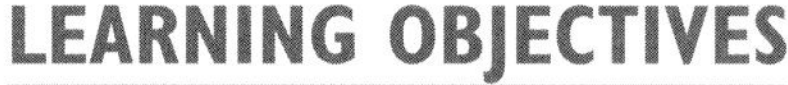

LEARNING OBJECTIVES

1. Explore the financial requirements of getting your business started
2. Introduce traditional and innovative ways of finding funding
3. Define bootstrapping and identify ways to cut start-up costs
4. Contrast the pros and cons of partnering for money
5. Examine the importance of separating personal and business accounts
6. Describe techniques to forecast profits
7. Introduce financial statements: cash flow, income statement, balance sheet
8. Define accounting for your business and assess the role of accountants
9. Define countertrade and examine the benefits and drawbacks of bartering your services

KEY TERMS

accountant *222*
accounting *222*
accounts payable *221*
accounts receivable *221*
angel investor *216*
balance sheet *220*
bartering *222*
bootstrapping *217*
breakeven *222*
collateral *215*
countertrade *222*
debt financing *215*
equity *221*
exit strategy *219*
financial statements *220*
fixed costs *213*
forecast *219*
grant *216*
income statement *221*
inflows *221*
outflows *221*
partnership *218*
profits *219*
recurring expenses *213*
revenue *219*
scale *212*
scope *212*
start-up costs *212*
statement of cash flows *221*
sweat equity *216*
variable costs *213*
venture capitalist *216*

MONEY MATTERS

> *In all realms of life it takes courage to stretch your limits, express your power, and fulfill your potential . . . it's no different in the financial realm.*
>
> —Suze Orman

In Chapter 7, you explored the basics of personal financial planning; this chapter will expand on that knowledge by delving into the financial aspects of your massage business. Financial management is the cornerstone of a healthy, thriving business. No matter what your business focus or professional goals, money matters. A business cannot start, grow, or survive if there isn't enough money to pay the bills and provide income to those involved.

It is true that there can be external challenges to small businesses that are beyond the control of business owners, and lately the uncertainties in the global economy have made many business owners (current or potential) quite anxious. According to a recent survey of the National Small Business Association, more than half of all small business owners listed financial uncertainty as one of the top challenges to their growth and survival.[1] But regardless of the external climate (which you ultimately cannot control), you can navigate the financial health of your business with a little foresight. This chapter will help you develop tools to keep your business on financial track.

In order to get any business going, it is imperative to spend some money first. **Start-up costs** are the initial expenses associated with starting any new business: leases or property purchase, deposits with public utilities, legal fees, licenses, permits, rental expenses and deposits, new equipment, decoration, marketing and promotion, and so on. Your start-up costs will be in direct proportion to the scale and scope of your operations. **Scale** refers to the size of your business—are you opening up a full-service spa with 15 employees or developing a solo practice where you will work a few days a week? **Scope** refers to the breadth of the focus of your services and products. Will you be forgoing an office for a mobile office or home visit-based practice, or will you be leasing a 10,000 square foot professional space to provide 10 different styles of body–work? Of course business scale and scope exist along a continuum, and your financial requirements will vary along that range.

FINANCIAL REQUIREMENTS: WHAT IT TAKES TO GET STARTED

One of the biggest mistakes entrepreneurs often make is failing to grasp the actual financial needs of starting their business. Experts will tell you that one of the main reasons for the failure of new businesses is the underestimation of capital needs.[2] Getting too little financing is obviously a leading cause of most early business failures, but so too is getting too much.[3] Is there such a thing as too much money? Sure there is—especially if you are borrowing it. Some companies actually require very little money to get started. Stacey Saggese of Rocky Mountain Microfinance Institute claims that for most service-based businesses (such as a massage practice), $5000 can go a very long way.[4] Remember what you learned in Chapter 7 on personal finances about bad debt: overestimating and overspending in the beginning can cause you and your business major problems down the road, just as underestimating expenses can.

So how do you know what your exact financial requirements will be? You may not be able to arrive at an exact number without a crystal ball, but you can certainly do some educated calculating. As Tama McAleese, the author of *Get Rich Slow* advises, "Overestimate your expenses and underestimate your revenue."[5] There are usually some fairly predictable start-up costs, such as the things mentioned previously and later in the chapter that you may need to pay for to get started (see Figure 13-1 ■). But it is also important to keep your eye on expenses beyond just initial ones. How will you keep the lights on and the rent paid once everything is in place?

As discussed previously, the start-up costs for your company will vary significantly based on your size and scope. A person opening a 4,000 square foot sports massage complex will have a very different picture of financial requirements than someone turning a spare bedroom into a work-from-home

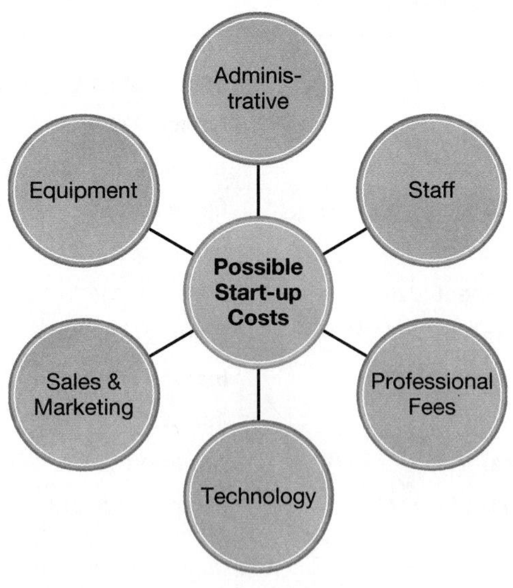

FIGURE 13-1

Possible start-up costs for a new business can include staff expenses, professional fees, technology outlays, sales and marketing expenses, new equipment investments, and administrative costs. Can you think of any others?

practice. Here's a glimpse at some of the costs that you may encounter:

- Professional fees: Trade association and professional memberships, establishing legal structure (LLC, S corp., etc.), consulting fees, legal fees, and licensing fees.
- Technology costs: Computer hardware and software, Internet access, website development and maintenance, cell phone, BlackBerry, etc.
- Sales and marketing costs: Business cards, brochures, stationery, gift certificates, advertising, retail product packaging, trade shows, website set up and maintenance.
- Administrative costs: Rent, parking, licenses and permits, office supplies, business insurance (often included in massage trade association memberships), utilities, desk, filing cabinets, postage expenses, accounting, and other things that will keep operations running smoothly.
- Massage equipment: Massage table, massage chair, sheets, lotions, creams, linens, t-bars, liniments, aromatherapy oils, hydroculator, hot stones, paraffin treatments, body treatment products, table warmers, and other things you will incorporate into administering massage services.
- Interior decoration: Paint, wall art, plants, candles, objets d'art, furniture, shelving, storage, new carpet, textiles, and other objects to create the desired atmosphere for your business.
- Employee wages and benefits: Employee salaries, unemployment insurance, workers' compensation, benefits, incentives, payroll taxes (these things will be explored in detail in Chapter 14, "Managing Yourself and Others").

Take a very good look at your list of start-up items. Take some time to consider realistically the things that you are going to be including in your beginning expenditures. Use Table 13-1 to flesh out all the items you will have in your business, and what you estimate each item will cost. If you don't have a clue about some expenses or don't know what some items may cost, do a little research by asking around or looking online before you make a guess.

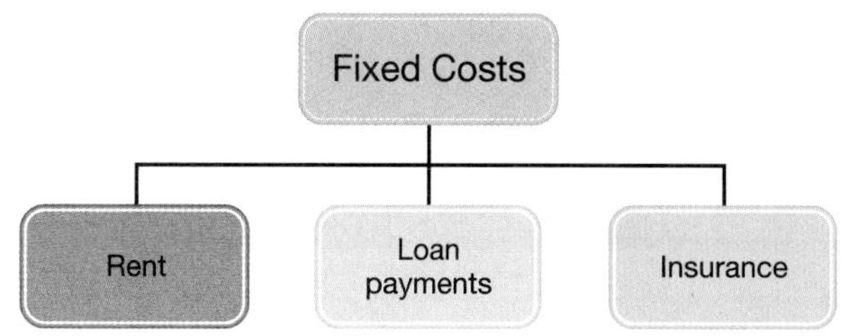

FIGURE 13-2

Fixed costs are consistent and must be paid regardless of changes in business volume, such as rent, insurance, or loan payments.

The list you made gives a very good idea of where you will need to make investments in the beginning. But as you know, all businesses also have recurring costs in addition to start-up costs. **Recurring expenses** are ongoing costs that require repeated commitment and fulfillment, whether weekly, monthly, annually, or every few years. Recurring costs include things such as rent expense, marketing collateral, insurance, loan payments, taxes, professional fees, payroll expenses, and so forth.

Some of these recurring expenses will be fixed. **Fixed costs** refer to expenditures that must be paid regardless of business productivity. In other words, you have to pay these no matter how many massages are given or how much money is made. Examples of fixed costs include rent, loan payments, insurance, or taxes (see Figure 13-2 ■). **Variable costs,** on the other hand, fluctuate based upon the volume of productivity and output activities of the business. For example, if you are giving twice as many massages in February than you did in January, you will double the costs for laundry and oils. Other examples of variable costs can include traveling expenses, or postage and printing for a Valentine's Day marketing campaign (see Figure 13-3 ■).

PUT IT IN WRITING

Start-up Costs

With all the work you've done thus far to creatively visualize the business you are trying to create, you should have a pretty solid vision of how you want it to look. Now what are all the tangible factors that are going to turn that vision into a reality? Will you have a hydraulic table? Where is your office? Is there paint on the walls? What kind of linens will you use? Will you have employees? A filing cabinet? A computer? Write down things you currently own and things you will need to acquire. Take a moment to write out as many material things as you can possibly think of to support your business vision. This is your dream wish list:

______________	______________	______________
______________	______________	______________
______________	______________	______________
______________	______________	______________
______________	______________	______________
______________	______________	______________
______________	______________	______________
______________	______________	______________

PUT IT IN WRITING

Would Like/Must Have

As you continue on with your financial planning, you may find it necessary to pare down expenses to fit within your financing options. To help you out later, Table 13-1 ■ has a "would like" and "must have" section, so you can distinguish between items that are essential or would just be nice to have.

TABLE 13-1 Would Like versus Must Have Items

Item	Cost	Would Like	Must Have

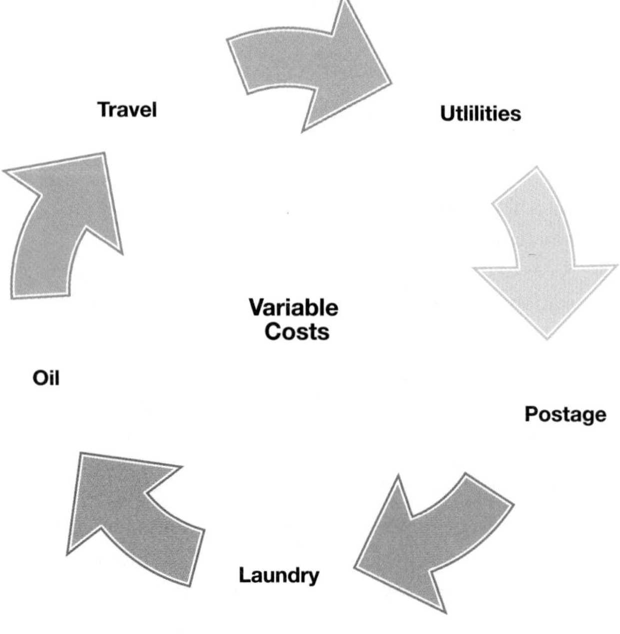

FIGURE 13-3

Variable costs rise and fall based on the amount of business productivity and output, such as laundry, travel, or seasonal marketing.

Considering the size and scope of your operations, what will your expenses look like? Which costs are fixed, and which are variable? You will find a full monthly expense worksheet with an extensive list of potential costs in Appendix B, but for now, take a moment to jot down what might be foreseeable expenses, as well as ballpark figures of your outlays.

Reviewing and revising the lists you have created of all the things you will need to acquire for your new business, as well as the costs that will be associated with keeping it running, will help give you a better picture of what your start-up costs will be. This understanding will put you in a better place when you seek funding for your new business.

PUT IT IN WRITING

Estimating Monthly Expenditures[6]

Expense	Projected Monthly Cost	× 12 months	Fixed	Variable
Rent	$1800	$21,600	✔	

Total: ______________________

GETTING ORGANIZED

Once you have filled out the Would Like/Must Have form and the Estimated Monthly Expenditures exercise, file these away in your *Business of Massage Therapy* notebook so you can better distinguish necessities and luxuries when the time comes to make purchases for your business. This will help you to tame splurges and tailor unnecessary costs. You will find a blank Would Like/Must Have table and Monthly Expense worksheet in Appendix B.

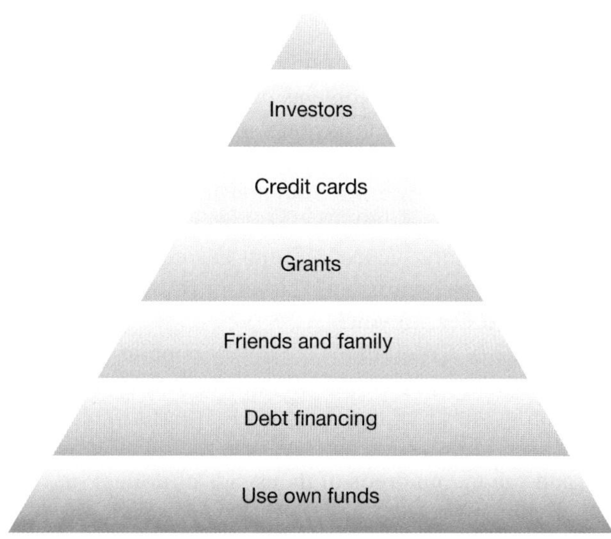

FIGURE 13-4

There are many sources of funding that may be available for your business, and you want to find those that work best for you.

SOURCES OF FUNDING

Now that you have a handle on your start-up costs and a reasonable budget for maintaining your business, it is time to find the money to pay for it all. Whether you have concluded that you will need $500, $2,000, $10,000 or $1,000,000 to create the business of your dreams, it has to come from somewhere. Many sources of capital exist, but most have strings attached in one form or another.

Unless you have a wellspring of money bursting the seams of your bank account, you will likely have to tap some sources to fund your new business. However, you will want to do this strategically. When you are frantic about finding financial backing, it may seem counterintuitive to start being picky. But the truth is, it is very important to find and pursue the type of funding that is appropriate for you and your business's needs. Check in with local economic development centers, Small Business Development Centers, or local business incubators to get more insight on optimal choices for your unique situation. They usually offer free (or very inexpensive) small business counseling and financial management advice.

Figure 13-4 ■ gives a few typical channels that entrepreneurs use to fund their ventures:

- *Use your own funds:* Many business consultants will tell you that you should not even consider going into business unless you can front 50 percent or more of the costs. There are several reasons for this. First of all, if you are putting a substantial amount of money on the line, you will be all the more motivated to see your business succeed. Second of all, bankrolling yourself puts you in a far less risky position if things don't go according to plan; you will not be beholden to a bank, an investor, or your mother-in-law. And finally, very few financial sources will even consider lending money to someone who doesn't believe in their own idea enough to put their skin in the game. Of course you take on great personal financial risk when you put your nest egg on the line—but with great risk often comes great reward.
- *Debt financing:* **Debt financing** is when you fund your business with money borrowed from an outside source, with the promise to return the principal sum and the interest on it. Although there are many complex ways to do debt financing, such as issuing bonds, the scope of a new massage business is most likely going to require simpler debt financing, such as bank loans. Remember from the personal finance chapter that not all debt is bad; like school loans, business loans are part of "good debt." Many entrepreneurs maintain that their relationship with their bank is the key to their success. The Small Business Administration (www.SBA.gov) works as a guarantor of loans by private lenders, and building a relationship with your bank in the beginning can help you secure financing down the road should you chose to expand your business. There are, of course, downsides: interest rates may be high, and many banks require that a business show at least two years of history and credit. It may also be necessary to provide personal collateral to the bank.[7] **Collateral** is an asset that is held as a guarantee for repayment of a loan by the lending institution to insure against potential loss. A common example of collateral is one's house.
- *Friend and family plan:* Maybe you don't have 50 percent of the money you know you will need sitting under your mattress, but you don't feel comfortable going through a bank or SBA for a loan. Another popular source of funding for new businesses is typically found in those nearest and dearest to you. Though technically a form of debt financing, borrowing from friends and family has a unique dynamic that is absent when borrowing from a bank, and so you might consider it as a separate option. The upside of this is that you are leveraging relationships and usually don't have to have as much collateral as you would with other types of loans. In addition, the

money is usually available more quickly, and grandma may be willing to give you a better interest rate than a corporate bank would. But be careful—money can cause problems quickly in personal relationships. Treat this as you would any other contract, with specified payments and interest agreements *in writing*. And consider seriously the consequences on relationships if your business does not ultimately succeed. If your business goes belly up, will it jeopardize a relationship with someone near and dear to you?

- *Charge it:* Credit cards are a very popular but highly risky approach to financing. It is not uncommon in entrepreneurial circles to hear tales of brazen impresarios that leverage their credit cards and run up hundreds of thousands of dollars in credit card debt to finance their ventures. Even financially cautious business owners often use their cards to ramp up their businesses in the absence of other alternatives. But tread cautiously here. Remember the bad debt concern you explored in Chapter 7? Because of the incredibly high rates on most cards, credit card debt can zap the life out of your massage start-up and get your business trapped in a debt cycle. If you do use credit cards, do so conservatively and establish a workable repayment plan early on, being sure to stay on top of all payments. Make it a priority and a habit to pay down balances as swiftly as possible.
- *Grants:* Some small business owners have claimed great success with using grants to fund their startups, particularly for women and minority entrepreneurs. A **grant** is a form of financial endowment that is typically given to a recipient by a foundation, a corporation, an individual, or the government. Companies and individuals typically apply for grants through written proposals or submissions. Many cities have grant money for start-up companies, particularly for minority- and women-owned businesses. The wonderful thing about grants is that they are essentially free money on which you do not have to pay interest. The hard part is that the competition for grants is very stiff, and many of those giving grants have strict requirements on who can receive them (those with tax-exempt status, for example). Do some good research here before deciding if this funding method is appropriate for you and your massage business.
- *Angels and capitalists:* Although they are not common in the world of massage therapy, there are those holistic entrepreneurs whose scale and scope make it appropriate to approach angel investors and venture capitalists. An **angel investor** is usually an affluent individual who invests his or her own money in startup companies by providing capital in exchange for ownership and a stake in the company. An angel typically helps bring your business along in more ways than just financially by providing mentorship and contacts. However, don't approach an investor for amounts less than $25,000 to $1 million—they are hard to find and they are almost always expecting a high financial return from your company. A **venture capitalist** is an individual or investment firm that manages the pooled money of others, and they can provide a huge financial boon to a new company.[8] However, the stakes are incredibly high with venture capitalists, as they give a lot (usually $1 million +) and expect very high returns on their investment. The kind of financing required for massage businesses is well below what is typically sought with angel investors or venture capitalists. While it is good to know of the option, unless you are considering the next Massage Envy or SEC-filed franchise, angel investors and venture capitalists may not be right for you.

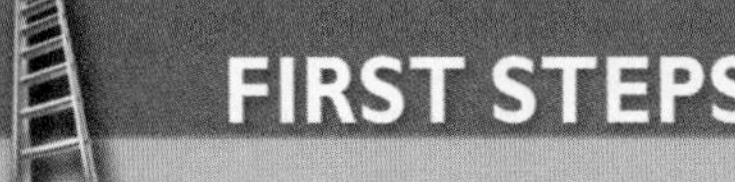

FIRST STEPS

Surely you know someone (or several people) who has started a new business: perhaps friends, family members, neighbors, or colleagues. Find a few people whose opinions you respect and ask them what financial approaches they took when starting their business. Why did they seek the funding they did? What worked for them? What do they wish they had done differently? Be respectful and sensitive when approaching this subject, as people can often be very touchy talking about finances.

Remember, no matter what venue you pursue in obtaining your financing, you need to be prepared to present hard numbers and compelling reasons to invest in you and your business. Later in the chapter you will learn about financial documents such as cash flow (profit and loss), balance sheets, and income statements. These can be helpful, if not expected, to have in hand when approaching a funding source. One important thing to keep in mind, and something that is often a challenge to quantify, is the value of your sweat equity. **Sweat equity** is the unpaid physical and mental labor of the owner of a business that increases the business's worth. It is your unique contribution and commitment to your business that makes it valuable, especially in the beginning. All the time that you spend crafting business plans, working on marketing strategy, painting walls, and networking to build clientele goes into the sweat equity of your business. You can quantify this by assigning an hourly wage to your time spent on the business and factoring it into your assets, but you should also be able to communicate to potential funders that your energy contributions and role in the organization are

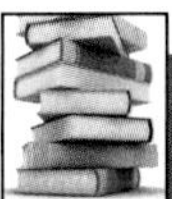

HELPFUL RESOURCES

One of the best resources out there for learning more about financing and starting your new business is the Small Business Administration website, www.sba.gov. In addition to tools on marketing, legal aspects, and market research, the SBA can help steer you towards financing options that are available to you. Also check out local economic development centers and local business incubators in your area to discover more resources.

larger than the sum of their parts. This is true in most new businesses, but especially so in massage businesses, where the service is so personally driven.

BOOTSTRAPPING

It is very important to be aware of different sources of funding, particularly as your business grows and your needs change. However, most entrepreneurs and small business owners are very familiar with the need to self-sustain their business. This is particularly true in hard economic times, when traditional lending sources restrict credit to small businesses and friends and family are strapped for cash. **Bootstrapping** refers to starting a business entirely on self-generated sources for initial expenses, and being as financially conservative as possible. As the name implies, bootstrapping is pulling yourself up and being as self-reliant as possible in your financing. *Inc.* magazine reports that 82 percent of private U.S. companies had entirely self-financed funding, while Entrepreneur.com reports that nearly 99 percent of business owners incorporate a creative mix of personal finances, those of family and friends, credit cards, life insurance, home equity, and other financial resources more directly within their control in order to bootstrap.[9]

Regardless of the form your unique financing takes, one of the most important things to remember is that it helps to be conservative with spending, especially in the beginning. When you are a small business owner, every penny matters. This does not mean that you can't get what you want or have to severely sacrifice quality to start your business. It just means that sometimes it is advantageous to engage some creative frugality. Remember the importance of perceived value for your clients—if they won't be able to distinguish the difference in quality between a $20 lamp and a $100 lamp, is it justifiable to borrow the extra $80 to buy the more expensive lamp? At the same time, if it is evident that a less expensive item is substandard quality, you may want to invest in a pricier item that will reflect better upon your business and make operations more effective. The "Bright Ideas" box lists tips and tricks to save money when starting your massage business.

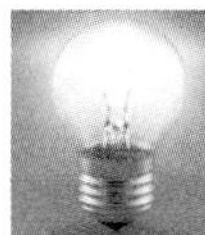

BRIGHT IDEAS

Tips for the Penny Pinching 'Preneur

If you are like most entrepreneurs, you don't necessarily have an abundance of capital behind you. Even though the list of expenses may seem overwhelming when you are just getting started, there are always creative ways to save on spending. Below are a few ideas of ways to cut start-up costs. See if you can come up with a few of your own!

- *Buy used equipment.* Check with local massage schools to see about buying second-hand tables or check *Craigslist* for a hydrocolator that has already seen a few hot packs pass through.
- *Buy in bulk.* Buying things like massage lotion, sheets, and even business cards can be much cheaper when you buy a large volume at once rather than making small periodic purchases.
- *Be realistic.* Don't start out of the gate spending lavishly. Do you really need to buy the latest state-of-the-art equipment or hire a couture interior designer, or will something more sensible be just as effective in your business?
- *Shop around for deals.* Take time to compare prices on the things that you need, from sheets to medicinal liniments to office space. Don't always snatch the first thing you see.
- *Negotiate.* As they say in business, everything is negotiable. From the rent on your new space to the credit terms on a small business loan to the price you pay the printer for your marketing materials, you can always ask for a lower price. The worst thing that can happen is they tell you no, but you won't know unless you ask!
- *Barter!* From equipment to marketing to getting the walls painted, barter is a great way to save money when you're getting started. See the bartering section of this chapter for more information.
- *Use credit cards cautiously.* Although it may seem tempting (and very easy) to pay for everything with credit cards, spending more than you can afford to pay off quickly can end up costing you considerably in the long run. Shop around for good interest rates, and when reaching for the plastic, ask yourself if the purchase is a *want* or a *need* for your new business. If it isn't something you have to have, give it a few days to think about it before you charge it.

Now you: what are some other great ways to save money with your start-up costs? Try and come up with a few more things that will help you to preserve your precious financial resources upfront.

____

____

____

____

____

TO PARTNER OR NOT TO PARTNER: EXPLORING THE PROS AND CONS OF BRINGING OTHERS ON FOR MONEY

One approach that many entrepreneurs take when starting a new venture is to enlist a partner or two. It is a common occurrence among students or recent graduates of massage school to gaze lovingly upon one or two of their favorite classmates and utter those five little words: "Let's start a business together." If you are entertaining this idea, read this section before you start drafting kitchen table contracts or scrawling napkin business plans with your buddies.

A **partnership** is a business relationship between two or more individuals who share risk, labor, cooperation, and responsibility. Typically all parties agree to provide financial, material, or knowledge capital for the business. One of the top reasons people partner is to increase their financial parameters and to minimize personal risk. However, like any business arrangement, there can be considerable pros and cons to entering a partnership. Sharing risk may sound good, but sharing profits, responsibility, and control is not for everyone. This section will help you weigh the benefits and drawbacks of bringing on partners, especially for money.

> *A friendship founded on business is a good deal better than a business founded on friendship.*
>
> —John D. Rockefeller

The SBA claims that businesses formed in partnership often have a better chance of weathering storms than do sole proprietorships.[10] Obviously, bringing in a partner often means more access to capital, but there are other benefits as well. Partnerships are typically very easy to form, and because they are a pass-through tax entity, filing taxes is often much simpler than for more complex business structures like S corps. or C corps. (refer back to Chapter 10 for more on legal structures in business). Partnerships allow the owners to share the burdens of running a business, as responsibilities are shared and tough times are endured together. Having more than one owner increases the knowledge and skill base of a company, which can benefit from the pooled ideas and productivity of more minds, more hands, and more points of view. Forming a partnership can help alleviate some of the fear of going it alone in business, and a partner can serve as a great source of support and inspiration through the ups and downs so common in the massage industry.

However, partnering is not for everyone, and it is not always an easier or more advantageous option. Though you do stand to have more money to start the business, your profits will be shared, which could significantly limit your income potential on the back end. Also, because partners are both individually and jointly liable for the activities of one another, if your partner disappears in the night, you will be responsible for all of the debts—not just half of them. Having a partner means you lose some control over how things are done, as decisions have to be reached together and compromise is inevitable. Finally, if you go into business with a family member or a close friend, partnership could have disastrous effects on the relationship if things go badly or if your operational styles differ substantially. Getting along and caring about one another is not necessarily the same as being good business partners.

If you still think you would like to partner with someone, be sure to have very clear expectations of one another's

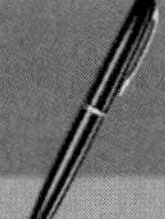

PUT IT IN WRITING

"Do You Take This Person to Be Your Business Partner . . ."

Forming a partnership can be a great way to start a new business, but without clear goals and understandings, it can be doomed to fail. Before you sign any documents or seal it with a handshake, ask yourself the following questions to see if you and your potential partner should go forward.

1. Do I like to be in control? Would it be hard for me to reach consensus before making decisions?

   ____

2. How do I handle conflict when misunderstandings arise? Do I face them directly, or do I avoid confrontation?

   ____

   ____

3. If someone else is not pulling their weight, how do I handle it?

   ____

   ____

4. Am I good at sharing responsibilities evenly, or do I have a tendency to ride in others' air currents sometimes?

   ____

If you have a specific person in mind that you are thinking of forming a partnership with, ask yourself the following questions:

1. Do we share a similar vision for our massage business?

   ____

2. From what I know thus far, how similar are we in work ethic, motivation, and values?

   ____

3. Is this a person I genuinely trust?

   ____

4. Do our strengths and weaknesses complement one another, or could they be problematic?

   ____

roles going into the relationship. Take time to get to know one another in a business context, and be sure that you have a clear understanding of what your relationship will look like. Get that understanding in writing, do your research into your prospective partners' backgrounds, and invite them to do the same by offering references and recommendations from people you've worked with in the past. It is highly recommended to create an exit strategy for all partners in the relationship. An **exit strategy** is an agreement about what will happen in the event that one of the partners decides to leave the business for any reason. Exit strategies outline transition of ownership between parties and help to plan ways for individuals to sell their interest, recoup their investment, or reclaim their assets in the business. Having a solid exit strategy is a bit like having a prenuptial agreement—it helps those involved understand the terms and expectations should the business relationship dissolve for any reason. A partnership can be a wonderfully rewarding business arrangement, but make sure you go into one with your eyes wide open.

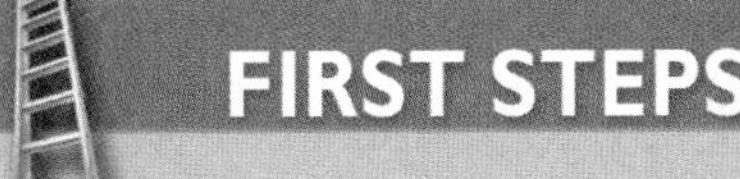

FIRST STEPS

Do a little online research and compare what local banks have to offer new business account holders. Also look at what they require to open a new account (some banks may want to see a business plan, certificates of incorporation, financial forecasts, and so forth).[13] When you find a banker that looks like a good match for you, make an appointment to set up your new business bank account.

DRAWING A BOUNDARY BETWEEN PERSONAL AND PROFESSIONAL FINANCES

A common financial mistake that many novice entrepreneurs make is to blur the boundaries between their personal and business finances. This is especially true for individuals who establish their business as a sole proprietorship or as a single-owner LLC (see Chapter 10 for more on these). It can be very easy to buy something for the office with your personal credit card, deposit a client check into your own bank account, or use business funds to pay for a shopping trip.

However if you are going into business for yourself, it is imperative to draw a clear boundary between your personal and professional finances. The foremost reason for this is taxes. Individuals and businesses are entitled to different deductions and responsible for different tax liabilities; separating accounts will help ensure you follow the tax laws and benefit from any applicable tax advantages.[11] Keeping your personal and business finances from intertwining will streamline the process should you ever be audited by the Internal Revenue Service.

You may also be required to demonstrate the profitability of your business to get a lease, apply for a loan, or request a grant. You could gum up your chances of securing any of these things if you don't have a clear paper trail or if your business expenses are peppered with personal expenditures. Keeping the two areas of your life compartmentalized and organized will make things easier for you, and as a business owner will help clarify and demonstrate financial strengths and weaknesses of your business to others.[12]

An easy way to start the separation is to immediately establish a business bank account. Take whatever funding you have and set up a business checking account in the name of your business. You can use this to pay yourself a paycheck, paying yourself weekly, biweekly, monthly, or whatever works best for you. This money will of course then go into your personal accounts, and will make your personal income taxes much easier to account for.

WHAT IS THE FORECAST? TOOLS FOR FORECASTING PROFITS

Nearly all funding sources will want to take a look at your financial forecasts, as they want to ensure that your business will be viable and able to pay back any borrowed funds with interest. A **forecast** is a researched, calculated, and carefully formulated projection of the expected financial situation of a business. It estimates a company's revenues, and subtracts from these all estimated expenses to reach an estimated profit. Forecasts are generally based on the current understanding and future expectations of many internal and external conditions. Forecasts help to demonstrate how your business will be sustained over time, and whether you will generate enough money to support operations. Most people who look at financial forecasts are interested in seeing your bottom line: the profits.

Profits represent the money you have left after you have paid all your costs. The simple equation for profits is your revenue minus your expenses. You've already spent time exploring your projected expenses, so now take some time to think of your potential revenue (which is much more fun to think about anyway). **Revenue** is the total amount of money generated by the company for all goods and services sold. In order to estimate your revenue, figure out the number of clients you are seeing (or would like to see) in a typical week. If you are just getting started, how many clients do you think you will be able to attract in the first six months? The first year? You established your price points in Chapter 11, and evaluated your approach to discounting for special events, promotions, or even special clients. Take the average

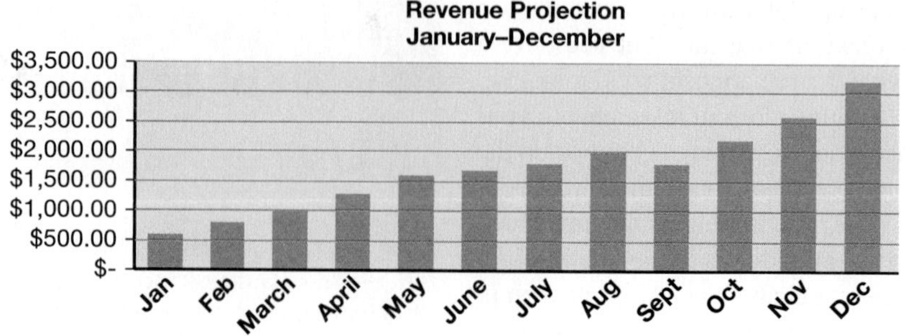

FIGURE 13-5

A massage therapist's projection of revenue for the coming year.

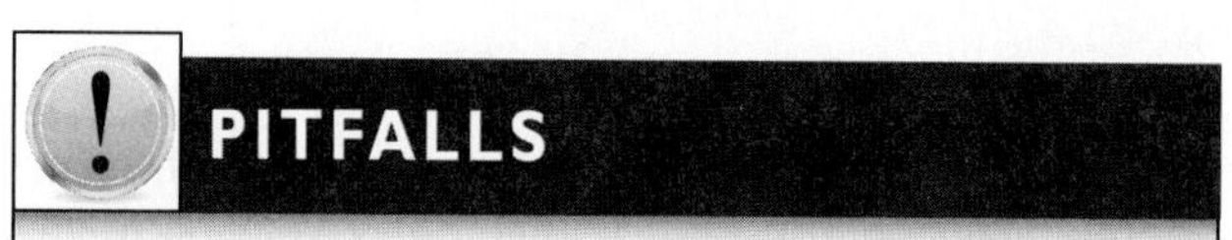

Don't forget that a financial forecast is just that—a projection. Just as the weatherman is never 100 percent accurate, very few businesses hit their estimates dead-on. Projections are helpful tools for a business, but don't be so number bound you let the figures command you. Don't feel bad if you fall short, and don't feel limited if you see that you could surpass your own financial predictions.

amount you will charge clients and multiply it by the amount of people you feel confident you could attract and service each week. This number is your projected revenue, and will help you get an idea of how much your business can realistically expect to make based on the information at hand. Now, take your projected yearly expenses and subtract them from your projected revenue: this is your profit forecast for the year (see Figure 13-5 ■ and Figure 13-6 ■).

MAKING A STATEMENT: BALANCE SHEET, INCOME STATEMENT, AND STATEMENT OF CASH FLOWS

While profit forecasts are helpful, they only offer a potential sketch rather than the whole financial picture. Thinking you know your whole financial picture from a forecast is like thinking you read a book because you glanced at the cover. This section will explain basic business **financial statements,** the documents that provide a more thorough outline of your business's financial health from a short- and long-term view. Financial statements include the balance sheet, income statement, and the statement of cash flows. In the beginning, you can do these as pro formas, or documents that are based on assumptions, as were your forecasts. However, you will want to replace the assumptions with real numbers as your business starts generating real revenues and expenses.

A **balance sheet** (Table 13-2 ■) gives the details of a company's liabilities, assets, and equity in order to understand its financial condition at a specific point in time. Remember how you calculated your net worth in Chapter 7? A balance sheet is similar to this, as you are subtracting your liabilities from your assets. However in financial statements, net worth is better known as a company's equity.

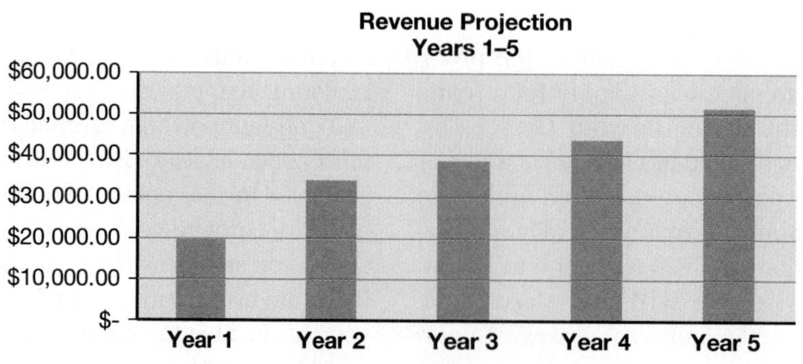

FIGURE 13-6

A massage therapist's projection of revenue for the next five years.

TABLE 13-2 Balance Sheet, Therapeutic Hands Massage

Assets		Liabilities		Owners' Equity	
Cash	$35,700	Accounts payable	$7,000	J. Clever, Capital	52,900
Accounts receivable	7,000	Salaries payable	0		
Inventory	50,000	Loans	35,000		
Supplies	2,200	Total liabilities	$42,000		
Total assets	$94,900			Total liability + owner equity	$94,900

On the balance sheet, **equity** equals total assets minus total liabilities. Conversely, total assets equals liabilities plus equity. Notice how the total assets equal total liability plus owner equity. This should always be the case. There may be some terms in Table 13-2 that you don't recognize. You don't have to master accounting lingo, but you may want to familiarize yourself with a few key financial terms. For example, **accounts receivable** refers to money that is owed a company in exchange for goods or services that were extended on credit rather than on a cash basis. For example, if you give a client a massage three times a month, but she doesn't give you a payment for the massages until the last day of the month, the money she owes you goes into your accounts receivable. Conversely, **accounts payable** is money that a business owes to vendors, suppliers, or creditors for goods or services that they have extended on credit rather than cash. For example, the money you owe the utility bill for the month's electricity is part of your accounts payable.

The next famous financial statement is the income statement (Figure 13-7 ■). The **income statement** summarizes a business's revenues, expenses, and profits over a period of time (usually an accounting quarter). Income statements are also known as profit and loss statements, or PNLs. The income statement helps you (and others) to see if the company made or lost money from its business activities and operations.

J. Clever Massage
Income Statement
For Quarter Ended 12/31/12

Revenues	
Massage services	$17,500
Product sales	2,000
Gross Revenue	$19,500
Expenses	
Lease	$6,250
Advertising	600
Licenses	0
Linen cleaning	140
Professional fees	176
Salary	11,000
Supplies	180
Interest expense	300
Total Quarterly Expenses	**(18,646)**
Net Income	**$ 854**

FIGURE 13-7

This income statement shows the business revenues, expenses, and profits for J. Clever Massage.

The **statement of cash flows** gives an account of a company's cash activities, particularly as they relate to operations, investing, or financing. The statement is divided into those three functional areas as well (Figure 13-8 ■). A statement of cash flows usually gives a snapshot of a period in time (usually a quarterly accounting period), similar to a balance sheet. Money that comes into the business as a result of operating, financing, or investment activities is known as **inflows:** product sales, services rendered, rent income, or investment dividends are all examples of inflows. **Outflows,** of course, represent all the money that goes out of a business to sustain operating, financing, or investment activities. Examples of outflows include utilities, mortgage payments, or loan payments.[14] Of course, inflows and outflows are relative, as one business's expense is another's income. Formats may differ, but general accounting procedures (GAP) usually illustrate outflows within brackets or parentheses, and inflows as normal numbers.

GETTING ORGANIZED

All of these financial statements are available for you in Appendix B. Now that you have created some basic financial statements for your business (even pro formas), you know what comes next! File them away in your *Business of Massage Therapy* notebook. When you are ready, you can formalize and polish these documents when it's time to ask for a loan, apply for a lease, or impress your in-laws with your amazing business acumen.

The Fountain of Youth Day Spa Statement of Cash Flows For Quarter Ended 12/31/12	
Operating Activities	
Cash received from massage services	$180,000
Cash received from sale of products	30,000
Cash paid for lease expense	(28,785)
Cash paid for salaries	(90,000)
Cash paid for other operating items	(19,000)
Cash provided by operations	$72,215
Investing Activities	
Cash used to buy property (PPE)	(65,000)
Cash used to buy fixed assets	0
Cash provided by investing	(65,000)
Financing Activities	
Cash paid for interest expense	(5,000)
Cash Increase/Decrease	$ 2,215
Cash at Beginning of Quarter	$142,000
Cash at End of Quarter	**$144,215**

FIGURE 13-8

This statement of cash flows shows the incomes and outflows of cash for operations, investing, and financing for the Fountain of Youth Day Spa.

ACCOUNTING FOR THE BUDGET, AND BUDGETING FOR AN ACCOUNTANT

Many small business owners feel bogged down or overwhelmed by all that is entailed with doing all the financial accounting on their own. **Accounting** is the consistent recordkeeping, verification, interpretation, and reporting of a business's assets, liabilities, expenses, cash inflows, cash outflows, and financial activities. It is also known as bookkeeping. As you saw in Chapter 10, you will likely be responsible for filing estimated self-employment and business taxes quarterly. Even with the best of financial acumen, it can be cumbersome to do all of your bookkeeping on your own. Many massage therapists have found it incredibly advantageous to hire an accountant, particularly as their business grows.

An **accountant** is a professional who help individuals, groups, and businesses to track and accurately report financial information. Accountants are highly versed in the often complex tax codes, and can help you clarify and demystify your tax liabilities. Whether you work with or without an accountant, you will always want to keep all your records and receipts for all business transactions.

Accountants can also help you keep your eye on the big picture by illuminating the true financial situation of your business. They can help you move beyond **breakeven,** the "just-scraping-by" point where profits and expenses are the same and there is neither profit nor loss. Some small business owners stay at the breakeven point for a very long time without knowing it or seeing how to move beyond it. Accountants can also help your business handle payroll, and help you find other helpful professionals, such as attorneys, realtors, or insurance agents. The right accountant can be an ally in your financial success over a lifetime. Even if you think you might not want to keep an accountant over the long term, it is advisable to work with an accountant during the first few years of your business. This can help you learn the accounting process, avoid costly mistakes, and build a relationship with an accountant with whom you can consult down the road. Some massage therapists maintain that finding a good accountant was one of the most important things they did for their businesses.[15]

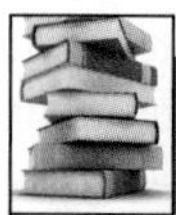

HELPFUL RESOURCES

Want to learn more about financial statements for your business? Check out *Small Business Financial Management for Dummies* by Tage C. Tracy, CPA (2007, Wiley) or *Balance Sheet Basics: Financial Management for Nonfinancial Managers* by Ronald Spurga (2004, Penguin). There are financial statement templates for you in Appendix B. You can also go to www.sba.gov/tools to access a multitude of financial forms for your business.

THE BEAUTY OF BARTER

It is not always possible for companies to get everything they want or need by direct cash payment. It has long been a practice in domestic and international business and government to use **countertrade,** the exchange of goods or services paid for in whole or in part with other goods and services. There are many manifestations of countertrade, but the one most familiar and most often seen in small businesses circles is barter.

Savvy entrepreneurs have long used the art of bartering to start, grow, and propel their business while preserving their cash. Used throughout human history, **bartering** is the exchange of goods or services without the use of money. Bartering is one of the most popular and well-known aspects of countertrade. It is the oldest exchange method of record, but bartering isn't just swapping wampum and shells these days. The International Reciprocal Trade Association (IRTA) estimates that 470,000 U.S. companies participate in barter, averaging $12 billion in "swapped sales" each year. Of the corporations listed in the New York Stock Exchange, 65 percent use barter, and IRTA calculates that at least 25 percent of world trade involves barter or countertrade of some kind.[16] In recent economic times, recessions, layoffs, and financial hardships have made individuals and businesses more concerned than ever about preserving cash and more apt to barter goods and services. In March 2009, community board websites like Craigslist reported a 100 percent annual increase in listings for barter.[17]

Ideally, a bartering relationship brings added value to both parties, and is mutually beneficial. As a massage therapist, you have an incredibly helpful, valuable, and portable skill that others want, and you can utilize that skill to help you build your business without exhausting a lot of cash outflows. Perhaps you are just getting started and you want to develop new business cards for your business. Maybe you have a good friend who is gifted at design and print who would be happy to trade out for massages. Or maybe you know of an interior designer with TMJ problems, which just happens to be your area of specialization. Suggest a barter of their services for yours. One massage therapist trades her services for monthly carpet cleaning, while another has a plumber on call to fix his office's pipes. The options are limitless.

As you begin to cultivate your barter garden, you will want to do so strategically. Just as with business partners, you will want to barter with people you trust. One thing you will want to be aware of, of course, is the value of each individual's time. Direct trades are not always equitable.[18] For example, if you charge $90 per hour for your massage, but a graphic designer charges $5000 to create a logo and brand image, the inequitable value transfer could complicate a strict barter relationship. In these instances, you might consider a partial barter to reduce fees, other countertrade arrangements, or just submit to a cash outlay. You also want to be careful that you aren't paying more through barter than you would with cash; don't do an hour-for-hour exchange with someone who charges $10 for their service when you charge $65. Sit down and discuss an equitable exchange that works for both parties *before* you enter into a trade relationship.

If you don't know of any professionals with whom to barter your services, or if you just don't know where to start, there are several online resources for you. There are commissioned barter brokers and commercial barter clubs online. The National Association of Trade Exchanges (NATE) is a clearinghouse for barter members across the United States, and there are worldwide organizations such as BXI and ITEX. There is a host of barter sites available, such as Exmerce, barter.net, U-exchange, and TradeAway. Of course, you can't FedEx a massage to Dublin or Dubai in exchange for financial services or legal advice. Due to the rather geographically limited nature of your service offering, you might want to stick to community bulletin boards and Craigslist to tap into local barter scenes. And of course, exercise all common sense and safety precautions when developing any kind of relationship with individuals online (refer to Chapters 2, 6, and 15). You can always go to your networks or draw on word of mouth to find good referral partners as well.

As great as bartering and countertrade can be in business (and personal life), you should be aware of some of its limitations, as well. Bartering is not a tax loophole, and you are responsible for reporting all bartering activities as taxable income. You can typically report this income on Schedule C, Profit or Loss from Business Form 1040 or 1099-B from the IRS (more on this in Chapter 10). In addition to tax liability, you will have to evaluate the time-money equation. It can be hard to collect on a barter exchange if you are dealing with an individual or company who is less responsible, overly committed, or headed for bankruptcy. Therapists often report that they have rendered services from other professionals (and often other massage therapists) but never received their end of the bargain. Your time is valuable, and in certain instances it may just make more sense to pay for things in cash rather than lose a lot of your time chasing your benefit from exchanges.

PUT IT IN WRITING

Becoming a Barterista

As a massage therapist, you are well positioned to engage in barter relationships to get what you need or want without spending cash. Your skills are highly desirable (who can't use a massage?), and can be used to help you preserve your money as you build your business. Refer back to the Would Like/Must Have exercise you did at the beginning of the chapter. In the left-hand column, write out five things you "must have." In the right column, write down as many corresponding professionals or companies who might be willing to do some barter or countertrade with you for the things you want. Estimate the dollar value of the good and service, so you can get an idea of how much time you'll need to invest in bartering.

Product/Service	Dollar Value	Possible Barter Partners

CHAPTER SUMMARY BY LEARNING OBJECTIVES

1. **Explore the financial requirements of getting your business started** Financial management is the cornerstone of a healthy thriving business. A business cannot start, grow, or survive if there isn't enough to pay the bills and bring income to those involved. Start-up costs are the initial expenses associated with starting any new business, and will be in direct proportion to the scale and scope of your operations.
2. **Introduce traditional and innovative ways of finding funding** There are many ways to get funding for your business. You can use your own money, get debt financing through a bank, borrow from friends and family, get grant money, use credit cards, get venture capital, or bootstrap your business. Check in with local economic development centers, small business development centers, or local business incubators to get more insight on optimal choices for your unique financial situation.
3. **Define bootstrapping and identify ways to cut start-up costs** Bootstrapping refers to starting a business entirely on self-generated sources for initial expenses, and being as financially conservative as possible. Buying secondhand equipment, buying in bulk, shopping around, and bartering are good ways to bootstrap a new business.
4. **Contrast the pros and cons of partnering for money** A partnership is a business relationship between two or more individuals who share risk, labor, cooperation, and responsibility. Typically all parties agree to provide financial, material, or knowledge capital for the business. One of the top reasons people partner is to increase their financial parameters and to minimize personal risk. However, like any business arrangement, there can be considerable pros and cons to entering a partnership. Sharing risk may sound good, but sharing profits, responsibility, and control is not for everyone.
5. **Examine the importance of separating personal and business accounts** A common financial mistake that many novice entrepreneurs make is to blur the boundaries between their personal and business finances. But keeping the two separate is important for tax purposes, streamlining audits, staying organized, and assessing your business's true financial picture.
6. **Describe techniques to forecast profits** A forecast is a researched, calculated, and carefully formulated projection of the expected financial situation of a business. Forecasts are generally based on the current understanding and future expectations of many internal and external conditions. You can forecast your profits by estimating your revenue, and then subtracting your estimated expenses.
7. **Introduce financial statements: cash flow, income statement, balance sheet** Financial statements are documents that provide an outline of your business's financial health from a short- and long-term view. Financial statements include the balance sheet, income statement, and the statement of cash flows.
8. **Define accounting for your business and assess the role of accountants** Accounting is the consistent recordkeeping, verification, interpretation, and reporting of a business's assets, liabilities, expenses, cash inflows, cash outflows, and financial activities. An accountant is a professional who helps an individual, group, or business manage its books. Many massage therapists that run their business maintain that their accountant is one of their most valuable financial allies over time.
9. **Define countertrade and examine the benefits and drawbacks of bartering your services** Countertrade is the exchange of goods or services paid for in whole or in part with other goods and services. Bartering, a subset of countertrade, is the trade of goods and services with no cash exchange. Bartering can be very beneficial to a business, as it helps secure valuable goods and services while preserving cash. However, all barters are taxable, and you must be vigilant about engaging in trades that are both equitable and value-adding for you and your business.

ACTIVITIES

Quiz: Financial Management Review

1. ______________ fluctuate based upon the volume of productivity and output activities of the business.
   a. Variable costs
   b. Fixed costs
   c. Countertrades
   d. Loan obligations
2. The ______________ gives an account of a company's cash activities (such as operations, investing, or financing) in a period of time.
   a. forecasted profits
   b. balance sheet
   c. income statement
   d. statement of cash flows
3. If you are in a business partnership with Kate, and Kate skips town to move to Kauai, you are legally responsible for ______________ of the business debts.
   a. none
   b. 50 percent
   c. 80 percent
   d. 100 percent
4. Breakeven refers to:
   a. the phase when both partners are contributing equally.
   b. the point where revenues and expenses are equal, and there is no profit or loss.
   c. the perfect wave.
   d. the point where profits are greater than losses.
5. ______________ is the unpaid physical and mental labor of the owner of a business that increases the business's worth. It is your unique contribution and commitment to your business that makes it valuable, especially in the beginning.
   a. Exploitation
   b. Sweat equity
   c. Barter
   d. Inflow
6. Your bank wants you to show collateral for a loan. An example of what you could use is:
   a. your business plan
   b. your financial statements
   c. your house
   d. your friend's car
7. True or False: Most entrepreneurial massage therapists receive their funding through venture capitalists.
8. True or False: While it is possible to use credit cards to build your business, the typically high interest rates can zap your business's financial health if you do not repay the balances quickly.
9. True or False: Bartering is a great way to build your business under the table and off the radar.
10. True or False: Once you get beyond the initial start-up costs for your massage business, you don't really have to worry about spending much to keep it going.
11. True or False: If you do not perform exactly as your financial forecasts indicate, you will have to give your money back to the bank.
12. True or False: It is possible to borrow too much money when starting a new business.

Financial Scavenger Hunt[19]

People have all kinds of experiences related to finances for their business; you may be surrounded by a wealth of financial resources and not even know about it. Pair up and use Table 13-3 ■ as a scavenger hunt list to find as many people as you can who have done the things below. Start with classmates, teachers, friends—anyone! The team that finds the most matches wins (and remember people's experiences; you might be able to ask them for help with your own financial management).

TABLE 13-3 Find Someone Who . . .

• Has employed others and paid payroll taxes	• Has had a business checking account	• Has started a business on credit cards	• Knows an angel investor or venture capitalist
• Is a member of local chamber of commerce	• Made money on the Internet	• Has taken a company public (and sold stock)	• Has been on the floor of a stock exchange
• Borrowed money from friends and family	• Has formed an LLC	• Is a Certified Public Accountant	• Has gone bankrupt
• Has bootstrapped a company	• Likes to make financial statements	• Has done financial forecasting	• Knows someone at the Small Business Administration
• Has been audited by the IRS	• Has received a grant	• Has more than five credit cards	• Has an accountant

Case Study

Athena

Athena wants to open a massage business, and she knows she needs to figure out her start-up and maintenance costs to gauge her financial requirements. She has come to you, her business coach, for some help. At your first meeting, the two of you explore the things that she will need to support her dream business. This is what Athena tells you:

> I have just finished massage school, and I want to open up my professional massage business in the historic storefronts near my house. There are two currently available, and the one I like most rents for $1,000 per month. I have been using my massage school's table, so I don't currently have one. I would like to get one of those hydraulic tables so that I don't have to adjust it, but only if I can find a used one that is affordable. As far as marketing materials, my friend is a graphic designer and designed my cards and brochures as a gift when I graduated. I don't have a website, though I believe I definitely need one. My student membership in my massage organization is expiring now that I'm graduating, and I need to get a professional one, as well as all the licenses, permits, and fees for my business. I have talked with another designer friend who estimates that the furniture and decorations I want can be obtained for about $500. I don't anticipate hiring anyone at this point.

Help Athena fill out Table 13-4 ■, based on what she has told you.

TABLE 13-4 Athena's Would Like versus Must Have Items

Item	Cost	Would Like	Must Have

CHAPTER 14

Managing Yourself and Others

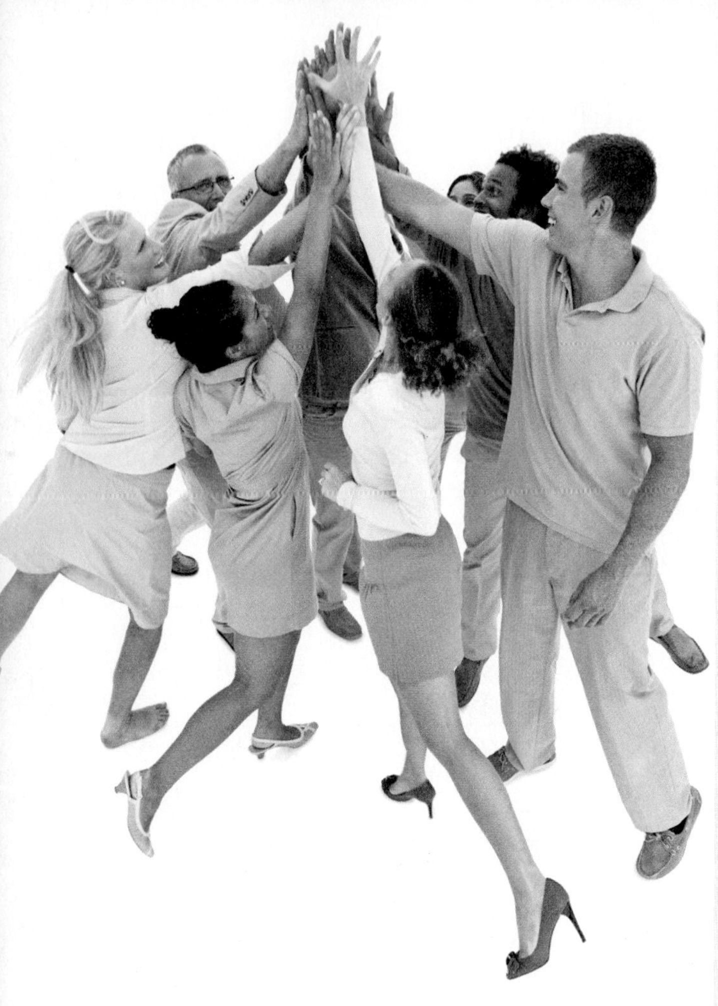

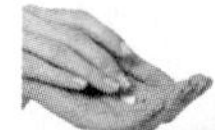

CHAPTER OUTLINE

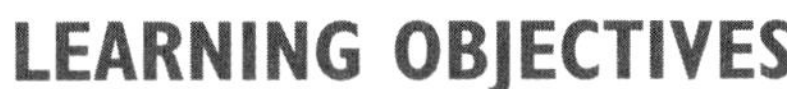

LEARNING OBJECTIVES

1. Explore aspects of yourself as a manager
2. Introduce different management styles
3. Evaluate the difference between management and leadership
4. Explain how to budget and pay employees, and introduce employment contracts
5. Describe the process of staff selection and interviews
6. Define retention and explore ways to keep people on board
7. Explain the components of creating and branding culture
8. Analyze staff handbooks and basics of employee training
9. Research techniques for scheduling employees
10. Identify ways to develop great customer service from all employees

KEY TERMS

autocratic manager *231*
branded culture *237*
contract *233*
customer satisfaction survey *241*
customer service *240*
democratic manager *231*
employee benefits *233*
empowerment *232*
intern *232*
interview *234*
job description *234*
knowledge management *238*
laissez-faire manager *231*
leadership *232*
learning culture *239*
management style *231*
manager *230*
mixed management style *231*
non-compete agreement *233*
onboarding *237*
paternalistic manager *231*
payroll *233*
reference *235*
retention *235*
staff handbook *238*
standard operating procedures *238*
training *239*
turnover *236*

BEING IN CHARGE

> *The conventional definition of management is getting work done through people, but real management is developing people through work.*
>
> —Agha Hasan Abedi

Perhaps you have employees already, or know that a time will come when your business will grow to the point of needing to bring in some help. Or perhaps you will design a business model that involves employees from the beginning. Suddenly you are not only the business owner, you are the manager as well. A **manager** is a person who has authority to administer and supervise the affairs of others. Many of the chapters in this book have revolved around the skills to manage yourself and your business, but this chapter will focus on some of the main skills you will need to manage other people (note: throughout thc chapter, the term "employee" will be more commonly used. This is for simplicity, and does not intend to ignore the distinctions between employees and independent contractors; see more on this topic in Chapters 2 and 10).

As you saw in Chapter 2, it is not uncommon for managers of massage therapists to have little or no background in massage. This chapter focuses on you, a therapist, having the additional role of manager, a situation which puts you in a good position to be an empathetic and supportive boss. Perhaps you already have some experience in supervising others, or have administered a large staff before. Or perhaps you have never been in charge. Either way, this chapter aims to help you be the best manager you can be.

NOT ALL MANAGERS ARE CREATED EQUAL: LOOKING AT THE DIFFERENT MANAGEMENT STYLES

No matter how good you are at wearing every imaginable hat in your business, no business owner can do everything alone. Regardless of your business model or where you are conducting your services, a growing business relies on its

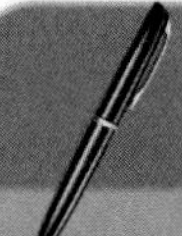

PUT IT IN WRITING

Let Me Speak to Your Manager

Functioning as a manager can be both exhilarating and intimidating. Take a few moments to explore your thoughts and beliefs about managing others. Write out your responses and put them in your *Business of Massage Therapy* notebook.

1. When I think about sharing key business information with others, I feel
____
____
2. I realize that when there are problems, people will come to me for solutions. When I think of that, it makes me
____
____
3. It is said that a good manager is able to inspire and motivate others. When I think about myself in this role, I
____
____
4. When it comes to delegating tasks, I am typically
____
____
5. It is possible that there will be times when people on my staff are angry or confrontational with me. I usually handle these situations by
____
____
6. If someone does something that is against the rules or that I do not like, I will generally
____
____
7. Workforces can be very diverse; when I think of managing many different people with many different personality types and backgrounds, I
____
____
8. A lot of effective management can hinge on good communication. When I think about communicating openly with staff, I
____
____

As with so many of the other self-explorations in this book, there are no rights or wrongs to the questions above. However, do take a moment to reflect on your answers, and see where your management strengths and weaknesses may lie as you go forward.

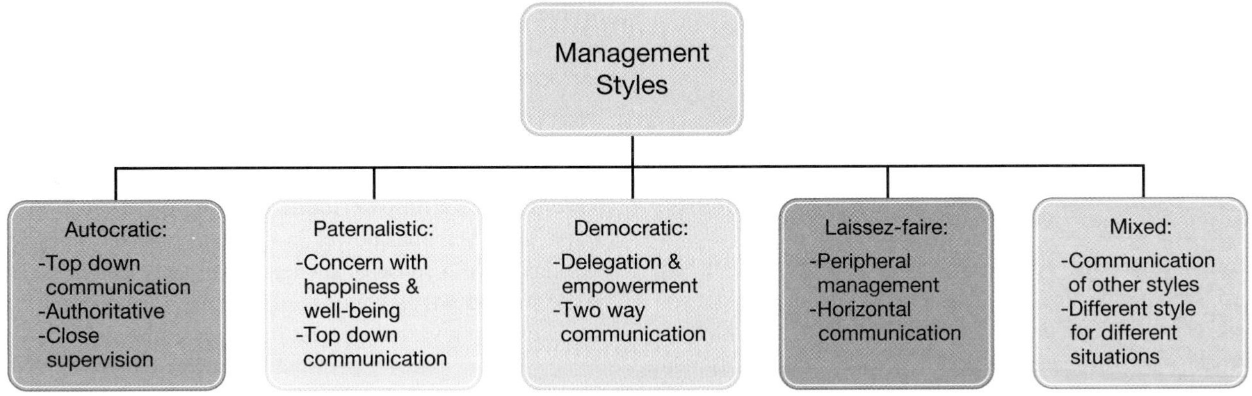

FIGURE 14-1

The most common management styles include autocratic, paternalistic, democratic, laissez-faire, and a mixed style.

employees. The kinds of people you hire and the way you manage them can have a tremendous impact on your company's overall success. It will also impact your own experience within your business, as anyone you bring in and the relationships that develop become a major part of your life.

Before you even begin to think about putting out a want ad, take some time to really consider what it takes to manage not only yourself, but others. Write down a detailed list of things you hope for and expect of potential employees. Think how effectively you can oversee operations, and consider your own management style. A **management style** is the approach you take to interacting with and directing others. Experts maintain that there are generally five different management styles: autocratic, paternalistic, democratic, laissez-faire, and mixed[1](Figure 14-1 ■).

An **autocratic manager** tends to restrict information, make all the decisions, and retain all the power. Communication is top-down, and employees are expected to follow the directives of the manager. This is typically referred to as the "classical management style." While this can be effective in consistency of operations, many view this style as very authoritative and find that it can create dependency or decreased motivation in subordinates. Many studies have shown that this management style often results in higher absenteeism and employee turnover.[2]

A **paternalistic manager** is one who tries to operate as a parental figure, factoring the needs and happiness of the workers into management decisions. Still a top-down management style, paternalism is often described as a more "touchy-feely" form of autocratic management (think Michael Scott from the TV show *The Office*). *Pater* is Latin for father—however, women can operate from this management style, too. This style can foster loyalty for some employees, and often results in less turnover; however it too can result in a dependency and decreased initiative.[3]

> *A good manager doesn't fire people. He hires people and inspires people. People, Ryan. People will never go out of business.*
>
> —Michael Scott, *The Office*

A **democratic manager** is one who allows consensus in decision making, and permits a great deal of interaction between management and employees. Communication is both top-down and bottom-up, and information is openly shared. This works particularly well in situations that require more empowered decision making from employees. It can often result in more job satisfaction and work performance, as employees gain a sense of ownership in their work. However, without a solid company culture this management style can result in company inconsistency and slow decision making.[4]

With what is often called the "hands-off" management style, a **laissez-faire manager** is typically on the sidelines while other staff run the business. The term comes from the French expression used to describe a strategy of allowing events to run their own course. Communication is often much more limited and horizontal in laissez-faire management than in other styles, and employees are given the authority to determine their own objectives and resolve their own issues. This style can lead to high levels of autonomy and creativity in employees; however, it can also result in lack of direction and focus, and a sloppy business presentation.

A **mixed management style** occurs when a manager utilizes different management styles for different people or different situations, blending autocratic, paternalistic, democratic, or laissez-faire methods. This can also be a result of a manager's own diverse background. While it can be very effective to adopt different aspects of the different management styles, it can confuse both employees and clients if a manager changes styles frequently. In general, consistency and cohesiveness are best in business.

MANAGEMENT VERSUS LEADERSHIP

> *The world is full of managers but desperately short of leaders.*
>
> —Jack Welch

Before you ever bring in anyone else to work for you, it might help you to spend some time reflecting on what kind of manager you would like to be. Your unique style will be rooted in the way you approach others in general. A person who sees workers as mere interchangeable workhorses or fuel for the fire of their business will manage people quite differently from someone who sees them as integral, invaluable members of a team. Most people who gravitate toward holistic practices tend to be more interpersonally empowering, with an intuitive nature and an emotional openness. Though many holistic practitioners still operate business in an old-school manner, most tend to reject the fear-based management patterns that can be common in other industries. Because they are called to help others, they are often very focused on the satisfaction and happiness of other people, including those working for them. In addition to wanting to provide a space of healing and retreat for their clients, many holistic business owners are also compelled to provide that environment for individuals in their employ as well. In an ideal holistic work environment, everyone is happy: the community, the clients, the employees, and the boss. However, people-pleasing alone is not enough to manage successfully or to inspire others.

A lot of management literature talks about leadership, as many leaders are also managers. However, not all managers are cut out to be (or desire to be) in a leadership position. **Leadership** is the process of guiding others in the accomplishment of a common objective or goal. It is about rousing others to the point that both you and they can align around purposeful business pursuits and inspired action. Managers provide resources, but leaders provide vision.

In addition to the personal gratification and fulfillment of positive leadership, it is becoming increasingly evident that happy employees are much better for your bottom line. Over years of research, leadership consultants Jackie and Kevin Freiberg have found again and again that managers who successfully provide an environment and context where people can work hard, love what they do, be grounded in values and authenticity, and find balance in their lives often outperform those in the industry who do not.[5] Their consistent findings show that companies that provide their employees a sense of ownership and empowerment have lower turnover rates and higher productivity (two very good things for any bottom line).[6] **Empowerment** supports others to find and assert their personal power in the workplace. Empowered workers have a sense of ownership in your business, and, while maybe not as committed to it as you yourself, definitely exhibit a vested interest in things going well.

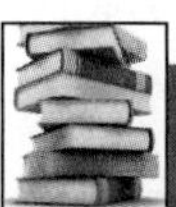

HELPFUL RESOURCES

Approaching your role as a manager *and* a leader can be a wonderful way to maximize your experience as a business owner. There are many terrific books on leadership available. Check out *Guts: Companies that Blow the Doors Off of Business as Usual* by Kevin and Jackie Freiberg (2004, Random House) or *The 21 Irrefutable Laws of Leadership* by John C. Maxwell (2007, Yates & Yates).

PAYING THE PIPER: TAKING CARE OF YOUR EMPLOYEES

There are many reasons you might elect to bring employees or independent contractors in to your business: perhaps you need support with administrative tasks such as answering the phone, managing client appointments, or filing SOAP notes. Perhaps you would like to bring in someone with a lot of marketing experience to take over promotional activities. Or perhaps your own schedule is getting so full that you simply need other therapists and bodyworkers to help you meet the demand.

Some holistic practitioners have had success with bringing in an apprentice or an intern. An **intern** is a person who works temporarily in a capacity that focuses on on-the-job training. Because the focus is on gaining experience and knowledge, and often exchangeable for school credit, internships are typically unpaid; however, some businesses pay their interns for their time. If you decide to bring in an intern, know that the U.S. Department of Labor has outlined a list of criteria that must be met in order for an internship to be unpaid legally. Unfortunately, many employers abuse intern relationships as a source of free labor, particularly during hard economic times.[7] If you bring in an intern, make sure you are following legal guidelines and providing real value to him or her.

Many massage students get valuable training and hands-on experience through internships. They are also able to fulfill their schools' hands-on hours requirements while being exposed to new techniques and skills. You will want to check with your local laws regarding massage regulations if you intend to have an unlicensed student intern performing massages—many cities will not allow this. However, massage therapist interns who can't perform massages yet can benefit from learning the administrative aspects of running a massage business, and can help with business-specific tasks such as marketing or client management.

In Chapter 10, "Organizing and Legal Structures," you learned a great deal about the responsibilities as an employer, the forms you will need to fill out, all about workers' compensation and unemployment taxes, and the withholding taxes you will need to pay. Don't forget that you have different responsibilities if you claim people as employees or independent contractors. Although many business owners in the massage, spa, and wellness industries still greatly misclassify employees as independent contractors, the IRS is very clear on the distinctions. In fact, it is increasingly cracking down on business owners in these industries, so remember to be very cautious on how you make your designations.[8] Remember that if the IRS establishes that you have been classifying workers as independent contractors yet treating them like employees, you may be subject to large penalties and fines (see Appendix B for the 20 factors the IRS utilizes to determine employee versus independent contractor status).[9]

In addition to all of those logistics, there is one other very important element of having employees: ensuring that you have enough money to consistently make payroll! **Payroll** is all wages, salaries, bonuses, benefits, or other compensation that is paid to employees or independent contractors for services rendered. Employee-related costs are usually the largest line item expense for any company's budget.[10] When you are the boss, you are responsible for making sure that everyone else gets paid. In many cases, you won't pay yourself until everyone else is taken care of (which can really hurt in lean times). Some holistic business owners have reported that they didn't take any money out of their own business for a year or more to ensure that their employees were taken care of first.

When you are creating a budget for employees, make sure that you include all of the hidden costs of employee benefits. **Employee benefits** are any non-wage or salary-related compensation given to employees. For example, if you provide employees with health insurance, matched retirement contributions to a 401(k), sick leave, or vacation time, these are all employee benefits. You might offer your employees discounts on products or services, or provide additional trainings for continued skill-building. While many employers in the massage industry are increasingly doing away with these benefits, and while most part-time employees do not qualify for them, if you are a business owner who plans on providing these benefits, you want to ensure you have enough cash flow to cover the comprehensive cost of an employee.

In general, it is a very good idea to draw up contracts or agreements with anyone who is working for you. A **contract** is an exchange of agreements between two or more parties, wherein promises are made about what will and will not be done. Contracts, whether verbal or written, are legally binding; however, written contracts are much more easily enforced in a court of law. Although massage therapists, by nature, often tend to be more trusting and less preoccupied with legal contracts, they are becoming increasingly common in the industry. In an often very labor-friendly, litigious society, employers have to be very careful to protect themselves against any legal action. But contracts are not just for the sake of the employer. A good contract supports and protects both employers and employees. In addition to pre-empting problems, good contracts can also serve to help resolve misunderstandings or clarify relationship terms and goals. Contracts are usually negotiable. Depending on your operating model, your management style, and your company's vision, you should leave some room for adaptation and negotiation down the road.

The complexity of contracts can vary significantly, from a standard boilerplate form from an office supply store to a unique 40-page document drafted by your attorney. There are many software products on the market that are designed to help you tailor your own contracts. The level of complexity of your contracts will be a function of your own specific needs, including the scope and the scale of your business. Some of the common components and themes for written contracts include:

- Full names, addresses, contact information of all parties
- Company mission statement
- Employee-employer relationship definition and expectations
- Obligations of both parties
- Fees and terms of payment
- All services to be provided
- Expense reimbursement
- Benefits
- Disputes and relationship termination policies
- Signatures and dates

It has become increasingly common to include non-compete clauses in a contract, or even to have new hires sign a stand-alone non-compete agreement. A **non-compete agreement** is a binding contract wherein one party (usually the employee) agrees to avoid certain behaviors or activities that would be in direct competition against another party (usually the employer). Examples of stipulations in non-compete agreements include working for competitor companies, starting a similar business, soliciting clients for personal business, stealing trade secrets, or using other proprietary company information for personal gain.

In the massage industry, it is incredibly common for therapists to substantiate their income by working for multiple employers, or by supplementing income from their own practice by working for another. Thus, it can be completely crippling to one's livelihood to create a non-compete agreement that prohibits an individual for working for anyone else. However, it is completely within your rights to want to retain the clients, trade practices, and business systems that you have worked so hard to create for your company. A good and realistic non-compete agreement can help you be protective of these things without mercilessly tying the hands of the individuals working for you.

GETTING THE RIGHT PEOPLE ON YOUR TEAM: HOW TO ATTRACT, SELECT, AND KEEP GREAT PEOPLE

Now that you have a good idea of your management style and have thought about some of the logistics of bringing people on board, take some time to really think about what you want from an employee and to be strategic in obtaining it. The people you hire can be a major factor in determining the success of your business, and the importance of hiring decisions are magnified in small companies.[11] Anyone who works for you will become an ambassador of your business, and you want to attract and select people that will represent your business in the desired way. In addition to the impact workers have on your external market, they have a substantial impact on your internal one. Many management experts advise business owners to hire for culture and with the company mission at the forefront of the attraction, selection, and retention systems.[12] You will be spending a lot of time with the people working for you, and they will have a large impact on your company culture (review Chapter 2 for more on company culture).

Think about it: there are vibrant, enthusiastic, optimistic people who can find opportunities in any challenge. These people emanate enthusiasm and have a contagious passion for the work that they do. People generally like to be around these kinds of people. There are also the negative, cynical, pessimistic people who complain about everything and drain the energy from a situation. This may seem like a no-brainer, but which type of person would you rather have working in your business?

Now that you have the *kind* of person in mind, take a moment to get clear on your goal for hiring them. Figure out what exactly you want them to do, and the skills required to do those things. Then take the time to craft a comprehensive job description. A **job description** is a written explanation of expectations that accompanies a job, including duties, responsibilities, working relationships, desired outcomes, and materials to be used. With a good picture of the kind of person you are seeking and a clear job description in mind, it will be easy to start the hunt for the right person or people. You may want to create an enticing recruiting ad and run it through public listings, or perhaps you prefer to recruit through the grapevine. Asking around and letting people know you are looking for help is a great way to attract quality candidates. Go to your networks and put the word out.

FIRST STEPS

As you go about your life in the next few days, try this exercise. Observe the employees working in the places you frequent and take note of the exchanges you have with them. Does the cashier make you feel special? Does the bank teller act nasty? Does the barista at your favorite coffee spot snap at her co-workers? Is there a playful atmosphere among the employees at your favorite restaurant? From these experiences, write about the kinds of interactions you have had and the kinds of people you would and would not like to have in your business.

____

____

____

____

____

____

GETTING ORGANIZED

If you decide to post an employment ad, there are many ways to go about it. Many holistic employers post ads on targeted websites, such as Massage Jobs.com. AMTA, NCBTMB, and other trade organizations offer online job boards. Craigslist is an incredibly popular (and relatively inexpensive) place for job listings, and can help you attract people to fill different kinds of roles within your business. Depending on the level of skill you are looking for, you might post a listing on the job board of local schools.

While it isn't always common (or necessary) to post commission or salary structures in an employment ad, you will want to be clear on the amount of money you will are willing and able to pay people ahead of time. Deciding how much to pay people will have a lot to do with your geographic area, your business model, and the standard rates of pay in the industry. There can be a wide range in compensation for massage therapy, so you might find it helpful to ask around about what other similar businesses in the area are paying their employees.

Once you start getting resumes, you will want to start scheduling interviews. As you learned in Chapter 2, an **interview** is a formal meeting that is designed to gauge the qualifications, skills, and fit of a potential employee by an employer, and vice versa. You will need very different skills to be the interviewer than you may have used in the past as the interviewee. While your goal as a job seeker is to sell yourself and gauge the company's fit with your goals, your goal as an employer is to find top talent to represent your business. As a manager, your role in an interview is to be a bit of an investigator, while at the same time facilitating a smooth social exchange and processing a lot of information.[13] Preparation is key.

Before any interview, you will want to come up with a list of questions that will determine whether an individual has the qualities and skills you are looking for. If you are interviewing multiple candidates, you will want to be consistent and ask the same questions of all applicants. If you are looking for information about cultural fit and qualitative factors, you might ask for examples from past work or life experiences that illustrate desired traits. Because so much of what makes a good massage therapist is nonverbal, it is very common to divide the interview process between a face-to-face conversation and a hands-on demonstration. If you are very interested in the quality of skill and technique, have candidates give you a massage. This is beneficial because there is no other way to gauge a person's touch (and, it goes without saying, because you get a massage!).

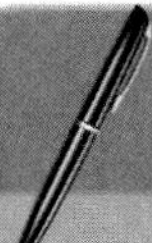

PUT IT IN WRITING

Who Is Interviewing Who?

The hot seat isn't just the one that the interviewee is sitting in—you have a lot of responsibility in the hiring situation as well. As you learned in Chapter 2, an interview is a chance for both parties to suss out a mutual fit. Expect (and hopefully invite) the candidate to ask questions of you and the business. To help you think of ideal comportment in an interview, think back to one of the better interviews you can remember as an interviewee, and answer the following questions:

1. When you think about the person who interviewed you, what do you remember?

   ____

   ____

2. What things did the interviewer do to put you at ease at the beginning of the interview?

   ____

   ____

3. Who directed the flow of conversation?

   ____

   ____

4. Were there things that you did not like about what he or she did?

   ____

   ____

5. What would you do differently if you were in charge?

   ____

   ____

6. What things would you like to do the same or similarly?

   ____

   ____

Of course, go with your gut instincts. If someone looks great on paper but gives you a bad vibe in person, trust yourself and do not bring them on to work with your team. It is also a good idea to ask for and check references. A **reference** is a contact person that has a relationship with the candidate, and can vouch for him or her in some capacity. References are typically personal or professional, and their name and contact information is supplied to you by the candidate. They can provide a lot of background scoop on an individual's character. Checking references can also help you find out about some of the more abstract qualities of candidates, such as loyalty, reliability, and/or employment longevity. Here are a few more tips for interviewing and selecting great people:

- Do your homework. Most hiring managers do internet research on prospective candidates. See if you can learn anything about the individual before they come in for an interview. You might be surprised at the things (good, bad, and ugly) that you may find.
- Take notes during the interview, so you can remember highlights and record likes and dislikes.
- Take your time. Don't feel pressured to give someone a job just to fill the position or make them happy. You want the fit to be the right one for both your sake and the candidate's. Honor the importance of this decision and the impact it will have on you and your business.
- Keep it legal. Don't ever ask questions that are not job specific. Asking about a candidate's religion, age, sexual orientation, marriage status, or any other questions that do not relate directly to the position could lead to a discrimination charge and even a lawsuit.
- Have fun! Interviews don't have to be somber events. Set a professional but relaxed tone up front.

KEEPING EVERYONE ON BOARD: THE IMPORTANCE OF EMPLOYEE RETENTION

In earlier marketing chapters, you learned that it is more expensive to attract a new client than it is to keep them. The same is true when it comes to human resources and retaining your employees. **Retention** is the intentional and ongoing practice of maintaining and holding on to staff. This is often done by measures such as providing a harmonious work environment, creating programs that boost motivation and morale, providing clear expectations and objectives, emphasizing good work/life balance, and being a good leader. Employee retention should start in the initial attraction and selection process, where you first begin to gauge a match. It should then continue on throughout the employer-employee relationship.

If you factor in the resources and expenses involved with having a position vacant, advertising, interviewing, training, replacements costs, and so forth, hiring people can be very expensive. The Society for Human Resource Management reports that the average cost of replacing an \$8.00 per hour worker was \$3500.[14] As the amount that an employee earns goes up, so do your replacement costs. In general, hiring and retaining massage employees or contractors is not typically as expensive as in other industries that require intensive training or complex operations. However, replacing people is still costly and employee retention is a major factor for your business's bottom line and the cohesiveness of its culture. Every time a new person is brought on or a team member leaves the organization, the dynamic is impacted. This is particularly true in small businesses, where changes in personnel are not as quickly absorbed as in large corporations.

According to the U.S. Department of Labor, the average person in America changes careers three to six times in a lifetime. However, people in the Generation Y age group (born between the early 1980s and mid-1990s) are only expected to stay in any given job for one or two years.[15] Of course, people start and leave jobs all the time and for innumerable reasons; many of those reasons have nothing to do with the company. However, the vast majority of reasons people leave a position is employer-related.[16]

Turnover is the rate at which a company obtains and loses workers. As you have seen, when all of the expenses involved in recruiting, training, retaining, and replacing workers are considered, the cost of turnover can be quite high. Turnover costs can involve investments of time, money, resources, and energy (see Figure 14-2 ■).

While turnover rates can often be quite high in the massage industry when compared to others, some conditions lend themselves to higher turnover rates for some massage companies over others. There are plenty of massage businesses that operate from the cheap labor model, and do not spend much time, energy, resources, or money on the hiring or retaining process. Due to the low pay scale and lower employee investment, turnover rates in these businesses can be very high. There is nothing inherently wrong with a low-cost model, and if this is your model, that is perfectly fine. However, if you are interested in retaining high-quality help and want to minimize turnover, here are a few helpful tips to guide you through.

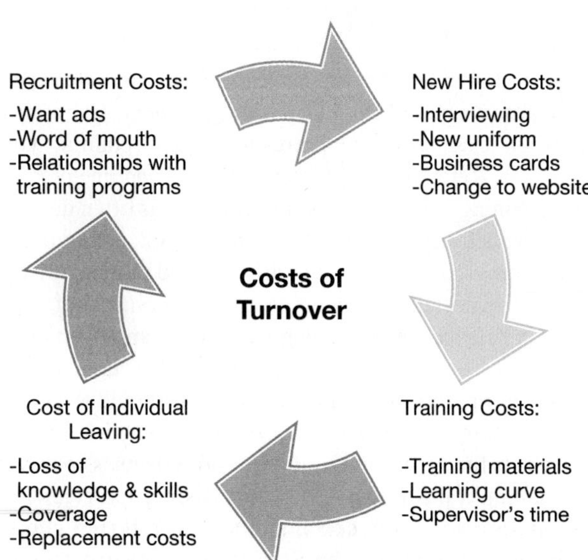

FIGURE 14-2

There are many hidden costs of employee turnover, such as loss of interpersonal dynamics and knowledge capital of departing employees, recruiting new employees, and management's time spent interviewing and training new employees.

- *Be the change you wish to see:* When you are modeling great customer service, ethical practices, and high standards, it is much more likely that people will respect and want to work with you over the long haul.
- *Keep it interesting:* People like to stay engaged and even challenged in their work, and stagnant work environments can zap people's motivation. Create a contest, organize events, offer professional development workshops, or anything else you can think of to keep people engaged and keep the work interesting for everyone involved.
- *Treat everyone like a CEO:* Of course you want your clients to feel important and cared for. Aim to take great care of your clients *and* the people working for you. Treating employees like guests will carry exponentially into the care and service your paying clients will receive.
- *Be consistent:* As much as possible, stay steady in the way you deal with people and the way that things operate. Having an employee manual, standard operating procedures, or other recorded systems helps this consistency.
- *Be clear:* People often report a lack of clarity about expectations as a major source of anxiety in their work environment. Make sure that you explain objectives and expectations, and leave room for people to ask questions if they do not understand anything.
- *Communicate:* Keep in touch with your people. Even if you are all very busy, take time to touch base with internal meetings, newsletters, e-mails, or other communications. Keep people posted about important information—especially the kind you don't want them hearing from someone else.
- *Train:* A major cause of frustration and turnover is insufficient training. If people are going to be expected to have specific knowledge, such as how to use a computer scheduling system or how to perform a spirulina body wrap, make sure they get the training necessary.
- *Provide the necessary materials and resources:* Nothing is more frustrating than work slowdowns that are caused by faulty or insufficient materials. Of course, computers will go down and laundry may get backed up, but try to stay on top of ensuring that everyone has what they need to do the job.
- *Recognize achievement:* Everyone likes to feel valued for the contribution that they are making, and

PUT IT IN WRITING

I Quit!

Chances are good that you have left a job or two in your day. Write down your reasons for leaving here. Then write down the things that you would have done as your manager in that situation that might have made you stay.

Job	Reasons for Leaving	What I Would Have Done as Manager

working hard without recognition can make people want to leave. If someone makes a great marketing piece or begins to develop a steady following of clients (bringing you consistent business), acknowledge the importance of their contribution.

- *Have realistic workloads:* People can burn out in any industry, and massage is no different. The physical and emotional demands of the work can lead to burnout quickly. Make sure employees have sufficient breaks—even when it gets busy, try not to schedule people so tightly that they don't have time for a snack or a trip to the restroom.

CREATING AND BRANDING CULTURE

One of the main reasons reported for leaving a job, particularly early on, is insufficient assimilation into the company culture. This is often due to a lack of training, accommodation, explanation, or general feeling of welcome for new employees. This can be avoided with a strategic plan for onboarding new people. **Onboarding** is the process of helping a newcomer adjust and assimilate into the culture and operations of the business. The way in which you onboard new employees can make a big difference in how long they stay in your company.

You have heard a fair bit about culture in this book. You have also heard a lot about branding—mostly in the marketing context. Now you are going to hear about branding culture. A **branded culture** is a company culture where members of the organization are enthusiastically devoted to the values and mission of the organization to the point where company culture becomes an integral part of company image. Companies that have been successful with branding their culture include Southwest Airlines, Kimpton Hotels, and Enterprise Rent-a-Car. You may say to yourself, "But those are all huge corporate companies—what does branding culture have to do with *my* small business?" The quick answer: a lot! Even if you only hire one person, there will indeed be a company culture. What is more, there will be a great opportunity to make that culture a major contributing factor to your success.

Having a company that is known for its great working culture does tremendous things. First of all, it promotes an environment of enthusiasm and commitment, where people are there for much more than a paycheck. Branded cultures of all sizes are magnets for attracting the "right kind" of people—both clients and employees—to their business.[17] Not only do people want to patronize places where the workers are genuinely passionate and truly happy, but great people always want to work there. The word of mouth buzz for both employees and clients is incredibly powerful when it comes to a strong company culture.

> *People will work very hard for money, but they will give their life for meaning.*
>
> —David Pottruck, CEO of Charles Schwab

Sounds great—but how do you get there? Like everything, branded cultures occur through intentional strategy and clear vision. And shaping culture can take time, especially if you are trying to change an existing one. The best place to start is with an end goal in mind. What kind of organization do you want to have, and what kind of a culture will help you achieve your goals? And what will people need to accomplish *their* goals in that culture? People are motivated by innumerable reasons, and their needs vary along a continuum (refer to Chapter 12 to learn more about Maslow's Hierarchy of Needs). If you already have people working for you, take the time to inquire about what they need, what motivates them, and what would make their job more meaningful. If you have yet to hire someone, put yourself in the role of an employee in your company and answer the questions yourself.

Another important tip is to remember that building a culture is not a one-time deal: cultures are intentionally

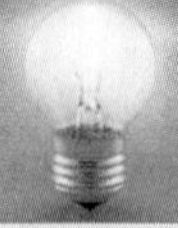

BRIGHT IDEAS

Sara is the owner of a wellness center, and knew that culture was so important from the beginning that she wrote about it in her business plan. Sara offers generous benefits, provides free child care to her employees (and clients), and coordinates frequent team-building events. She also hosts an annual weekend retreat for all her staff, giving everyone a chance to come together, unwind, and enjoy one another outside of the work environment. Sara's center is known throughout the community for its great service and culture. Not only do clients rave about it and provide endless referrals, Sara gets a stack of new job applications every week!

crafted and maintained on an ongoing basis. Culture isn't something that is created once and then goes on autopilot, but rather something that requires vigilance and commitment. If it is something you value, keep culture at the forefront of your planning efforts as a manager. If you provide any kind of training to new people, be sure to talk about culture in training material and handbooks. Kimpton Hotels spends a great deal of time talking about their "Culture of Care" throughout their training program, understanding that their branded culture is the cornerstone of their success. Many companies that brand their culture offer employee referral programs, as most fabulous people know other fabulous people. Depending on your scale and scope, you might offer people financial or service incentives for bringing on other great team members.

And finally, believe in the culture, the vision of the business, and ultimately the people in it. As Dave Liniger, founder of REMAX International, maintains, "Believe in your employees (or potential employees) more than they believe in themselves. They will rise to your expectations."[18]

PITFALLS

Many holistic entrepreneurs have made the mistake of confusing their role as managers. There is a very fine line between valuing your employees while creating a great culture and trying to be close friends with people that work for you. Remember that your role as a manager is to be a manager, not a buddy. While you can have a great working relationship with everyone, be cautious of your boundaries.

BY THE BOOK: CREATING STAFF HANDBOOKS AND TRAINING STAFF

You have heard about the importance of systems for simplifying business operations and making your life as a manager and business owner much easier. One way to do this is to create materials that support consistency of business activity. For example, if you are verbally communicating expectations to everyone you manage, you will spend a lot more time and energy than if you were to put it all in writing. Not only does this make things easier for you, it contributes to the constancy of the information. This is a form of **knowledge management,** the practice of identifying, collecting, organizing, and circulating the collective knowledge and experiences of an organization and its people. Strong company communication can be a major part of knowledge management. The more efficient the knowledge management process, the better the application and leverage of internal knowledge.

Although there are many sophisticated technologies available for knowledge management that you might be interested in for your business, one tried and true form of knowledge management is the staff handbook. A **staff handbook** provides general information on guidelines, expectations, requirements, policies, resources, and procedures for a business (Figure 14-3 ■). Handbooks are a wonderful part of onboarding new employees, as well as a source of support throughout the employer-employee relationship. Similar to a contract, a staff handbook helps clarify roles for both managers and staff, promotes consistency, and protect parties from legal disruptions.

In addition to general policies, handbooks often include standard operating procedures. **Standard operating procedures** (or SOPS) are sets of instruction for handling regular

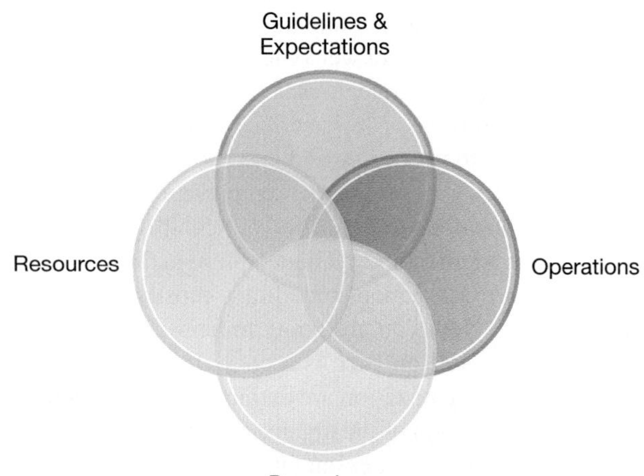

FIGURE 14-3

Although staff handbooks differ, an effective one usually includes general information on such things as guidelines, expectations, requirements, policies, resources, and procedures for a business.

business activities in a way that leads to the consistency and efficiency of operations. For example, the specific process for filing receipts, filling out insurance paperwork, managing e-mail marketing campaigns, or even answering the telephone can all be standardized and recorded into SOPs. This can be particularly helpful for new employees who want to learn quickly the unique systems in your business.

A few more tips for writing your own unique handbook:[19]

- Making a handbook does not have to be complicated. There are employee handbook templates and software available.
- If you have a standard contract, take out key information (things such as benefits, requested time off policies, termination policies, etc.) and include it in the handbook.
- Avoid jargon—keep the language in the handbook easily understood. The point is to make things clear, not to leave them open to interpretation.
- If you are hiring a multilingual staff, do your best to translate the materials in the handbook into the languages people know best. This can be time-consuming and costly, but it can save you a lot more time and money down the road.
- If you already have people working for you, ask them what kinds of things would be helpful to include in the handbook. Are there pieces of information that they feel would make their jobs easier?
- Have people sign a form saying they have read and understand the information provided, and that they agree to the terms of the handbook. Doing this gives people an incentive to actually read the information, and offers you one more buffer against legal action later. If someone on the staff says they were never informed of the company policy on missing work without notice, you have a signed form saying that the person received, read, and understood that policy.

Providing a good staff handbook does not necessarily replace adequate training. **Training** is the process of imparting the necessary skills and knowledge to perform a particular job or project. Of course, most of the technical training that massage therapists working for you will need has been acquired through a formal training and licensing process before they come to you. However, many management experts maintain that successful businesses (particularly those with a strong customer service component like massage) train *every* individual who deals with customers to some capacity.[20] While the resources in small business can only go so far, it is highly recommended that you devote at least some time to training people who will be dealing directly with your customers.

In a business world that is rapidly changing, many businesses have found it advantageous to adopt a learning culture. A **learning culture** is an environment in which everyone is invested in teaching, learning, and enhancing their exceptional abilities. In today's fast-paced economy, if a business isn't learning and adapting, it can quickly fall behind. Creating a work environment that encourages and supports learning for all its members can be incredibly good for business.[21] Regular training is a part of this culture, although you can encourage people to take initiative in developing themselves outside of the organization as well.

Here are some helpful tips for training programs:

- *Clarify your desired goal for training.* Get clear on what you hope the group and the business will get out of training. Do you want people to learn specific online scheduling systems? Are you trying to improve customer service? Are you wanting your team to get specific hands-on training on a new bodywork modality? Make sure you know what your goal is before you start a training session.
- *Train employees to train coworkers:* If you train people well enough, ideally they will be able to turn around and train others. Maybe someone on your staff has advanced training in a modality others might want to learn—offer to pay them training pay to teach the rest of the team.
- *Keep it going:* Just as with the crafting of company culture, training and professional development should be an ongoing process.
- *Set metrics to gauge success:* In the absence of measurement, perpetual training can feel like a nice exercise but not necessarily a sound return on investment. Implement ways to measure training outcomes and share the progress with your team.

GETTING ORGANIZED

As you begin to brainstorm ideas and create your own handbook, make sure to keep all the components together in your *Business of Massage Therapy* notebook. This will make it almost effortless to create a real handbook when the time comes!

EVERYTHING ACCORDING TO SCHEDULE

You learned about time management in Chapter 3; this subject gains an additional dimension the more responsibility you have for others' schedules. In a holistic business that is appointment-based, maintaining a schedule is a crucial part of your business. When you are running your own practice, this can be tricky enough. You can't answer the phone when one client calls to schedule an appointment if you are giving a massage to another client. And in a world with increasingly abundant choices for bodywork, missing an incoming call can cost you business. When you are managing the schedules of other people, this becomes increasingly complex (especially if you are still seeing clients yourself while managing all the other aspects of the business).

For years, holistic business owners have dealt with this problem through the use of a receptionist or an administrative assistant to manage incoming calls and arrange client appointments. In the last several years, this complex issue has become much less complicated with the advent of online scheduling services and automatic arrangement and confirmation software. People are becoming increasingly conditioned to expect to be able to schedule appointments online. In addition to client convenience, using an online scheduling service has many benefits: it frees you and your staff up from the time it takes to make appointments and confirmations in person. It also streamlines scheduling communication within the staff, as instant notifications are sent out by e-mail and anyone who has access to the Internet can look at up-to-the-minute schedules. Keep in mind, however, that many clients are still much more comfortable speaking with a person directly than using an online scheduler. Evaluate the appropriateness of this technology for your unique business.

If you are careful to synchronize online and offline scheduling activities, this combined approach can often help eliminate scheduling mistakes and double-bookings, and helps to minimize no-shows (see Chapter 3 for other tips on minimizing cancellations and no-shows). In a service-based business such as massage therapy, where income is based on hands-on delivery, no money is coming in unless clients are being seen. The way in which you organize your payment structure for employees and contractors adds another level of complexity onto your scheduling considerations. For example, if you are paying employees by the hour, regardless if they are working on clients, you might be more conservative with employee scheduling than if all of your employees work on commission.

Regardless of the way in which you coordinate your scheduling systems for your staff, be sure to keep a few things in mind. As you saw in Chapter 3, scheduling adequate time between sessions is an important aspect of time management for massage therapists. To the degree possible, allow sufficient break time between your therapists' appointments—time before and after sessions to greet clients, see clients off, change sheets, take care of physiological needs, and so forth. This not only helps avoid burnout in the people working for you, it helps to create a less stressful environment for everyone involved. Even if your practice is slammed, try to schedule enough time for room preparation and client transition. You may also have legal requirements on how many hours therapists and staff can work at a time, or how much break time is required in between appointments.[22] Check with your local labor authorities to learn more about the specific regulations in your area.

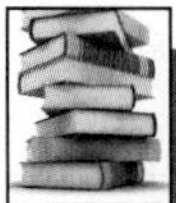

HELPFUL RESOURCES

There is a wealth of online scheduling options available, and the cost is usually fairly nominal. Common scheduling providers for holistic practitioners include Schedulicity MINDBODY, North American Studio Alliance (Namasta), My Receptionist, Time Center, and Appointment-plus. Most of these services allow for multiple practitioners' schedules, allowing you to outsource the management of everyone's bookings.

HOW TO GET EMPLOYEES TO GIVE GREAT CUSTOMER SERVICE EVERY TIME

While good training, ongoing learning, and sophisticated scheduling systems are great drivers for good management and successful business, it is excellent customer service that leads to client loyalty and strong referrals, as you saw in the earlier marketing chapters. **Customer service** is the combination of activities that enhance client experiences and develop relationships between a business and its patrons. It used to be said that customer service was about meeting a client's need; that then evolved into anticipating a client's need. Now great customer service is about anticipating, meeting, and exceeding a client's need, and doing so consistently.

Surely the importance of customer service is not a new concept for you, but consider this: a recent study by Pew Charitable Trusts found that 45 percent of customers had walked out of a business within the last year due to poor customer service, while another consumer behavior study found that 73 percent of consumers buy for reasons that have less to do with price and more to do with relationships.[23]

While customer service is important in any business, it is vital in a massage business, where your people are often alone with guests for long periods of time and in a very personal context. As a manager, you will look to hire people that will fill this role naturally, but even the most enthusiastic and passionate people can fall into professional ruts or become complacent about delivering the best service possible. Even though the world of bodywork creates boundless opportunities for new approaches and innovative experience, most therapists report times of lackluster performance and mediocre engagement. So how do you guide your team away from the "broken record" and into the "opening night on Broadway" mentality to customer service?

Experts agree that one of the best ways to ensure great customer service is to communicate the importance of it—not just for the health of the business, but for the benefit of the client. Empathy and compassion are intertwined with the emphasis on customer service, and you can encourage your workers to think like clients. Typically, people coming through the doors will be looking for relief from something, whether pain, stress, loneliness, or any other ailment they would like to escape. Keeping that fact in the foreground can do wonders for the group's commitment to great service.

Creating an environment where *everyone* is valued (not just the people with the checkbooks and credit cards) is an essential component of a great service culture. Through your own behavior and actions, model an environment where every individual is valued and absolutely everyone who comes through the door is a CEO. Encourage others to do the same, and acknowledge it when they do. Demonstrate and communicate that great customer service is a long-term investment in deep satisfaction in the work environment and for life in general.

With all the front-end encouragement of customer service, how do you gauge effectiveness of initiatives or know how good your customer service actually is? It is very common practice in many high-end spas to hire third-party "secret shopper" services. These services send an incognito representative into a business with a specific list of criteria of customer service behaviors and activities; the representative evaluates your staff along every point of client contact (from first phone call to check-out). The list of criteria is typically generated by the spa or wellness center itself, and is designed to evaluate how well employees are performing. The philosophy behind the secret shopper approach is that observation of employees when they do not know they are being evaluated (or at least don't know when) provides a more authentic picture of employee performance.

However, one of the best ways to get information on performance and customer service is to simply ask clients directly! A **customer satisfaction survey** is a written or verbal assessment of client experience with your business, as well as a measure of his or her overall approval and an opportunity to provide feedback. Ideally, surveys are provided immediately after a service while the experience is still fresh in the client's mind. Surveys can be done through the traditional paper and pen technique, or they can be done through an online service such as SurveyMonkey. The usefulness of these surveys lies in the questions you ask and what you do with the feedback you collect from clients.

While most satisfaction surveys are aimed at customers, some holistic managers develop internal and external satisfaction surveys. Internal surveys are designed to measure employee satisfaction with customer service and their overall experience in your business. This helps provide valuable information about how to improve your management style, and can include questions such as "what do you like most/least about working here?" and "what would you do differently if you were in charge?" Typically, such surveys are the most useful when those surveyed are allowed to remain anonymous (allowing them to be more candid about their responses).

Well done! You have learned a lot of great management and leadership ideas in this chapter, and are in a great position to start building and overseeing a fabulous team to support your business. Managing other people and bringing them together around a common goal can be a wonderfully rewarding experience. Remember, even if you hire only one person, you are still a manager and you can still benefit from all of the strategies and techniques in this chapter. The more you are able to systematize your operations, the easier running your business will be. And the more you are able to create an environment of harmony, learning, and respect, the happier your clients, team members, and you will be, too.

HELPFUL RESOURCES

For more books on inspiring great customer service, check out *Guts: Companies that Blow the Doors Off of Business as Usual* by Kevin and Jackie Freiberg (2004, Random House) and *Customer Service Training 101* by Renee Evenson (2005, Amacom).

CHAPTER SUMMARY BY LEARNING OBJECTIVES

1. **Explore aspects of yourself as a manager** No matter how good you may are at multitasking, no business owner can do everything alone. Regardless of your business model or where you are conducting your business, a growing business relies on its employees. The kinds of people you hire and the way you manage them can have a tremendous impact on your business's overall success. It will also impact your own experience within your business, as anyone you bring in becomes part of your life.
2. **Introduce different management styles** Experts maintain that there are generally five different management styles: autocratic, paternalistic, democratic, laissez-faire, and mixed. An autocratic manager tends to restrict information, make all the decisions, and retain all the power. A paternalistic manager is one who tries to operate as a parental figure, factoring the needs and happiness of the workers into management decisions. A democratic manager is one who allows consensus in decision making, and involves a great deal of interaction between management and employees. A laissez-faire manager has more of a "hands-off" management style, and is typically on the sidelines while other staff run the business. A mixed management style occurs when a manager utilizes different management styles for different people or different situations, blending autocratic, paternalistic, democratic, or laissez-faire methods.
3. **Evaluate the difference between management and leadership** Leadership is the process of guiding others in the accomplishment of a common objective or goal. While many leaders are also managers, not all managers are necessarily leaders. The main difference lies in the philosophy one has towards management, the ability to inspire and motivate others, and the capacity to unite people around a common goal or vision.
4. **Explain how to budget and pay employees, and introduce employment contracts** Employee-related costs are usually the largest line item expense for any company's budget. Before you bring on other individuals, you want to make sure that you have enough cash flow to make payroll consistently. When you are creating a budget for employees, make sure that you include all of the hidden costs of employee benefits. A contract is an exchange of agreements between two or more parties, wherein promises are made about what will and will not be done. Contracts, whether verbal or written are legally binding; however, written contracts are much more easily enforced in a court of law. Good contracts protect the interests of both employer and employee or contractor.
5. **Describe the process of staff selection and interviews** The people you hire can be a major factor in determining the success of your business and the importance of hiring decisions are magnified in small companies. With a good job description, you can begin to attract candidates through online and offline job boards or through word of mouth. During the interview process, you will need very different skills as the interviewer than you did as an interviewee. Take time to prepare questions that will help you investigate and determine a good fit. Pay attention to nonverbal cues, check references, and go with your gut instinct.
6. **Define retention and explore ways to keep people on board** Studies show that it is incredibly costly to have high staff turnover, and can adversely impact your company's culture. Retention is the intentional and ongoing practice of maintaining and holding on to staff. Many things can be done to increase happiness and boost retention, such as consistency, clarity, communication, training, a good work environment, a commitment to professional development, and a learning culture.
7. **Explain the components of creating and branding culture** Branded culture is a company culture in which members of the organization are enthusiastically devoted to the values and mission of the organization to the point where company culture becomes an integral part of company image. Even if you hire only one person, there will be a culture and an opportunity to make that culture a major contributing factor to your success. Great cultures are magnets for attracting both great clients and great employees.
8. **Analyze staff handbooks and basics of employee training** A staff handbook provides general information on guidelines, expectations, requirements, policies, resources, and procedures for a business. A great method for knowledge management, staff handbooks help clarify roles for both managers and staff, promote consistency, and protect parties from legal disruptions. Training is the process of imparting the necessary skills and knowledge to perform a particular job or project. Creating a learning culture, where teaching and expanding knowledge are valued, is a great way to continue training.
9. **Research techniques for scheduling employees** In a holistic business that is appointment-based, maintaining a schedule is a crucial part of your

business. Scheduling can be done personally through a manager, receptionist or administrative assistant; it can also be done through an online scheduling service. Schedules should balance the needs of the business, the needs of the employee(s), and all applicable labor laws.

10. **Identify ways to develop great customer service from all employees** While good training, ongoing learning, and sophisticated scheduling systems are great drivers for good management and successful business, it is excellent customer service that leads to client loyalty and strong referrals. This is true in any business, but especially massage therapy. Hiring people with inherent customer service skill, communicating its importance, and modeling behavior that treats every individual as a CEO are good ways to instill a customer service ethic. Customer satisfaction surveys can help identify areas that need improvement.

ACTIVITIES

Quiz: Identifying Management Words and Concepts

1. ______________ is the process of helping a newcomer adjust and assimilate into the culture and operations of the business.
   a. An exit interview
   b. Onboarding
   c. Hazing
   d. Indoctrination
2. A major cause of employee frustration and resignation is:
   a. insufficient training
   b. no onboarding process
   c. unclear expectations
   d. all the above
3. An example of an employee benefit is:
   a. paid sick leave
   b. wages
   c. matched retirement contributions
   d. a and c
4. A ______________ is an environment in which everyone is invested in teaching, learning, and enhancing their exceptional abilities.
   a. fear-based culture
   b. hierarchical culture
   c. learning culture
   d. bacterial culture
5. A manager who tries to operate as a parental figure, factoring the needs and happiness of the workers into management decisions, is likely operating from a ______________ management style.
   a. autocratic
   b. laissez-faire
   c. mixed
   d. paternalistic
6. ______________ is the rate at which a company obtains and loses workers. It can be very costly and have an adverse impact on company culture.
   a. Turnover
   b. Churn and burn
   c. Retention
   d. Termination
7. True or False: Nearly all cities will allow interns to provide massage therapy to clients.
8. True or False: A manager and a leader are the same thing.
9. True or False: In the massage industry, any good non-compete agreement should stipulate that employees neither have their own practice nor work for any other massage establishment.

Discussion Questions

1. Think of the managers you have worked for in the past, and choose one that sticks out in your mind. It doesn't matter if he or she stands out for good reasons or bad, but just that this person is memorable to you. What kind of management style do you think he or she had? What kinds of things did he or she do that you liked? What kinds of things did you not agree with and might have done differently?
2. In today's world, what do you think the three biggest challenges are for managers in general? How about for

managers in holistic businesses? What qualities do you think a good manager needs to overcome these challenges?

3. You have heard several times that managers and leaders are not necessarily the same thing. What do you think about that idea? When you think of a leader, who comes to mind? What qualities does that person have? Do you see any of those qualities in yourself?
4. One of the assumptions made in the section about turnover was that companies that pay their workers less typically have higher turnover than companies that pay more. Do you agree with this statement? What are your opinions about a low labor cost model in the wellness industry? Do you have any experience working in one?
5. Thinking as a manager or business owner, what do you think about "secret shoppers"? Do you think this is a good idea? Would you ever want to use one of these services? What do you think about "secret shoppers" as an employee or independent contractor?

Beyond the Classroom

Customer service is a very important element of client attraction and retention, especially in North American culture. Poor customer service can be very detrimental to business, and even people with natural service skills can grow complacent. As a manager and business owner, you will be tasked with trying to deliver great service both to and through your people.

Create a customer satisfaction survey or list of criteria for a good experience, based upon the things that you look for as a consumer. Maybe you love the way they remember your drink order *and* your name at your favorite coffee shop. Maybe you like the way everyone is smiling and making jokes with one another behind the counter, and getting customers in on the fun whenever you come into your favorite rental car chain. Jot these criteria down in the Figure 14-4 ■ (the first few fields have been filled out for you to give you a head start). Now make copies of this form, and carry blank surveys with you wherever you go. You are now the "secret shopper" for every place you are visiting. How do they rate in your book?

As a bonus assignment, try this. Any time you see really great service, tell the person and ask him or her what is motivating such great service? If you are feeling even more adventurous, ask to speak with the manager. When the manager comes out, tell him or her how great your experience has been as a customer, and inquire into what he or she is doing to inspire such a great team. Most managers will be completely flattered by this, and delighted to share with you their secrets of success. Take notes—you may be including their tips into your own managerial repertoire soon!

	Excellent	Very Good	Good	Poor
Phone was answered before third ring. Warm and professional reception.				
Ensured all of my questions were answered.				
Service provider was friendly and professional.				

FIGURE 14-4

Customer service is an important aspect of client attraction and retention. As a customer yourself, what is important to you, and how to other businesses measure up?

CHAPTER

15 Leveraging the Internet

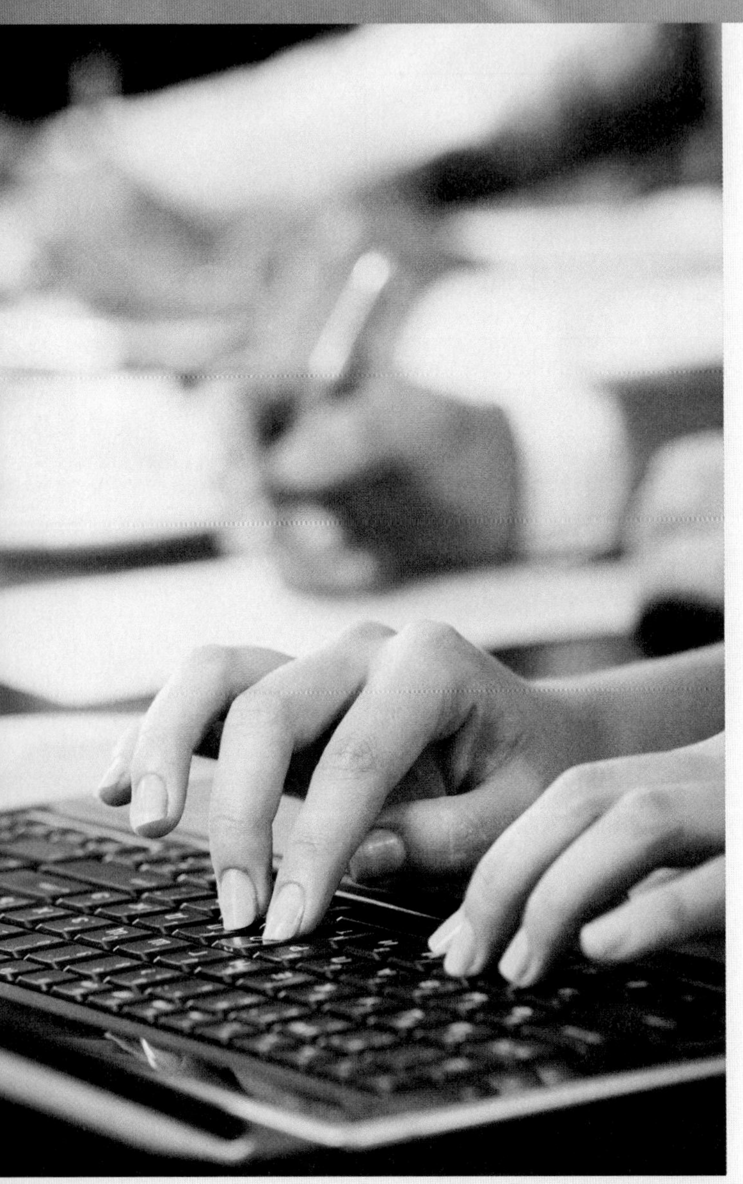

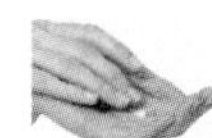

CHAPTER OUTLINE

LEARNING OBJECTIVES

1. Assess the benefits of technology and the Internet for your business
2. Examine the process of developing and maintaining a website
3. Define the anatomy of a website
4. Explain search engine optimization and explore optimizing techniques
5. Identify link partners/reciprocal links
6. Define blogging and e-zines, and assess their role for your business
7. Uncover ways to streamline your valuable information to target audiences
8. Explore the benefits of online product sales and online scheduling
9. Examine security, legal, and privacy issues

KEY TERMS

affiliate programs *260*
blog *256*
cookies *260*
copyright *261*
domain name *250*
e-commerce *248*
e-mail marketing *257*
e-zine *257*
firewall *260*
home page *253*
HTML *252*
HTML document *252*
hyperlink *253*
identity theft *260*
intellectual property *261*
Internet *248*
key words *254*
lead generation *258*
libel *261*
off-site page optimization *255*
on-site page optimization *254*
open source shopping cart *259*
organic search results *255*
pay-per-click advertising *255*
reciprocal links *255*
RSS *258*
RSS reader *258*
search engine *253*
search engine optimization *253*
search engine results page *253*
site map *253*
spam *257*
subscriber list *257*
third-party merchant sites *259*
URL *251*
web authoring software *252*
web crawlers *254*
web developer *251*
web hosting *251*
website *250*
website templates *252*

The Internet is just a world passing around notes in a classroom.

—Jon Stewart

I have an almost religious zeal . . . for the Internet which is for me, the nervous system of mother Earth, which I see as a living creature, linking up.

—Dan Millman, author of *Peaceful Warrior*

LEVERAGING TECHNOLOGY

In the last 20 years, the landscape of business has changed dramatically with the advent of the Internet. Small business owners around the globe have found ways to incorporate new technologies to boost their sales and expand their marketing inexpensively. New technologies are constantly arising to make running a business more efficient and affordable. As a general rule, many massage therapists and holistic practitioners have traditionally shied away from technological applications, usually to the detriment of their business and overall success. As Eric Brown of Massage Therapy Radio (www.massagetherapyradio.com) asserts, the massage industry has typically been "high-touch and low-tech." But as you begin to recognize the many benefits of technology for your business, you might find new and exciting ways to apply it to your operations.

As was touched on in Chapter 3, technology is a key component in time management. It can save you ample energy and help you stay organized. Moreover, it can be a strong competitive advantage in your marketing mix. It can help therapists target their intended market and help people to find you that otherwise may not. When used appropriately, technology can serve to differentiate you from other therapists and propel your business forward.

Of all the technologies out there for you to consider for your holistic business, one of the most important is the Internet. The **Internet** is a global system of interconnected computer networks where individuals, governments, academics, and businesses all come together to share information, resources, and conduct commerce. Millions and millions of people come together online via electronic mail, file sharing, streaming media, social networking, and many other applications.[1] Businesses of all sizes, structures, scopes, and specialties utilize the Internet to maximize business functioning.

PITFALLS

As much as technology can be a blessing for small businesses, it can also be an albatross if applied incorrectly. Adopting technologies blindly without adding true value to your business can be time consuming, frustrating, and very expensive. When you are considering different technological approaches, be focused and strategic, and make sure that you aren't making things more costly or complicated than they ultimately need to be.

As systems have grown more sophisticated and users more familiar with shopping online, electric commerce has exploded. **Electronic commerce,** or **e-commerce,** is the buying and selling of products and/or services over the Internet. Many businesses have no brick and mortar storefront but exist solely through the Internet, where all marketing, communication, payment transfers, customer service, and product/service delivery occur. In addition, the Internet has become one of the primary marketing avenues for businesses of all sizes. Research indicates that 75 percent of consumers have turned away from traditional phone books and yellow pages and opt instead to get their information and to do their purchasing research online.[2] Figure 15-1 ■ shows the

% of US Internet Users in 1990 = 0%

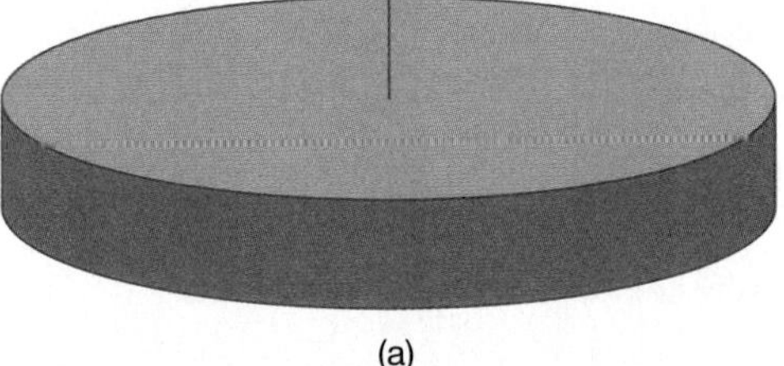

(a)

% of US Internet Users 2000 = 43.9%

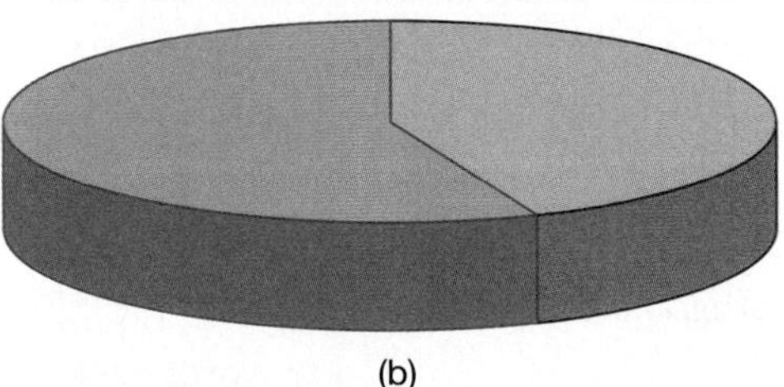

(b)

% of US Internet Users in 2009 = 72.4%

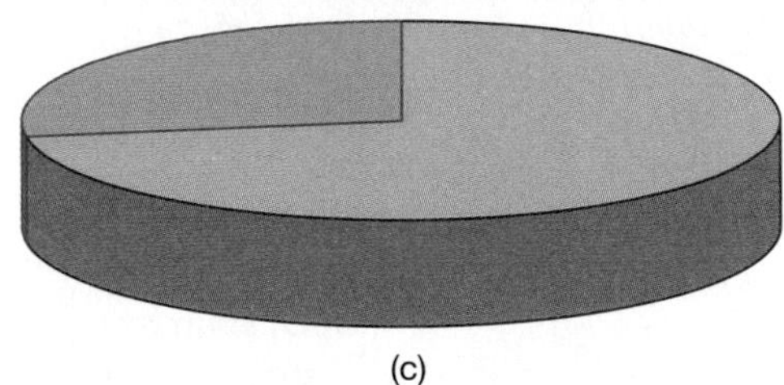

(c)

FIGURE 15-1

a. In 1990, 0% of Americans were actively using the Internet.

b. In 2000, less than half of Americans were actively using the Internet.

c. In 2009, nearly three out of four Americans were actively using the Internet. This represents a dramatic cultural difference in the way business is now done.

Source: World Bank Development Indicators, 2009.

dramatic rise of Internet use by percentages of U.S. population over the last 20 years.

Naturally, as massage is a personal service–based business, the Internet will never replace the inherent importance of direct contact and relationship building between therapist and client. But this does not mean that its importance as a business tool should be overlooked. In fact, the ability for clients to find you online and to use your website can be a "make it or break it" factor for a massage business. Research indicates that a company's presence on the Internet and its website can influence purchasing decisions more than most any other marketing approach, a finding that was the same in all industries and across all product/service categories.[3] Savvy massage therapists who recognize this truth about today's business landscape and do their best to leverage existing technologies position themselves for greater success than those who try to run an old-school business. What's more, the Internet can be an amazingly easy and low-cost tool to build your business.

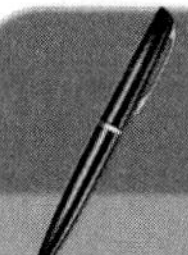

PUT IT IN WRITING

Gauge Your Technology Comfort Levels

With the omnipresence of the Internet and the unthinkably huge number of online users at any given moment, it can be a foregone conclusion that everyone is Internet savvy. However, this is hardly the case, and many people are all but flummoxed by the latest technologies. All manner of factors can influence one's comfort level, from barriers to access, lack of exposure, relevance to daily life, or even outright personal rejection. Whether you are a net newbie or a web wunderkind, take a moment to explore your own knowledge and comfort levels with using online technologies.

1. When my favorite singer puts out a new CD and I want to buy it, I:
   a. go to my favorite music store—I don't feel safe buying things online.
   b. order the CD from an online store, either direct from the artist or through an online big box store.
   c. don't want to pay for the whole CD—I'll just download my favorite songs from iTunes, buymusic.com, or Rhapsody.
   d. What is a CD? All my favorite music is on vinyl.

2. Cookies:
   a. are used to track and maintain information about website visitors, such as user preferences and recent searches.
   b. have something to do with how Amazon knows I love Thai cookbooks. How do they know that?
   c. are so sweet and delicious!
   d. sound a little too Big Brother to me.

3. When someone says they "caught a virus," my first thought is:
   a. They must not have any kind of Internet security.
   b. I better take some vitamin C—I don't want to catch it!
   c. They were obviously looking at some shady sites online—for shame!
   d. That's too bad. Even with standard preventative measures, viruses are ever more sophisticated. Perhaps I could tell them about the multipronged prevention/defense approach that has been useful for me.

4. A hyperlink is:
   a. an over-caffeinated sausage.
   b. a web address.
   c. underlined and usually a different color from other text on a site that someone wants me to click.
   d. a redirect encoded in a site that navigates to another location, either in the same document or a different one.

5. What is the name of the language that most websites are written in?
   a. WWW
   b. HTMM
   c. HTML
   d. Swahili

6. I keep hearing that social networking sites can be beneficial for my business. I think:
   a. Of course—I started using Classmates and Six Degrees back in the 1990s.
   b. I guess I better get out my suit and tie and hit the Rotary Club network events.
   c. I'm already on Facebook and LinkedIn and am interested in learning more about using these kinds of sites to leverage my business.
   d. I keep getting all those invites from friends to join those sites, but I just ignore them because it seems too strange to me.

7. One of my friends from school told me she has been using blogging to boost her new massage business. I told her:
   a. That was nice, and then changed the subject.
   b. I would like to start a blog, too, and asked her for some pointers.
   c. I didn't know what a blog was.
   d. I write a blog, too, and would love to talk about becoming link partners.

8. When I think of the relationship between the Internet and a massage business:
   a. I think it sounds nice in theory, but the Internet really isn't applicable or affordable for a small massage business like mine. It would be better for a big spa, a medical massage complex, or a massage franchise.
   b. I think it is completely inappropriate. Massage is very relationship-driven and practices are only built slowly via word of mouth. No one looks online to find massage therapists.
   c. I know that is has already been a fairly inexpensive and powerful driver in my massage business, and a great way for me to educate people on the benefits of massage while positioning myself as an expert in my trade.
   d. I think it's wonderful. I see competitors using it all the time with great results, and I'd love to get a website up and running to boost my bookings and propel retail sales.

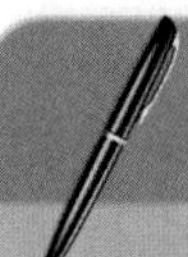

PUT IT IN WRITING

Gauge Your Technology Comfort Levels (continued)

9. I typed "massage, (my city)" into Google search, and over a million results were generated by the search engine. Obviously, the top five companies displayed in the results have great _____.
a. therapists
b. overall search engine optimization
c. websites that are strategically organized
d. online demand

10. I was online looking at jet skis when I saw a small ad for Lake Powell vacations. I clicked on it, and it took me to the vacation website. I was told that the Lake Powell company had to pay because I clicked on the link. This is an example of:
a. pay-per-click advertising
b. bait and switch
c. online marketing
d. fraud

Answer key

1) a = 2 b = 3 c = 4 d = 1 6) a = 4 b = 1 c = 3 d = 2
2) a = 4 b = 3 c = 1 d = 2 7) a = 2 b = 3 c = 1 d = 4
3) a = 3 b = 1 c = 2 d = 4 8) a = 2 b = 1 c = 4 d = 3
4) a = 1 b = 2 c = 3 d = 4 9) a = 1 b = 4 c = 3 d = 2
5) a = 2 b = 3 c = 4 d = 1 10) a = 4 b = 2 c = 3 d = 1

34–40: *Guru Geek*. Congratulations—you speak geek! Perhaps you sold your dot-com start-up to go to massage school, and now you are ready to start leveraging the amazing power of the Internet to propel your business forward. In fact, you might even consider a sideline business getting other massage therapists up and running online!

26–33: *Internet Intermediate*. You might not know every HTML tag on the block, but you know your way around the Internet. You grasp the potential it offers your business, and are ready to learn more. This chapter will help you polish your skills so you will be able to position your business online for optimal success!

18–25: *Lightweight Luddite*. You are still a little overwhelmed by the fast pace of technology, and are not necessarily aware of the full gamut of what the Internet has to offer you and your business. This chapter will help demystify some of the steps so you can begin embracing useful applications.

10–17: *Data Dinosaur*. You mourn the days of the abacus and thought technology reached its apex with Eli Whitney's cotton gin. You habitually shy away from technology and don't really see what the Internet has to do with a massage business. After reading this chapter and understanding how easy and exciting it can be, you may reconsider your phobias.

Like most of the chapters in this book, this chapter provides an overview. It takes a basic approach to some fairly baseline Internet technologies in an attempt to introduce and explore useful ones for your massage business. You are, of course, given many outside resources and encouraged to continue expanding your knowledge on this powerful tool for your business.

WEAVING A WEBSITE

> *We have technology, finally, that for the first time in human history allows people to really maintain rich connections with much larger numbers of people.*
>
> —Pierre Omidyar, founder of eBay

The most common way for clients to find you online is through your company's website. A **website** is an interconnected set of web pages that are furnished and supported by a host. It typically includes a home page and several other pages of interest through which visitors can navigate. Basic websites typically reflect information about your business, the value you create for clients (such as the benefits of massage), and your contact information. A good website is typically easy to read, engaging, aesthetically pleasing, well organized, and interactive. Optimally, your website will invite the client to take action and do business with you. Ideally, your website should mirror the look and feel of the rest of your marketing collateral and the rest of your business image (see Chapters 11 and 12).

In today's business world, having a website has almost become as expected as having a business card, regardless of the business you are in. A 2007 study by Pew Internet and American Life Project found that 71 percent of all Americans use the Internet daily.[4] Internet use spans the boundaries of age, race, education levels, socioeconomic status, and cultural backgrounds.[5] Having a website has become the cost of doing business. However, Massage Therapy Radio reports that less than 10 percent of practicing therapists have one.[6] Many therapists are discovering that not having a website can be leaving money on the table for their business.

One of the first things you will want to do is to explore the availability of and secure a domain name. A **domain name** is the unique address of your website, and it provides the recognizable calling card for a business. Domain names are like prime real estate, and popular ones can be very valuable due to their marketing and traffic potential. Picking an available, suitable, and memorable domain name can be a big part of establishing and building your brand. In order to secure an original domain name, you will have to find an

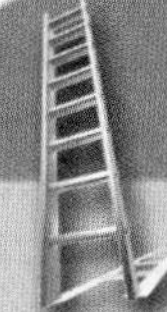

FIRST STEPS

Chances are you've already seen your fair share of websites and maybe even have a pretty good idea of ones you like. But if you've never had a website of your own before, this exercise is a fun way to get started conceiving and creating one. Identify five different massage therapist or spa websites (if you don't know of any offhand, just use a search engine like Yahoo or Google to find some). Go online, and take a look at what other people are doing and what you like about their sites. Maybe you notice the use of color, the ease of scheduling, the use of photography or images, the helpful tips, and so on. Take some time to really reflect on the aspects of the sites that appeal to you, and write down five of those things you like here.

1. ______________________________
2. ______________________________
3. ______________________________
4. ______________________________
5. ______________________________

Now take a moment to come up with ways you could get started creating something similar or implementing some of the five things you liked above. For example, if you liked the aesthetics or the imagery, you might start scanning some website templates for imagery that you love, or contact a graphic designer for a consultation. Brainstorm an action step for each thing you just listed, and write them here.

1. ______________________________
2. ______________________________
3. ______________________________
4. ______________________________
5. ______________________________

Now perhaps you also find things you do not like on these sites. Are there too few graphics, is the site hard to navigate, or does it contain so much information that you find yourself losing interest? It's important to have a handle on things you don't like, too, as you want to avoid creating a site that others might not like. If you can find them, write out five things you notice that you would do differently.

1. ______________________________
2. ______________________________
3. ______________________________
4. ______________________________
5. ______________________________

File your responses away in your *Business of Massage Therapy* notebook. Now when you are ready to create your own website, you will have a pretty good idea of how you would like to structure it, and a pretty good idea of things you can leave out.

available one, and pay to register and reserve it before you can use it exclusively. In contrast, a **URL** (Uniform Resource Locator) is the encoded address that designates where the information is available and gives the proper Internet protocol for retrieving it. An example of a domain name is massagingsuccess.com, while a URL would be http://massagingsuccess.com. And of course, once you have a website created, you will also need to host it as well. **Web hosting** is the housing, data storing, maintaining, and servicing of a website, and what needs to happen to facilitate and connect your website online. Many of the domain sites give you a very good deal on registering your domain if you host your website through their service, and many website development options listed in the "Helpful Resources" box offer domain registration, site creation, and web hosting.

If you do not already have a website, there are several different ways you can go about developing one. One of the many ways to produce a site is to hire a **web developer,** a professional who designs, develops, and maintains websites for others. Also known as webmasters or web architects, web

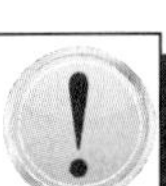

PITFALLS

ICANN, the Internet Corporation for Assigned Names and Number, can make it very difficult to transfer domain names from one host or registrant to another. You may have a rude shock if you register all your names through GoDaddy, for example, and then try and transfer your name to build your site with a developer host like SBI. Before you pay to reserve a domain name, check out what the policies are on domain transfers.

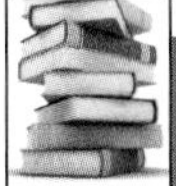

HELPFUL RESOURCES

There are many sites that help you research whether your domain name is available, allow you to reserve it, and even offer web hosting and website development. Popular ones include Network Solutions, Go Daddy, Yahoo Small Business, and many other services. All the companies have the same information on domain availability. If you aren't feeling ready or interested in signing up for web hosting, you can research availability of domain names for free and without any obligations to any company. But remember, even if you don't reserve it right away, someone else might!

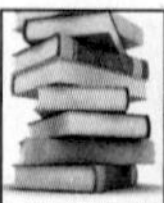

HELPFUL RESOURCES

In recent years, many companies have sprung up to provide website templates for small businesses. A few common sites that provide website templates are VistaPrint, Google, and Yahoo, and many of these templates can be obtained for free or provide a free trial. Some sites, such as Bodyworksites .com and Salonbuilder.com, specialize in websites for massage therapists and wellness practitioners. Do some research, and try and find a company that will provide you with good customer service and allow you to update and make changes as often as you need to.

developers are paid to create your website for you and to help you maintain your site so that it continues to add value to your business. The benefits of working with a web developer are that you can save a lot of time and hassle trying to learn everything about websites and developing one yourself. Skilled web developers can also produce quality websites that add to the credibility and appeal of your business to clients, and they provide support and answer questions when you need to make changes or adapt your website. The downside is that it can be a sizable up-front investment that is too costly for most people just getting started in business. Many people also find that working with a web developer makes them feel an ongoing dependence on the other person to maintain their website. If you do work with a web developer, make sure it is one who empowers you to understand and work optimally with your own site.

Another option is to work with an online company that offers easy site publishing through website templates. **Website templates** are mass-produced site layouts that can be purchased, downloaded, and used for any type of business. All the graphic design, layouts, and structuring are done for you, and often all you need to do is fill in your business's information and your site is done. There are even companies that specialize in massage-specific templates, which can be advantageous for getting quality massage related graphics. The benefits of using web templates are that you do not need to know anything about web design to have a website, and they can be relatively inexpensive to purchase and maintain through annual or monthly subscriptions. Templates are generally very big timesavers, too, and most can be set up very quickly, with most packages providing ongoing technical support. The drawbacks are that your website will be more generic and not customized for your business, which may present a problem in terms of cohesiveness with the rest of your marketing materials. This could also challenge your brand development, especially if many other businesses buy the same templates and create virtually the same website as you. Using templates can also hamper search engine optimization (discussed in a later section) in certain cases, making your site harder to find in online searches. There are many companies that provide template services, so really shop around and do your homework before you sign up with anyone.

Another option is to *do it yourself.* **Web authoring software** (also known as HTML editors) is any program that allows you to create your own web pages and interconnect them into a viable website. There is wealth of website-building software on the market, and most are pretty user friendly. Programs such as Adobe Dreamweaver, Microsoft FrontPage, GoLive, and CoffeeCup are popular with small businesses. This out-of-the-box software is typically not very complicated and does not require that you have any knowledge of HTML or other web-building languages (see the next section).

ANATOMY OF A WEBSITE

Whatever technique you use to develop your website, there are many characteristics that websites have in common, and this section will give you a brief overview on the composition of a typical website and definitions of common aspects. Remember, even if you decide to outsource web development to a professional or an online company, you will want to understand as many of the basics as you can to optimize control of your site.

One of the most important elements of a website is the language in which it is composed. Most websites are written in **HTML,** which is an abbreviation for HyperText Markup Language.[7] Sparing you a long, technogeek explanation, HTML is the basic and original language of the Internet. It is what formats your website so that it looks and behaves the way that it does. In the beginning, all web documents were scripted entirely with HTML, but as the Internet has matured and grown more sophisticated, other markup languages such as Java, JavaScript, and XML have emerged.[8] HTML is still typically the predominant language and one that is supported by all web browsers. An **HTML document** is a combination of plain text and HTML tags and codes; each document makes one web page. A group of associated and linked HTML documents is what constitutes a website.[9]

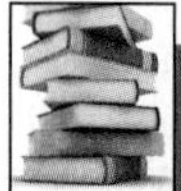

HELPFUL RESOURCES

Even if your approach to website development is more hands off, it will still behoove you to have a cursory knowledge of HTML. If nothing else, this will save you from being beholden to a developer. The wild world of HTML may seem a little daunting, especially if you are a newcomer to its ways. There are many helpful resources to help you navigate the Internet so that clients can navigate to you! Check out *The Really, Really, Really Easy Guide to Building Your Own Website (Step-By-Step Guide)* by Gavin Hoole and Cheryl Smith (2008, New Holland Publishers) or *Create Your Own Website* by Scott Mitchell (2009, Pearson Education). The *Dummies* books have a series of titles on HTML and web development that break the process down into digestible bits. If nothing else, your eyes won't glaze over when you talk to a developer or technical support.

PITFALLS

One mistake that many people make when designing their website is to try and include too much information on the home page. Nothing can be more irritating than a home page that reads like a novel. Few people will stick around to hear how the story ends. Remember that your potential clients likely lead busy lives, so cut them some slack (and don't scare them away) by keeping it simple and relegating longer content to subpages and on your blog (more on that later).

When a user visits your website, the first thing that he or she will see is your home page. A **home page** is the primary HTML document and the URL that all visitors will be guided to when they go to your site, whether through direct access or through a link from another site. This is your website's reception area, and you want all of your visitors to have a warm welcome! Studies show that many potential clients make purchase decisions based upon website presence and presentation.[10] Since the home page is often the first impression clients will have of your massage business, you will want to devote a lot of energy and intention to ensure its value. Good home pages usually make the purpose of the site (and the business) clear, demonstrate value to the visitor, and serve as a jumping-off point to navigate to other information on the site.

Home pages also typically display your website's site map. A **site map** (Figure 15-2 ■) is an overview of all the content on your website, and helps users connect to useful information on your website if it contains more than one page. In essence, it is a menu of all that your visitors have to choose from, and should be designed strategically to aid in search engine optimization. A good website will have a site map on every page so that visitors can navigate from any page to any other page. Nothing is worse than getting lost in someone's website because you don't know how to navigate back home. If that's happened to you, you probably just left altogether (which is not what you want your site visitors to do). Pages are linked to one another on your site map via **hyperlinks,** which are electronically embedded connections in a site that navigate to another location. Hyperlinks can connect a user to other pages within a contained site, or redirect them to another website altogether.

OPTIMIZING YOUR WEB PRESENCE

As the culture turns increasingly Internet dependent, it is becoming more and more important for massage therapists to have a way for clients to find them online. So how do users find information about products and services online? Typically, they find it through a search engine. A **search engine** is a system that mines and retrieves desired data, information, and resources found online. Popular search engines include Google, Yahoo, MSN, Bing, ask.com, and AOL.[11] More and more people turn to online search engines to find all kinds of information, from how to cook acorn squash to where to find the best eye doctor in town. Culturally, people are becoming conditioned to seek information, products, and services through these search engines (just think how ever-present the term "Google it" is). If your massage practice cannot be found online, it may end up costing you clients.

Look at the list you will create in the "First Steps" exercise on the next page. What you wrote down were the things that came up first on the **search engine results page (SERP),** the list of ranked web page results that are based upon key words or phrases entered by a user and generated by the search engine. But why did those companies come up first when you typed their name into the search engine? Surely they aren't the only ones out there. They came up first because they had *search engine optimization.* **Search engine optimization** is a way of getting your company priority in the listings of search engines in order to improve visitor traffic. Just like having the best massage skills in the land won't benefit you if no one knows about them, having the best website around won't matter if people don't find it. Typically, online customers will only look at the first few options that appear once a search has been generated, making it essential to land at or near the top of the result pile on any SERP.[12] Thus, optimization is a large part of an effective Internet marketing strategy.

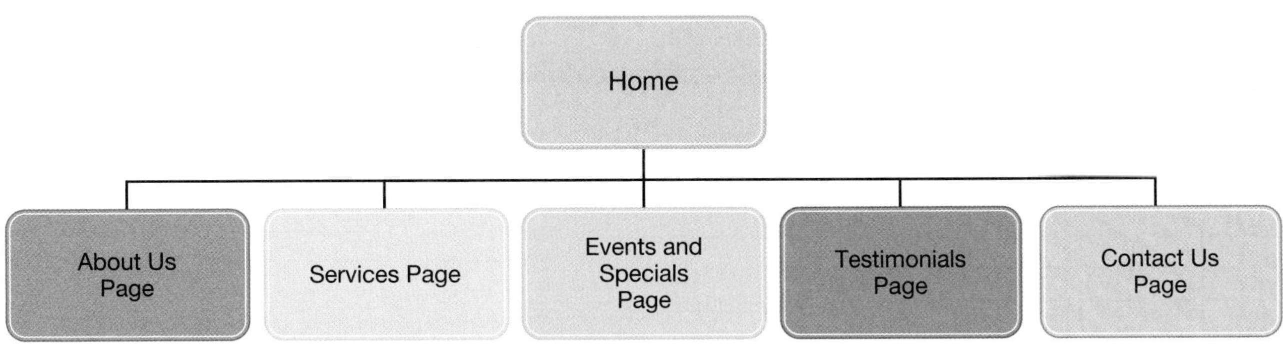

FIGURE 15-2

A sample site map that begins with a home page and branches into pages such as about us, services, events and specials, testimonials, and contact us.

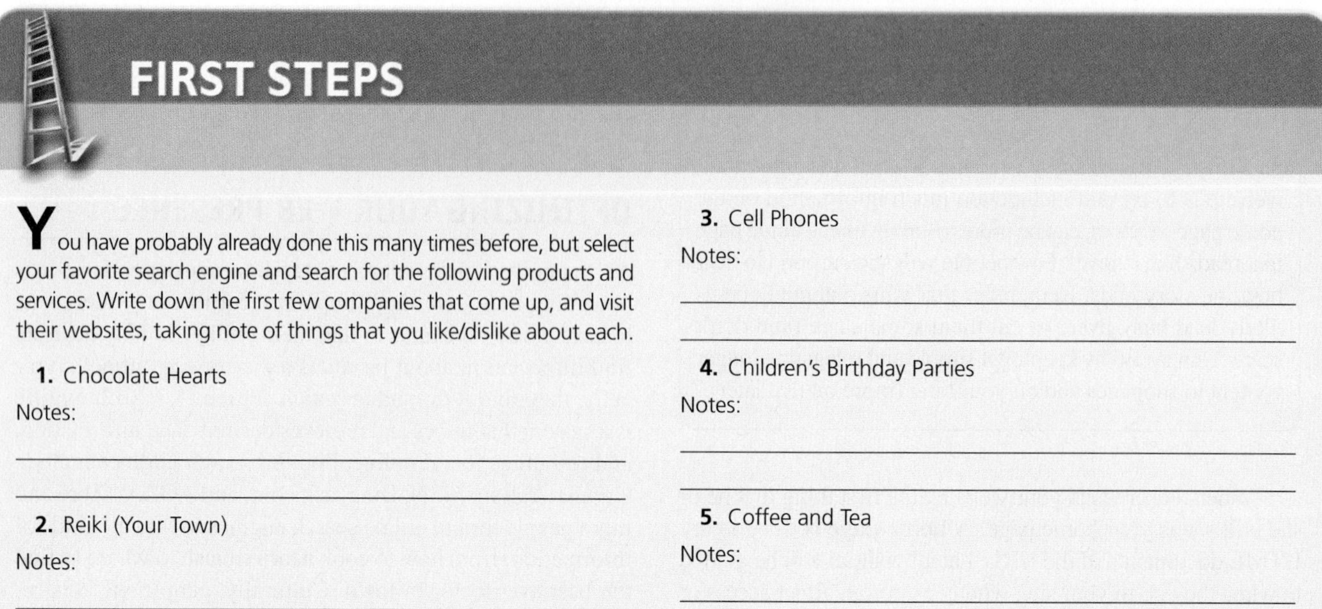

FIRST STEPS

You have probably already done this many times before, but select your favorite search engine and search for the following products and services. Write down the first few companies that come up, and visit their websites, taking note of things that you like/dislike about each.

1. Chocolate Hearts

Notes: ______________________

2. Reiki (Your Town)

Notes: ______________________

3. Cell Phones

Notes: ______________________

4. Children's Birthday Parties

Notes: ______________________

5. Coffee and Tea

Notes: ______________________

But how do you optimize your business's priority on a search engine anyway? In a nutshell—key words. **Key words** are words or phrases that relate to your business, and typically the words that people that are looking for businesses like yours are likely to type into the search engine to find what they are looking for. For example, if a man is looking for a place to stay during his family vacation to Mount Rainier, words like "lodge," "vacation," and "Mount Rainier" would all be key words he might enter to find what he is looking for. Especially with a location-based service like massage, it is important to have specific and geographic key words.

You may wonder how a search engine detects and connects to your chosen key words to ever drive anyone to your site. In the wonderful and wild world of the Web, there are creatures called web crawlers. Also known as web bots, web spiders, and web worms, **web crawlers** are automated programs that seek out information on the web. They scour through billions of web pages for data to use in search engines indices; because online content is constantly changing and being updated, web crawlers are always exploring to stay current.[13] It may sound incredibly creepy, but web crawlers can be great allies in the quest to optimize your website and draw clients to your business.

Now that you have a good handle on some of the key words you think would be advantageous for your business, use the "Put it in Writing" exercise below to help you brainstorm. Take a look at some ways you can incorporate them. **On-site optimization** is a way that you can directly influence your website's "findability," and it is typically done by creating all your web pages in such a way as to make them key word-rich, graphically appropriate, and search engine friendly. Your site map is actually a very large part of optimization, as it provides useful material for those web crawlers to "consume."[14] Making

BRIGHT IDEAS

Keep in mind that optimization is only one way for clients to find your website, and should never be your only strategy for building your online presence through your website. Other ways for clients to find your site include word of mouth, seeing it on other advertising or marketing collateral, or even getting it from you directly. Keep doing the footwork to get exposure for your site.

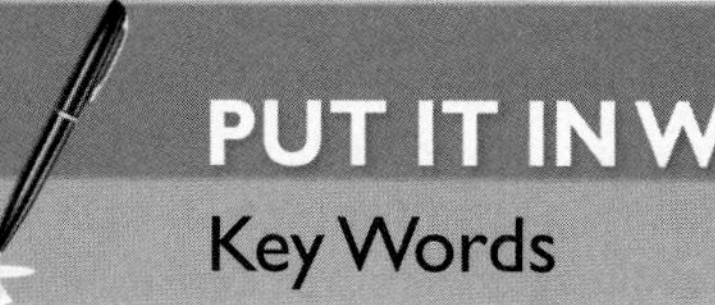

PUT IT IN WRITING

Key Words

Put yourself in the shoes of a potential client. If they were trying to find someone who was offering massage services just like yours, what would he or she be likely to use as key words in a search? Brainstorm some of those words here.

____________	____________	____________
____________	____________	____________
____________	____________	____________
____________	____________	____________
____________	____________	____________

Now, go online and type in those same key words. What do you find? Don't panic if your very brilliant blend of key words that you worked so hard on yields your competitors in the top spots . . . there is still hope.

PITFALLS

When making a first website rich in key words, many make the mistake of thinking more is better. Don't overload your site with key words, as excessive repetition of key words, or "stuffing," is something search engines don't like. Doing this may make you look like spam to a search engine, and may actually hurt your ranking.

your site map as descriptive and explanatory as possible will help web crawlers access your information and rank you higher in search results.

Off-site optimization refers to the outside sources that bulk up your websites "findability." For example, having hyperlinks on other websites that are relevant or complementary to your massage business is a great way to have off-site optimization that will improve visibility and give you priority in search engines. Some companies pay to place links on others' websites, but you can approach other local companies about building free link partnerships for mutual benefit (more on this later). You can often find link directories through your local chamber of commerce or local business associations. In addition, you can leverage off-site optimization by including a link to your website when sending out press releases or publishing articles online.

Remember, when you are creating a website, you always want to do it with search engine optimization in mind. Writing copy and content that is key word–rich, building a descriptive site map, and identifying off-site places for your site links are all important components of search engine optimization. When a company's website comes up because of all the above factors, it is typically known as an **organic search result.** This just means that a site gains priority naturally and by its own merit, and is not a paid advertisement.

Another way that many businesses have found to maximize exposure for their websites is by paying for it.

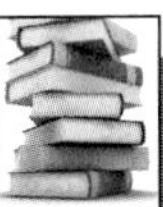

HELPFUL RESOURCES

Want to know if your key words are as good as you think they are? Google Adwords (adwords.google.com) has a keyword tool that can help you uncover how much search demand there is for any given keyword or key phrase. It will even tell you how much advertisers are paying per click. This will help you figure out the potential value for various key words, and to gauge if the ones you are considering are actually in demand.

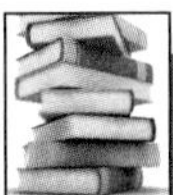

HELPFUL RESOURCES

To learn more about search engine optimization and how it can benefit your business, check out *Search Engine Optimization: An Hour a Day* by Jennifer Grappone and Gradiva Couzin (2008, Sybex) and *Search Engine Optimization for Dummies* by Peter Kent (2008, Wiley). If you have the money, it might be worth consulting with a professional. There are also many web consultants to help you out, and, of course, you can find one in your area by plugging key words into a search engine! See—works for everything!

Pay-per-click advertising (PPCA) is a promotional technique whereby an advertiser places an ad link on a given search engine or website, but only has to pay for it when users actually click on the link to the advertiser's own website. The advertiser is typically not charged to have their ad displayed in an organic search result. The popularity of this advertising/optimizing strategy has grown significantly in recent years.[15] Any individual or company that elects to use PPCA will typically select the key words they think will be popular with their target market and will thus drive more traffic to their websites (like the ones you identified in the last exercise). Then they will usually either bid on those key words, or pay a fixed price per click based upon the popularity of a word of phrase. For example, "massage therapy" might be a very expensive PPCA keyword, but "prenatal massage Detroit" might be much less expensive due to its specificity and lower demand. Geographically targeted key words are good for your business anyway, since you can likely only practice massage in a limited geographic area. There are many PPCA systems and sites to choose from, and popular ones include Google Adwords, Yahoo Search Marketing, and MSN AdCenter.

Yet another way that companies will optimize their web presence is through the use of reciprocal links. **Reciprocal links** are hyperlinks that mutually connect websites to one another. In exchange for having a link to your website on another company's website, you will display its link on your own. When identifying reciprocal link partners, you will want to find ones that are complementary to your business (Figure 15-3 ■). Then approach the company's owner and ask for a reciprocal link. You can do this by sending an e-mail, making a phone call, or walking into their business in person. Be sure that you are familiar with all the content displayed on partnering sites—you don't want to be associated with anything disreputable or any company that would not be a good affiliation for the image you are trying to present. Use links strategically, only partnering with sites that will lends yours value and credibility.

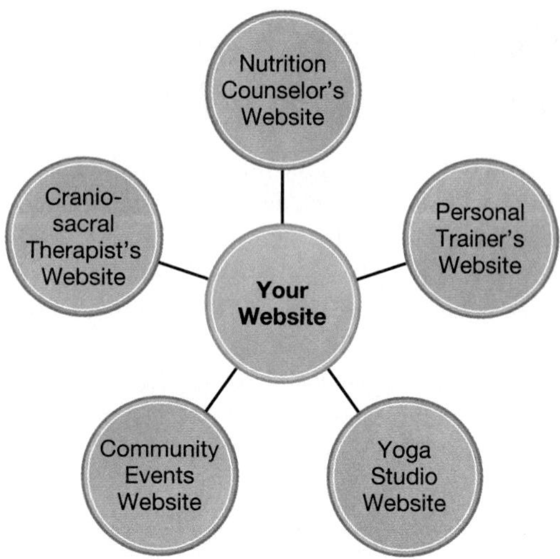

Examples of Reciprocal Links

FIGURE 15-3

Reciprocal links mutually connect different business websites to one another. Other holistic practitioners or good referral relationships would make good link partners for your business.

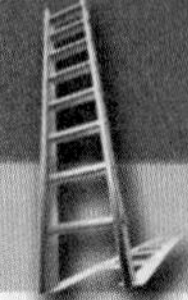

FIRST STEPS

To get a good idea of how other massage practices have leveraged reciprocal links for their business, find the top ranked websites for massage key words in your area. When you identify other local therapist or company sites, you can search their reciprocal links by going to Yahoo.com. In the search portal, write "link:www.competitorwebsite.com". For example, if www.knoxsvillemassage.com is one of the sites you identified, you would type "link:www.knoxsvillemassage.com" to find a list of their reciprocal links. Doing this will help you see how others are using this tool, and will also help you identify new potential link partners for your own business.

BLOGGING

Another way to optimize your site is with fresh content, something that search engines love. Many therapists find that maintaining a blog enhances their search visibility. A **blog** is a site that is devoted to an individual's or company's thoughts, reflections, commentary, or news. Blogs (a contraction of the original term "web log"[16]) are often compared to an online journal, and are kept updated with fresh original content on an ongoing basis. Though it may sound like a backlog of eggnog, the blog has become a very powerful tool for many small businesses and has grown exponentially in popularity.[17] This is due in part to the fact that blogs are typically free to set up and require little to no Internet savvy. They are a great venue for you to showcase your talents as an expert massage therapist and to reinforce the proficiency and skill associated with your business. Not just text entries, most blog sites typically allow you to upload photos, post videos and music, and create an integrated experience for your visitors. In addition, search engines typically love blogs (for they love fresh content), and they can help optimize your web presence even more.

Before you begin your blog, think strategically about what you would like to achieve with it. Because they are so easy to update, you can easily inform your readers of any new changes, additions to your business, and new products or services. Some hosting packages include a blog on your home website, but you can also blog through free sites. And, of course, you can have a reciprocal link between your blog site and your website, mutually increasing the visibility of both. Ideally, your blog's name will be a close facsimile of your company's name, or some variation of it. This will help leverage your blog to build your brand (see Chapters 11 and 12).

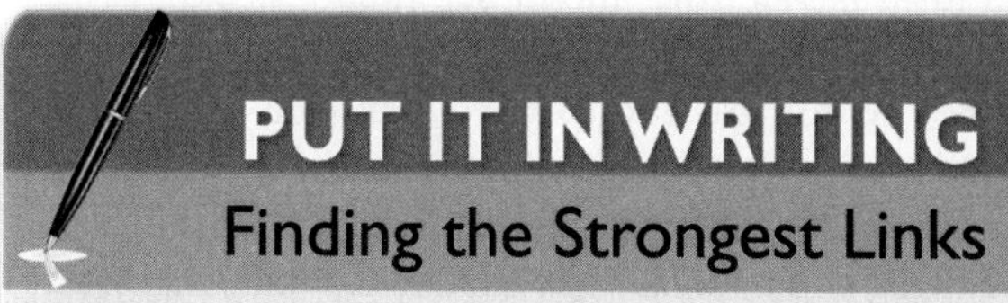

PUT IT IN WRITING
Finding the Strongest Links

Many massage therapists like to build reciprocal links with other germane practitioners such as chiropractors, acupuncturists, physical therapists, personal trainers, and so forth. Think of the people and the companies in your network, and write out some of the ones you identify as potential partners for reciprocal linking.

______________	______________
______________	______________
______________	______________
______________	______________
______________	______________
______________	______________
______________	______________

Once you've identified some companies, approach the owners and ask them if they would be interested in reciprocal linking. Be sure to explain all of the advantages and mutual benefits of linking with a quality site like yours.

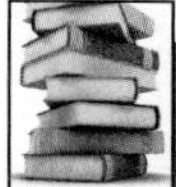

HELPFUL RESOURCES

So you have decided you want to start a blog. Where to begin? There are several free or inexpensive sites that will host your blog for you. Most sites have templates for you to fill out, and many provide tutorials on how to create and maintain a blog site. Generally, all you need is an e-mail address to get started. Popular sites include Blogger, WordPress, and Tumblr.

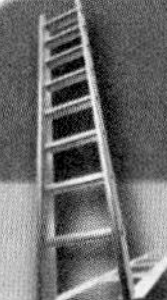

FIRST STEPS

Unclogging a Blog

Topics for blogs are as varied and diverse as the people who write them. Massage blogs often have themes such as health benefits, trends in the industry, local events, spotlights on other health practitioners, client success stories, and so forth. The world of massage is fascinating, wide-ranging, and topic-rich. If you have experience in other related industries, you can write about that as well, as long as it relates in a way that brings value to your readers. You can get creative—for example, if you used to be an accountant, write about the unique aspects of financial management for massage. Think about your own knowledge and all the fantastic experience you bring to the blogging table. Brainstorm some things that you could get started blogging about, and write your ideas below.

______________________ ______________________
______________________ ______________________
______________________ ______________________
______________________ ______________________
______________________ ______________________
______________________ ______________________
______________________ ______________________

Don't worry if you feel stuck or can't think of a lot of ideas at first. Blogging can be like exercising; the more you do it, the easier and more enjoyable it becomes. If it helps, check out other blog sites and read others' content. Not only can this help kick start your own creativity, you can typically leave feedback on another's posts which can guide readers back to your own blog and/or website. Now go flex those blogging muscles!

Blogging can be a great way to educate your clients and potential clients about all the amazing benefits of massage, while at the same time exhibiting your knowledge. Draw on the information you learned in school, as well as on the information from your personal experiences. Think about whom you are writing for, and the problems you and your business will solve for that person (think of sore muscles, stress-related discomfort, pregnancy strain, TMJ complications, and so forth). Look at what is going on in the world of massage and write about it. Even if you don't fancy yourself to be a world-class writer, you can still experiment with communicating all that you know and love about the world of massage.

GETTING THE WORD OUT

A close relative of the blog, an **e-zine** is a virtual magazine, article, or newsletter disseminated to clients or members of a target market, typically via mass e-mailings. E-zines are a key component of **e-mail marketing,** where a business promotes its products and services in electronic mailings to a target market. E-zines are sent out periodically and designed to inform and educate current and potential clients. The goal of any good e-zine should always be to focus on solving the problems of your target market, and to provide useful and good quality information to readers. Whereas blogs are typically actively accessed by visitors, e-zines are acquired passively. In other words, individuals will come to your blog, but e-zines generally come to individuals on your subscriber list.

> *There is so much media now with the Internet and people, and so easy and so cheap to start a newspaper or start a magazine, there's just millions of voices and people want to be heard.*
>
> —Rupert Murdoch

A **subscriber list,** or user list, is a collection of e-mail addresses obtained for the purpose of distributing information and communication.[18] It provides a way to communicate with clients on a different level, and to personalize those exchanges. Many massage therapists will tell you that their e-mail subscriber list is more important than their business card. Why? Because having e-mail addresses allows them to send clients periodic, value-adding e-zines or e-mails, which keeps them and their massage business fresh in clients' minds; business cards can be lost or discarded. When muscles ache, a client is more likely to think of you if your name resurfaces in their inbox then if your card is buried in a drawer. Sending out valuable content to clients also helps to establish and reinforce your role as a credible expert.

The methods that businesses use to acquire e-mails and grow a subscriber list vary, but typically people either get them from Internet users directly or obtain them from third parties. Ideally, you should be collecting e-mail addresses from every client who walks through your door. A good way to do this is to include it on your client intake form. It is typically always better to get e-mail addresses directly from individuals, as you want people to *actually want* the information you are sending them. This will also help distinguish your e-mails or e-zines from **spam,** the unsolicited e-mail advertisements that clog

PITFALLS

Even if a client gives you his or her e-mail address personally, treat that e-mail considerately. Be careful of the volume of newsletters/e-zines you send out. Most everyone is incredibly busy, and you do not want to annoy anyone by e-mailing excessively or sending useless content. Send periodic, concise, well-written, quality information that truly adds value to others. Be respectful, and remember that you are building trust with clients.

mailboxes and vex Internet users (who could be potential clients). Sending spam can seriously damage your business. When you send e-zines to people on your subscriber list, always be certain to include an *unsubscribe* option at the bottom of the page, so that people can opt out of receiving e-mails from you at any time (see Chapter 10 for more information on legal requirements in e-mail correspondence). You always want to be respectful of the people on your subscriber list, as they have entrusted you with their personal information; don't ever give out or sell their information to others.

Once your website is up and running, you can also use it as a way to grow your subscriber list. Create a clearly visible newsletter sign-up box toward the top of your website's home page. You might offer a free gift on your website that will entice them to fill out their information and build your database. This is **lead generation,** which is a way to market your business by generating interest in your product or services and by allowing you to develop an ongoing marketing relationship with someone via the contact information they provide. You can also encourage your readers to forward your e-zines or blogs to anyone else who might be interested or might benefit from the information you are providing.

As you begin to grow your subscriber list, remember to be patient. Keep in mind that you want a good quality list of contacts, not just a collection of e-mail addresses. Remember, you want your subscriber list to be composed of people who want the information you provide, and who will benefit from the knowledge and skills you have to offer. Quality of both the e-zine content and the subscriber list is the key to unlocking this powerful tool. Just like anything of quality, both can take time to develop. But when they do—look out!

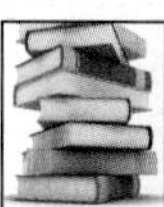

HELPFUL RESOURCES

Several free newsletter templates can be found online and sent from your e-mail, or you can design your own. Companies like Constant Contact and iContact can help you design and distribute your e-zine and e-mail communication to a large group of people, and typically charge a nominal fee. Chances are you may already be receiving these e-zines and newsletters from others in your e-mail inbox. Before you begin designing, take a look at what others have created and find out who is hosting the sites or providing the services you like the most. You can also turn favorite blogs and e-zines into Internet articles. Ezine.com is a venue where you can submit an article for Internet publication.

LOST IN THE LAND OF BLOGS

If blogs are something you think you would really like to use for your business, it is important to understand the volume of competition out there. Just like websites in general, blogs are an incredibly and increasingly popular communications medium. Technorati, a search engine just for blogs, maintains that there are currently more than 50 million blogs in the virtual "blogosphere," and the numbers are increasing.[19] With such overwhelming numbers, how can anyone keep up? More importantly, how can your target market find *your* wonderful blog (and business) amidst all the online noise?

Of course, just like for your overall website, key word rich content in your blog is always important to help search engines find it. Massage therapists who are really serious about broadcasting their blogs online and expanding their potential audience can set up an RSS feed for their blogs. **RSS** (Rich Site Summary) is a series of web feeds that are used to publish web content that is frequently updated. It is used to funnel content from everything updated online: blogs, news sources, podcasts, wikis, audio, and video streams.[20] RSS feeds help Internet users stay up-to-date with the ever-evolving information load online, while helping bloggers circulate their valuable information to more people without more effort (Figure 15-4 ■).

RSS feeds move your blogs from active to passive for your audience—in other words, rather than your visitors having to seek out your new blog entry, the updated content is automatically funneled to those who subscribe to your feed. As commoncraft.com explains, think of it as Netflix versus a video store, or Amazon versus your local bookstore. Things come to your home, rather than you going to get them. Users sign up with an **RSS reader,** a web-based or desk-based software that acts as a home for all the feeds that users are interested in receiving from their favorite websites. Think of readers as information mailboxes. Online readers are

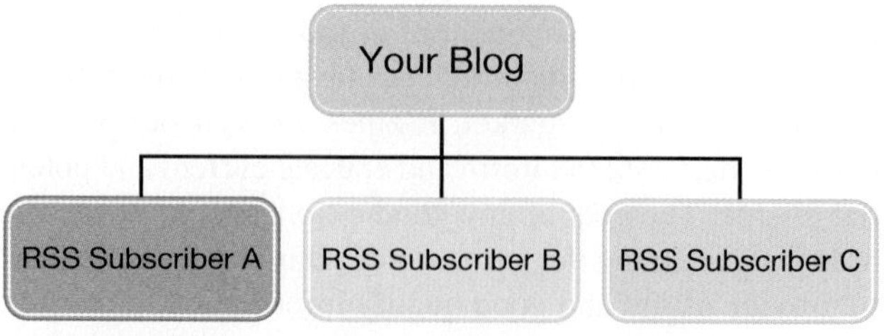

FIGURE 15-4

An RSS feed automatically funnels new content to your subscribers, rather than waiting for them to come find it.

PITFALLS

Information Overload

Because blogs and e-zines are so easy to maintain and update, and because they bear so many resemblances to a journal, some people fall into the trap of using these media for personal explorations. Keep in mind that you are ultimately responsible for any content that you include on your blog site or in your e-zine. Before posting an entry that rants about your political passion or uploading a photo from the bachelor party in Vegas, think back to the discussion of personal branding in Chapter 6. What image would you like to convey consistently about yourself and your business? As anything available online can either contribute to or discredit your personal brand, remember that blogs and e-zines are important ingredients in your professionalism. Create blogs and e-zines with your clients' needs in mind, not your own. You want these tools to position you as an expert and to strengthen your business, not to paint you as an amateur. Read more about this issue in the online security section of this chapter.

typically free, and popular ones include My Yahoo, Newsgator.com, Bloglines.com, and Google Reader. Users then subscribe to feeds by clicking on the icons on their favorite sites. These are often little orange squares, but can also be company logos. If your site has an RSS icon, your visitors can subscribe to a feed from your site and automatically receive your updated content.

CA-CHING: MAKING MONEY ON YOUR SITE WITH ONLINE PRODUCT SALES AND WEB SCHEDULING

Many massage therapists differ on the virtues of putting too much of their business online. Some prefer to have their websites be informational only, leaving most of the details to be done in person. Others, however, find that they have been able to increase their incomes and save themselves time by automating things like gift certificates, product sales, and client scheduling. Remember, there is no right or wrong way to do it—it is *your* business and it really should be whatever you are comfortable with.

In Chapter 9, you explored the ins and outs of selling products in your business, as well as developing your own private label. Earlier in this chapter you learned the term e-commerce. A lot of companies sell their products online to open their markets and boost their revenues. Some massage therapists have found great success in selling complementary health and wellness products on their sites, and have

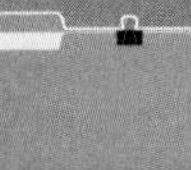

GETTING ORGANIZED

So you think you might like to include retail products on your website. Now it is time to do a little research. Although the Internet transcends all physical boundaries and jurisdictions, that does not mean that you aren't going to have to abide by regular retail regulations and laws when selling things online. Take some time now to investigate the common Internet trademark, copyright, tax collection, and liability guidelines. If you will be shipping overseas, you'll need to educate yourself on import and export regulations and restrictions. Some cities and states may even require you to get additional permits or licenses to sell some products online. Do your homework upfront, and document everything.

found that the income they generate really supplements their massage income nicely.

Some retailers elect to sell their goods through third-party merchant sites. **Third-party merchant sites** are usually the major e-commerce websites that, whether by auction or direct sale, act as a retail clearinghouse for every kind of product imaginable. Examples of this would be eBay, Amazon, or Half .com. Some people find third-party merchants to be an advantageous route because they don't have to spend as much time chasing clients or optimizing their sites to attract buyers—the buyers are already there looking (Figure 15-5 ■).

If you do decide you would like to sell products on your site or on a third-party merchant site, make sure that doing so fits within your overall business plan and really contributes value to your practice. While it can be lucrative, e-commerce is not a way to get rich quick, and you want to be sure you are willing to commit the time, energy, and resources it takes to make it. Do you have time to manage inventory and fill orders? Will it get in the way of the service-oriented side of your business if you are constantly running to the post office to ship foam rollers or your fabulous lavender lotion all over the globe?

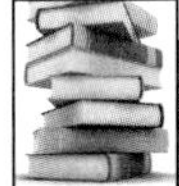

HELPFUL RESOURCES

If you want to sell things online, you will need shopping cart software for visitors to compile their purchases. **Open source shopping carts** are online systems that anyone can use and access for retailing products on their sites, often for little or no cost. At the time of this writing, Zen Cart, StoreSprite, and PrestaShop are all popular free open source shopping carts (read each site's copyright notices and terms before downloading).[21]

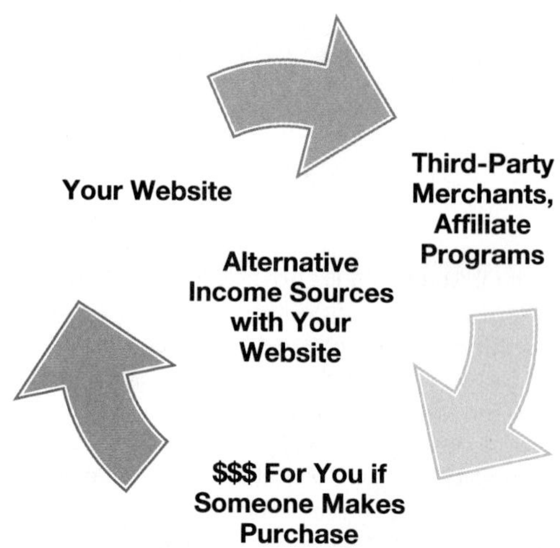

FIGURE 15-5

Many holistic businesses seek alternate income sources to supplement their service income. The Internet provides many ways to do this through your website, such as affiliate programs and third party merchants.

Some therapists have found a way to get around this dilemma through **affiliate programs,** in which they use their website as an intermediary for other vendors and ebusinesses. They park hyperlinks to other e-businesses on their site, promote their products, and collect a commission for any sales that are made through that click. In essence, companies pay website owners (you) to advertise and help sell their own product. The sales are then tracked back to the therapist's website via web cookies, and the therapist is able to make some passive income. **Cookies** are little packages of Internet information sent between the server and the client browser to help sites track user preferences, behaviors, and information.[22] A cookie is how Amazon knows what spy novels you looked at last week, how your bank can remember your user name, and how Facebook automatically goes to your profile page when you enter the generic address in your browser.

Client booking is another way to use your site to boost revenues for your business. This trend is no longer just for spas; as people are getting more and more accustomed to doing everything online, medical massage therapists, Reiki practitioners, rolfers, TMJ specialists, and so forth are adopting online scheduling. This can also make things easier for you, as you do not have to spend as much time making appointments and managing your calendar. There are several online services that help you do this through your site, such as TimeCenter, MindBody, SpaBooker, Appointment-Plus, and several other sites that have packages you can purchase. Comfort levels with this particular technology vary widely among therapists, and many people do not feel comfortable allowing complete strangers to book appointments without any preliminary screening processes. In the next section, you will learn more about security issues and protecting yourself and your business online.

SECURITY, PRIVACY, AND LEGAL ISSUES

Everyone knows that the Internet is an incredibly powerful and wide-reaching instrument. It is also common knowledge that it is not always a savory place, and that not all Internet users are reputable characters. Once you put something online, you do not have control over who accesses it. Thus, it is important to understand the need to protect yourself and others at all times when doing anything online.

In the blogging and e-zines section of this chapter, you read about the importance of maintaining your image. When you are writing blogs and posting pictures from the comfort of your home, it may seem hard to connect to the idea that others will see those things. But consider how hard you have worked in this chapter to find ways to *ensure* that people find you and your business, and you will understand the need to be all the more careful of what you put online.

It is not uncommon (and is entirely legal) for clients or potential employers to do background research on you before doing any business with you or giving you a job. Embarrassing photos, offensive remarks, or off-colored humor can end a professional relationship or cost you a job. Once something is put online, it is fair game for anyone with a computer. And once it is in the ether of the Internet, it cannot be retracted; it is there forever. This is something very important to keep in mind with sites like Facebook, MySpace, or any other social networking site.[23] A good gauge when posting anything is to ask yourself, "If I saw this, would I want to work with me?" (see Chapter 2 for more on this topic).

Of course, Internet security is not just about what you put out online, but also about what you have in your computer. Many individuals and small businesses do not think they are susceptible to threats or violations of Internet security, but in fact small businesses are often more vulnerable to threats than are large companies.[24] Any computer can be attacked by viruses, worms, spyware, or hacker attacks. And if you have client information stored in your computer insecurely, you could expose yourself and your valued customers to uncomfortable situations, or even fraud or identity theft.

Identity theft occurs when someone uses another individual's identifying information (social security number, birth date, address, credit card numbers) for his or her own benefit or profit. Identity theft is an ever-increasing problem that has devastating consequences for its victims, and its prevalence has skyrocketed as more and more sensitive private information is transmitted and stored electronically. Not only can having client information accessed by others destroy your professional relationship, it can open you up to legal liability. Your computer should have good Internet security such as antivirus software and firewalls. A **firewall** is a group

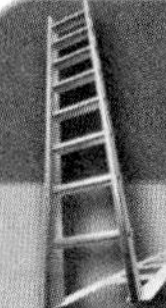

FIRST STEPS

If you are storing a lot of sensitive information in your computer, there are preventative measures you can take to protect yourself and your clients. The following checklist is adapted from the Federal Trade Commission's tips to help businesses protect themselves.[25]

1. Take inventory of what you have stored: Examine all your computers files to see where you have any personal information. You might be surprised at how much you have.
2. Clean house: Chances are good your computer holds a lot of information not necessary for your business operations. If you have unnecessary information on your computer, especially sensitive information, get rid of it. Make sure to dispose of it properly. Shred paper documents.
3. Safeguard it: Invest in good antivirus software and firewall protections to protect the sensitive information that is relevant to your business or personal life. There are many to choose from, such as McAffee and Norton Antivirus. Also, be smart with your passwords online, and don't use the same ones for all your accounts.
4. Preventative medicine: If a breach were to occur, how would you handle it? Having a plan for worst-case scenarios is a good part of prevention.

of security measures that assess the Internet traffic passing through your computer and prevents unauthorized access to it.

Beyond basic security measures, there are also legal issues to consider when posting online. Even though it may seem like the avalanche of information is a free-for-all that makes regular rules difficult to implement, easy access does not override offline laws. For example, many people get confused with rules of public domain and intellectual property. **Intellectual property** is an asset that is usually intangible and has been created by human creativity. Examples include music, writing, copyrights, trademarks, trade secrets, and patents. **Copyright** is the legal right to protect one's original works, and it is automatic as soon as the work is created. Most copyrights are not registered, but that does not mean the work is not owned by someone. If Person A writes content and uploads pictures for her website, that content becomes her intellectual property. If Person B cuts and pastes it onto her own website without permission, that is a violation of intellectual property laws and can be an infringement of copyright laws.

Another growing legal concern is Internet libel. **Libel** is a written defamation of another's character that falsely and harmfully impacts his or her reputation. If you break up with your girlfriend and write harmful things about her on your blog, she could take you to court for Internet libel if she could prove harm was done and information was knowingly falsified. As always, use your basic business ethics and strictest common sense when posting anything online.

PERSONAL SAFETY

Although the vast majority of Internet users are good people with benign intentions, unfortunately there are some less stable people out there. Some of the high-profile bloggers have had experience with hate mail and personal threats.[26] Experts believe that those threatening become emboldened by anonymity; many bloggers now preempt this behavior by posting a warning that they reserve the right to remove offensive posts or publish hurtful e-mails, as well as to expose the person's e-mail and information. People think twice about saying mean things when they know that their own information may be revealed.

All of the information thus far is relevant to any business that represents itself online. But massage is not just any business, and due to the personal and physical nature of the work it is important to also consider your physical safety when branching out into the Internet. The following are a few suggestions for preserving your well-being and safety online:

- Do not include too much personal information about yourself or your family on your website. It's generally best to make little mention of loved ones at all.
- For all the work that has been done to legitimize the massage profession, there are still some who continue to confuse its purpose and intent. Place a clearly stated policy about ethics, boundaries, and acceptable behavior for client/therapist in therapeutic massage.
- Implement a careful screening program for all new clients. This can be done automatically through a survey on your site, or done personally through a phone call to you.
- If you are working as a solo practitioner, you may not want to give your office or home location on your website. Have clients call to schedule an appointment, and give them your address only after they have been screened.
- Trust your instincts when creating content for your site. You know what feels safe and what doesn't. There is never a reason to put yourself at risk. Use the same precautions and common sense online that you would offline.

Congratulations! You have just covered a lot of information and learned a lot of ways to harness the Internet to benefit your business. Be creative in this process, and enjoy finding and tweaking ways to make your website, your blog, and your Internet experience uniquely your own.

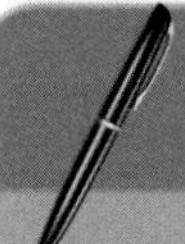

PUT IT IN WRITING

Safety Precautions

The suggestions given in this section is just a short list of precautions for protecting yourself online. Surely you can think of many other ways to keep yourself safe. Think of other suggestions you have heard, or other things you intuitively think would protect your safety. Write them down here.

CHAPTER SUMMARY BY LEARNING OBJECTIVES

1. **Understand the benefits of technology and the Internet for your business** Millions and millions of people come together on the Internet via electronic mail, file sharing, streaming media, social networking, and many other applications. Businesses of all sizes, structures, scopes, and specialties utilize the Internet to maximize business functioning.
2. **Explore the process of developing and maintaining a website** A website is an interconnected set of web pages that are furnished and supported by a host. Once you secure a domain name for your site, there are several ways to develop it. You can hire a web developer, pay for website templates, or design it yourself with website designing software.
3. **Define the anatomy of a website** A website typically includes a home page and several other pages of interest that visitors can navigate through. A site map charts all the pages available on a website, and pages are connected together with hyperlinks. Websites are typically written in HTML, the language of the Internet.
4. **Define search engine optimization and explore optimizing techniques** Search engine optimization is a way of getting a website priority in the listings of search engines in order to improve visitor traffic. Creating a key word rich website is a primary way to do this, though companies also use off-site optimization, reciprocal links, and pay-per-click advertising to get to the top.
5. **Define link partners/reciprocal links** Reciprocal links are hyperlinks that mutually connect websites to one another. Complementary businesses will post links to one another's websites for collaborative promotion.
6. **Define blogging and e-zines, and assess their role for your business** A blog is a site that is devoted to an individual or company's thoughts, reflections, commentary, or news. An e-zine is similar to a newsletter, and is sent periodically to people on a business's subscriber list. Blogs and e-zines provide fresh and valuable content to your clients, providing them with information that is beneficial. They also help to position the author/company as an expert, which in turn helps the business.
7. **Find ways to streamline your valuable information to target audiences** Subscriber lists, the unsubscribe option, and lead generation help to create an audience of people who want the information being provided in blogs and e-zines. Tools such as RSS feeds can help visitors be automatically updated of any new fresh content on a blog.
8. **Explore the benefits of online product sales and online scheduling** Many therapists use the Internet to increase revenues through direct online product sales, third-party merchant sites, and affiliate programs. Many find online scheduling to be a convenient time saver for themselves and their clients.
9. **Examine security, legal, and privacy issues** With the sheer numbers of people online that have access to anything that is posted, it is not possible to control who sees your content. Thus, it is very important to safeguard your private information, as well as that of your clients and family. It is also important to maintain professional privacy, as well as to adhere to governing laws whenever posting online.

ACTIVITIES

Quiz: Identifying Internet Words and Concepts

1. Max wants to get the latest information from his favorite online news source, but he doesn't want to have to keep checking for it. A solution for Max might be:
   a. getting cable
   b. reading the paper
   c. subscribing to an RSS feed
   d. using his time to volunteer
2. An example of a URL would be:
   a. www.stinkyshoes.com
   b. http://stinkyshoes.com
   c. <stinkyshoes.com/>
   d. stinkyshoes.com
3. Shelby works as a massage therapist in a hospice. Although she loves her clients, she does not like her boss or her coworkers. To vent her frustrations, she writes all about her irritations on her blog, exaggerating wildly at times. Which of the following could be a logical consequence for Shelby's choices?
   a. Her coworkers could see it and Shelby could be sued for libel.
   b. Her boss could see it and Shelby could be fired.
   c. Future employers could see it and not want to hire Shelby.
   d. All of the above.
4. Which of the following is *not* a way to develop a website?
   a. do it yourself with a web designing software
   b. pay a web designer to create it for you
   c. buy/lease a website template that you like online
   d. find a site that you like and borrow its graphics and content
5. Laisha started doing online booking for her MET practice. She was amazed at how many appointments she quickly filled, but grew concerned about who exactly might be coming in for a massage. What are some of the things Laisha could do?
   a. Implement a screening survey on her website before allowing anyone to schedule
   b. Post boundaries of treatment and rules of conduct on her site
   c. Create a system with her web developer where only clients that she has screened personally can book online; everyone else needs to call her directly for an appointment.
   d. Cancel an appointment with someone she does not feel comfortable with—after all, her personal safety overrides the money
   e. All of the above
6. HTML is:
   a. the IRS form for self-employed individuals
   b. the mainstream language of the Internet
   c. a poly-cotton blend
   d. the house that stores RSS feeds
7. Peach sent out a press release for her new holistic wellness center to local media outlets. The press release included the center's website address. This is a good example of:
   a. off-site optimization
   b. a shameless plug
   c. communications
   d. on-site optimization
8. In order to keep up with all of the new information available online and display relevant results, search engines send out _____ to "read" websites.
   a. crickets
   b. auditors
   c. spiders
   d. their minions
9. Rajiv stores all of his client files in his personal computer, as well as all of his own personal information and passwords. Rajiv might want to invest in:
   a. stocks and bonds
   b. continuing education
   c. antivirus software, firewalls, and other security measures
   d. pork belly futures
10. Emmy is passionate about the mind-body-spirit connection, and constantly reads books on the topic. She decided to include her favorites on her website, and includes links to some of her favorite authors' sites for clients. When clients purchase a book, Emmy gets 15 percent of sales. This is an example of a(n):
    a. third-party merchant site
    b. pay dirt
    c. manipulation of her clients
    d. affiliate program
11. _____ is the legal right to protect one's original work, even if it is not registered with the Library of Congress.
    a. Double indemnity
    b. Copyright
    c. Torts
    d. Punitive damage

12. Chris is a potential client who is directed to your home page by a friend. He wants information on your experience and the prices you charge. Where would he first look to see if you provide that information on your site?
    a. your blog
    b. your e-zine
    c. your site map
    d. your domain name
13. Blogs are popular with search engines because search engines love:
    a. cookies
    b. fresh and updated content
    c. reading about massage
    d. gossip
14. Eleanor is a prenatal therapist who has had great response to her personal line of pregnancy pampering products, and wants to start selling items online. Before she does this, she should do some preliminary research on:
    a. the laws of her city and state for online sales
    b. tax requirements for online sales
    c. copyright, trademark, import, and export regulations
    d. all of the above
15. _____ is unwanted, unsolicited junk e-mail.
    a. Bologna
    b. An e-mail from your ex
    c. Spam
    d. Any advertisement or e-zine

Discussion Questions

1. When you think about designing a website, what is most important to you? Convenience? Control? Cost? Look at all the options for developing and hosting a website, and discuss with other class members what is most appealing to you and why.
2. When you are shopping online or just surfing around, what kinds of sites catch your eye? What do you think is attracting you? The content? The graphics? The valuable information? The convenience? Now put yourself in the place of a potential customer. What sorts of things do you think they would be looking for in a website?

Case Study

Belle

Belle is a therapist who specializes in NMT and structural integration. She works in a business complex that has several other independent wellness practitioners: a nutritionist, a Swedish massage therapist, a psychologist, and a chiropractor. Lately she has seen the success that some of her colleagues were having with their own sites. Belle has never considered herself to be very tech savvy, but she decided she needed a website for her business.

Belle registers her domain name without any trouble, and starts to think about designing her site. She doesn't feel that she has nearly enough knowledge to go it alone, and doesn't have quite enough money to hire a web developer. So Belle decides to buy a website template online through one of the sites that specialized in health and wellness sites. She chooses a design that she likes, but not sure of what makes a successful website, Belle just creates one simple page. On it, she lists her name, her phone number, her credentials, and some of the benefits of her modality. Although she sells a few products from her office, she does not feel ready to sell anything online. Belle is delighted by the professional look of her page, and content that she now has a website. However, she is surprised when, after a few weeks, nothing has changed in her business. The people she has told about her website tell her it's quite lovely, but she has not received any new calls. She had hoped that the website would help increase her sales and increase her profits.

After a month, Belle has hired you, a massage therapy business consultant, to help her solve her problem. You hear her story and consider all of the diagnostic information.

1. Why do you think Belle's site has not generated any new traffic for her?
2. Belle asks you to help her start her website over from scratch. Knowing the value of on-site optimization, what would be the first thing you would ask Belle to identify and include in her web pages and web content?
3. You explain to Belle the concept of off-site optimization. What are some of the opportunities Belle might have for this option?
4. You see that Belle is very knowledgable and very passionate about structural integration. She gets very animated when talking about it, and truly believes in the way it helps her clients. Seeing this, what might be way Belle could leverage her website and play on this strength to benefit both her business and her clients?
5. Although Belle is not comfortable selling her own products online, she is interested to hear other ways that her site could make her money. What ideas might you share with her?

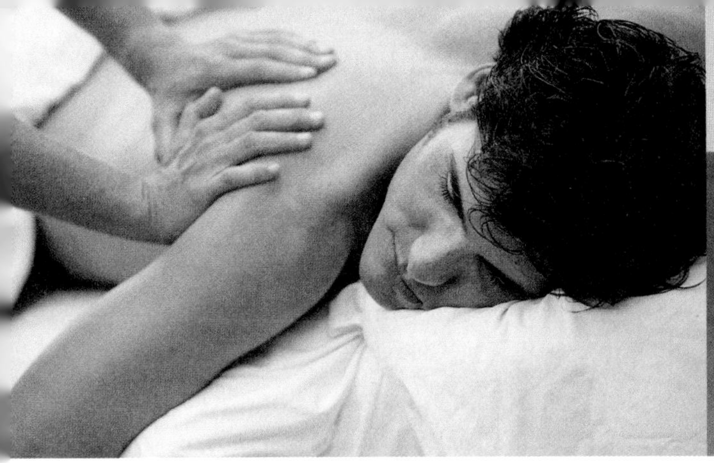

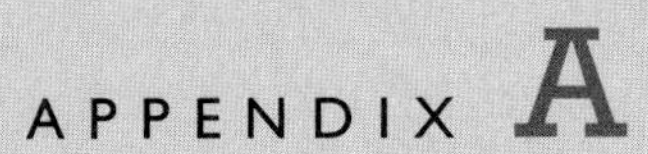

APPENDIX A

Answer Key

CHAPTER 1

Is a Massage Therapy Career Right for You?

None—all critical thinking exercises.

CHAPTER 2

Career Strategies and Professional Development

Quiz: Professional Development Review

1. b. STAR stands for Situation, Task, Action, and Result.
2. c. combination
3. a. nonverbal communication
4. d. cover letter
5. b. behavior-based interviewing
6. c. independent contractor
7. False. An employer is not responsible for paying taxes on a 1099 independent contractor.
8. False. Although geriatric massage is the overarching modality you would practice in either a retirement home or a hospice, the client need is not necessarily the same. Most people in hospice need end of life palliative care, while many retirement home residents are active, vigorous, and healthy individuals.
9. True.
10. False. Interview questions should relate only to your ability to do the job, and anything that does not reflect that is not permissible. Although it is not technically illegal to ask these "illegal questions," a discriminatory hiring decision based on these questions is illegal.
11. True.
12. False. Although it hard to erase information that is online, there are many proactive actions you can take to clean up your online image. You can tighten security settings on any social networking, and take steps to remove or preempt unfavorable photos of you on other people's pages. You can also write articles, press releases, or join professional social networks that project the professional image of a massage expert.
13. False. If you sign a contract that specifies the duration of time you are to work as an employee and quit before you have satisfied that time, you are liable for contract breach. Employment at will does not supersede a contract.
14. True.
15. False. Recruiters report that poorly crafted résumés will quickly excuse a candidate from consideration. This is especially true when there are many job applicants for one position, such as in a slack labor market. Regardless of market conditions, however, your cover letter and résumé are often your first point of contact and your essential marketing package. You always want to make a good impression with a polished, error-free résumé.

CHAPTER 3

Time Management 101

None—all critical thinking exercises.

CHAPTER 4

Professional Issues

Quiz: Identifying Professional Issues: Words and Concepts

1. a. an overstepping of a boundary that may or may not be harmful to an individual
2. d. privacy
3. b. intellectual, physical, emotional, sexual, and energetic
4. b. Financial boundary
5. c. a pledge taken by holistic and traditional medical providers
6. a. Subjective, Objective, Assessment, and Plan
7. c. National Certification Board for Therapeutic Massage & Bodywork (NCBTMB) and the Federation of State Massage Therapy Boards (FSMTB)
8. d. Confidentiality
9. d. dual relationship
10. False. Even with a business license, you may be required to obtain additional licenses specific to your jurisdiction's laws.

11. False. Sex with a client is strictly prohibited by nearly every professional organization, professional code, governing body, and licensure law. Violating this can result in loss of reputation, loss of licenses, and even a malpractice lawsuit.
12. True.
13. True.
14. True.
15. False. Both clients and therapists can project their past feelings onto the other through transference and countertransference.

CHAPTER 5

Self-Care

None—all critical thinking exercises.

CHAPTER 6

Networking

Quiz: Networking Review

1. c. The unique combination of the components that make up who you are and what you have to offer others
2. b. scam; contact the bank and the authorities
3. c. skill, image, exposure
4. a. feels energized alone and drained around others
5. d. an extrovert
6. b. strategic partners
7. d. Getting as many business cards as humanly possible.
8. c. By running away and not doing business with her.
9. a. Exposure
10. d. All the above
11. False. Always exercise common sense and professional boundaries in networking. While you want to remain honest and open to opportunities, you do not ever need to reveal any sensitive information to anyone.
12. True.
13. True.
14. False. A connector is a person in a community who knows people across a wide array of circles and makes a habit out of connecting individuals that can mutually benefit by association.
15. True.

CHAPTER 7

Abundance from Within: Personal Financial Planning Basics

Quiz: Financial Planning Basics

1. c. new iPod
2. b. His money is easily converted to cash.
3. c. Not planning, overspending, consumer credit, not planning for retirement
4. d. Moneta
5. d. All of the above
6. a. Net worth
7. d. new ski boots for her Aspen vacation
8. b. His estate will go through probate court, which will decide how to distribute his assets.
9. a. Her joy account
10. c. Equity on a home
    Case Study: Jean's Personal Financial Statement

Jean's Assets		Jean's Debts	
Home Equity	$58,000	Mortgage	$142,000
Checking Account	$800	Credit Cards	$12,000
Savings Account	$3,000	School Loans	$35,000
Emergency Fund	$8,000		
Roth IRA	$94,500		
Cash	$40		
Total Assets	$164,340	Total Debts	$189,000
Jean's Net Worth			
Total Assets	$164,340		
Total Debts	$189,000		
Net Worth	**$ −24,660**		

CHAPTER 8

Your Own Practice: Getting Started

None—all critical thinking exercises.

CHAPTER 9

Location, Location, Location

Quiz: Location Basics

1. b. location mix
2. d. b and c
3. c. can be very convenient and minimize operating costs
4. d. a and b
5. a. waiting for someone to ask you to join their wellness center
6. e. all the above
7. c. already furnished
8. b. professional ethics; scope of practice
9. False. Private-label products can either be made by the company selling them or by another company that sells to other companies for resale.
10. False. Most commercial real estate agents make their commission from the owners of the commercial buildings, not the tenants leasing them.
11. True.

12. False. Wellness centers are only one way to build your business collaboratively.

CHAPTER 10

Organizing and Legal Structuring

Quiz: Identifying Organizing and Legal Structuring Words and Concepts

1. b. S corporation
2. a. product liability insurance
3. d. trademark and trade name laws
4. e. both c (cybersquatting) and d (trademark violation)
5. c. creating your succession plan and exit strategy
6. c. CAN-SPAM Act of 2003
7. a. Employer Identification Number (EIN)
8. c. 4 years
9. d. all the above
10. b. deduction

CHAPTER 11

Marketing Fundamentals

Quiz: Identifying Marketing Words

1. b. publicity
2. b. product, price, place, promotion
3. a. internal
4. b. tactic
5. d. word of mouth
6. c. SMART (specific, measurable, attainable, realistic, timely)
7. c. cooperative marketing
8. c. opportunity
9. d. differential pricing
10. a. target market

CHAPTER 12

More Marketing for Massage

Quiz: Identifying Massage Marketing Words and Concepts

1. b. qualified prospect
2. a. skills, systems, and tools
3. d. Maslow's Hierarchy of Needs
4. d. all the above
5. d. both a and b
6. c. recession; discretionary goods and services
7. b. basic physiological needs
8. a. Viral marketing
9. d. marketing systems
10. False. The more specific you are about your target and niche markets, the easier your marketing efforts will become, and the more you will attract clients.
11. False. When the supply of a good or service increases, it often results in a decreased price or waning demand.
12. True. It can be a great idea to market collaboratively with or give referrals to other massage therapists, particularly if they specialize in different modalities or offer different skill sets.
13. True. During times of economic retraction, many people cut back or stop spending money on things they consider nonessential. Many people consider massage therapy to be a discretionary spending item.
14. Absolutely false. Many businesses of all kinds continue to thrive and grow during bad economic periods.
15. True.

CHAPTER 13

Abundance from Without: Financial Management for Your Business

Quiz: Financial Management Review

1. a. Variable costs
2. d. statement of cash flows
3. d. 100 percent
4. b. the point where revenues and expenses are equal, and there is no profit or loss.
5. b. Sweat equity
6. c. your house
7. False. Venture capitalists invest in businesses that will yield incredibly high returns. Most massage businesses are too small in scale/scope to generate any interest from venture capitalists.
8. True.
9. False. All bartering activities are to be reported to the Internal Revenue Service as taxable income.
10. False. Most businesses fail because they underestimate the recurring costs and expenses associated with keeping it running. Your business will always have fixed and variable costs, such as leases, equipment, taxes, and insurance.
11. False. Forecasts are only estimates. Most funders know that businesses rarely ever hit their financial forecasts targets dead-on.
12. True.

CHAPTER 14

Managing Yourself and Others

Quiz: Identifying Management Words and Concepts

1. b. Onboarding
2. d. all the above
3. d. a and c. Wages are not part of employee benefits, but are obligations of the employer for services rendered.
4. c. learning culture

5. d. paternalistic
6. a. Turnover
7. False. While it may be permissible (or simply not regulated) to have massage student interns provide manual massage therapy, more and more local authorities require that anyone providing massage must have completed an accredited program and be licensed with the state.
8. False. While many leaders are managers, not all managers are leaders. In addition to managing people and resources, leaders inspire, motivate, and unite people around a common goal or vision.
9. False. While you can create your contracts any way you see fit, and it is completely within your rights to want to retain the clients, trade practices, and business systems, many massage therapists work in multiple locations. Restricting employees or contractors could cripple their livelihood. Only include this requirement if you are able to provide enough work and income to substantiate such a constraint.

CHAPTER 15

Leveraging the Internet

Quiz: Identifying Internet Words and Concepts

1. c. subscribing to an RSS feed
2. b. http://stinkyshoes.com
3. d. all of the above
4. d. find a site that you like and borrow its graphics and content
5. e. all of the above
6. b. the mainstream language of the Internet
7. a. off-site optimization
8. c. spiders
9. c. antivirus software, firewalls, and other security measures
10. d. affiliate program
11. b. copyright
12. c. your site map
13. b. fresh and updated content
14. d. all of the above
15. c. Spam

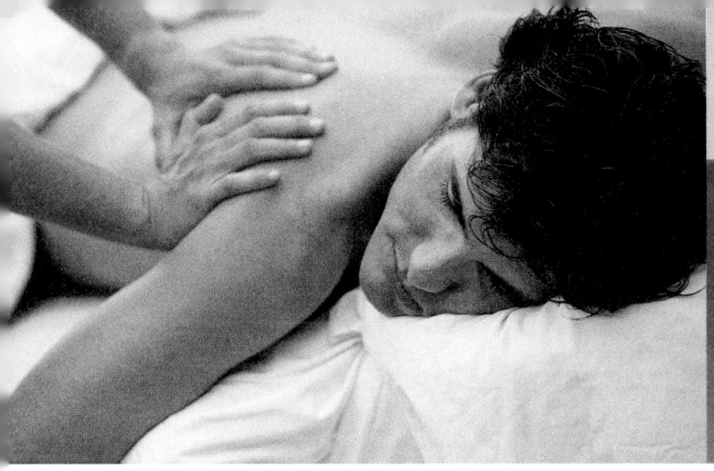

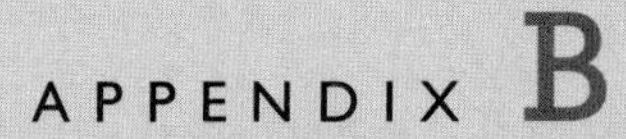

APPENDIX B

Documents, Samples and Activities

SAMPLE COVER LETTER

Charlie Chapstick, LMT

chuckchap@email.com | 522 Sugar House Lane, Nutbush, IA 22290
333-555-6644

December 18, 2012

Susan Pinckney
Sugar Cube Spa
7 Dixon Ave
Nutbush, IA 22290

Dear Ms. Pinckney,

In regard to the available position of **Massage Therapist** for the new Sugar Cube Spa**,** I am most interested in the opportunity. New to the Nutbush area, I have enjoyed watching the physical evolution of the Sugar Cube and would delight in joining my skill set with its certain success. A 2002 graduate of the distinguished Massage Therapy Institute of Savannah, I have been a massage therapist for nearly ten years. Having worked in both spa settings and in private practice, I am adept at blending therapeutic applications into luxurious experiences for clients and guests. I thrive at creating custom-catered encounters, and have traveled the globe to cultivate the aesthetic of escape and sanctuary via spas and massage. I feel confident that I will be an immediately effective contributor to the Sugar Cube spa, and a key player in ongoing development of the company brand.

Charlie Chapstick's Value to Sugar Cube Spa as Massage Therapist:

- 2002 Graduate of prestigious Massage Therapy Institute of Savannah—Honors.
- 2008 Graduate of International Training Massage Thai Program in Chiang Mai, Thailand—Honors.
- Experience at all levels along the spa value chain—therapist, reception, client, consultant, owner.
- Valued by clients, staff, and stakeholders as a trusted partner in development of an optimal environmental business culture and environment.
- Nearly a decade of involvement in the spa and wellness industry.
- Travel to over 30 countries researching, studying, and applying different spa/massage modalities.

I am most grateful to you for taking the time to peruse my information, and invite you to contact me for an interview to further expound on your needs and to outline my strengths in person. I warmly welcome the chance to explore a fit as a massage therapist at Sugar Cube Spa, and I sincerely thank you in advance for the consideration of my resume. I look forward to hearing from you.

Sincerely,

Charlie Chapstick
Charlie Chapstick, LMT
333-555-6644
chuckchap@email.com

SAMPLE RÉSUMÉ

987 Easy Street • East Orange, NJ 11190
Phone 771-222-0001 • E-mail scheese@email.com

Susie Creamcheese

Objective

To use my skills as a pre/post-natal massage therapist to assist women through the physical demands of labor and early parenting.

Work experience

January 2007–present

East Orange Fertility Clinic — East Orange, NJ

Pre-Post Natal Therapist

• Provide massage therapy to 20 pre-/post-natal mothers per week

• Help facilitate mothers' support groups

February 2003–December 2006

Eastern Community College — Eastern, NJ

Admissions Counselor

• Grew new admissions by 20 percent

• Integrated physical, emotional, and mental levels and personalities of all new students.

Education

El Reposo Institute of Mayan Massage — Antigua, Guatemala
Certificate Mayan Uterine Massage, 2008

New Jersey School of Healing Arts — Eastern, New Jersey
A.O.S. Therapeautic Massage, 2006

Professional memberships

AMTA, NCBTMB, Birth Transitions Support Group, Mayan Uterine Massage Professionals International

Volunteer experience

Support Volunteer, WIC (Women Infants & Children); Avon Breast Cancer Walk.

SAMPLE EMPLOYMENT CONTRACT

Cote D'Azur Massage, LLC Employment Agreement

This employment agreement, between Cote D'Azur Massage, LLC ("The Company"), located at 717 Foxspring Ct. Detroit, MI; and Mike Lehoya ("The Employee") is entered into this 24th day of April, 2011.

I. Performance of Duties of Employee
Employee agrees to perform massage therapy services within the scope of training and licensure. Employee shall also perform activities that support delivery of massage therapy services, such as linen maintenance, customer service, recordkeeping, maintaining a clean and safe environment for all clients and coworkers. The Employee may occasionally be called upon to assist in performance of basic clerical duties. Supportive duties are subject to change, as set forth in the provided employee handbook. The Employee also agrees to maintain the image put forth

by the Company, performing services in attire required. The Employee also agrees to fulfill the service schedule agreed upon by both parties, unless there is reasonable and just cause otherwise.

II. Performance of Duties of Company
It is the Company's responsibility to provide the employee with all necessary materials for the performance of massage therapy services, including (but not limited to): hydraulic massage tables, linens, stools, sinks, oils, lotions, audio system and music, adequate storage. The Company will also provide all marketing for the business, and will be responsible for administrative operations such as appointment scheduling and client billing.

III. Certification and Licensure
It is the Employee's responsibility to fulfill all local, state, and federal requirements and expenses for certification and licensure as a massage therapist, and to maintain currency of such certification and licensure.

IV. Compensation
The Employee agrees to the payment for service as follows: The Company will reimburse 45 percent of the fee for services rendered to clients serviced by the Employee. Gratuities will be reimbursed at 100 percent. Paychecks will be issued on the 1st and 3rd Friday of each month, and an itemized statement will be provided to the Employee for each pay period. These conditions are subject to change upon written and signed agreement.

V. Insurance
It is the Employee's responsibility to maintain a malpractice insurance policy of a minimum of $2,000,000 in coverage. It is the Company's responsibility to maintain all insurance of the business and facilities, including, but not limited to: fire, theft, flood, and liability insurance.

VI. Taxes, Worker's Compensation, and Unemployment Insurance
It is the responsibility of the Company to pay all required taxes, including local, state, and federal withholding, Medicare, and Social Security Tax. The Company will also supply the Employee W-2 and other forms for tax purposes. The Company will maintain Worker's Compensation and Unemployment Insurance.

VII. Confidentiality
During and after the employment period, the Employee will not divulge or reveal any secret or confidential information or knowledge relating to the Company. The Employee also agrees not to appropriate confidential information, material resources, or Company clients for his or her own benefit. Confidential and proprietary information shall include but not be limited to: client lists, personal information of clients, client assessment and treatment documents, company marketing plans, company business plans, and company paperwork.

VIII. Amendment and Termination of Agreement
This agreement may be amended by mutual agreement of both parties. As long as both parties are living, no persons other than the parties mentioned herein, shall have rights or responsibilities in this agreement. Without cause, either party may terminate this agreement at any time upon seven days of written notice. Immediate termination may be enacted by either party without mutual consent should the following events occur:

a. The Company's decision to terminate its business and liquidate assets.
b. Bankruptcy or Chapter 11 reorganization.
c. Employee being convicted of any felony or criminal charge.
d. Loss of requisite certifications or licensure by the Employee.
e. Material violations of the provisions included in this agreement and in the employee handbook.
f. Any activity that jeopardizes client or coworkers' health or safety.
g. Violation of ethical standards as defined by local and national associations or governments.
h. Employee's abuse of any chemical substance that negatively affects performance and/or the well-being of clients and coworkers.
i. Employee violating confidentiality or engaging in fraud, embezzlement, or similar behavior.

This constitutes the entirety of the Agreement between the two parties. This document takes precedence over all verbal or previously written agreements.

Signatures:

Employee: _______________________ Date: _______________

Company: _______________________ Date: _______________

SAMPLE INDEPENDENT CONTRACTOR AGREEMENT

Bioworks Health Center, LLC Independent Contractor Agreement

This contractor agreement, between Bioworks Health Center ("The Company"), located at 1010 Legare St. Charleston, SC; and Colby Danover ("The Contractor") is entered into this 20th day of September, 2011.

I. Status and Performance of Duties of Contractor
Following the proscribed status of independent contractor, the Contractor is not an employee of the Company. Thus, the Contractor has control of the means, manner, and method of services provided under the auspices of the Company, and can perform services for other unrelated businesses. The Contractor agrees to perform massage therapy services within the scope of training and licensure. The Contractor shall furnish all necessary supplies for delivery of services including but not limited to: linens, oils, t-bars, ointments, etc. The Contractor shall also perform activities that support delivery of massage therapy services, such as linen maintenance, customer service, recordkeeping, maintaining a clean and safe environment for all clients and coworkers. Supportive duties are subject to change, as set forth in the provided Company handbook. Due to the schedule structure of service, Contractor and Company shall mutually enter into agreements for scheduled service delivery. Within reason, the Contractor has control of attire during service delivery, as long as professional image of Company is maintained.

II. Performance of Duties of Company
It is the Company's responsibility to provide the Contractor with all essential and non-portable materials for the performance of massage therapy services, including (but not limited to): hydraulic massage tables, stools, sinks, oils, audio system and music, adequate storage, etc. The Company will also provide all marketing for the business, and will be responsible for administrative operations such as appointment scheduling and billing clients.

III. Certification and Licensure
It is the Contractor's responsibility to fulfill all local, state, and federal requirements and expenses for certification and licensure as a massage therapist, and to maintain currency of such certification and licensure.

IV. Compensation
The Contractor agrees to the payment for service as follows: The Company will reimburse 65% of the fee for services rendered to all clients serviced by the Contractor. 100% of all gratuities will be paid to the Contractor. Paychecks will be issued on the 1st and 3rd Friday of each month, and an itemized statement will be provided to the Contractor for each pay period. These conditions are subject to change upon written and signed agreement.

V. Insurance
It is the Contractor's responsibility to maintain a malpractice insurance policy of a minimum of $2,000,000 in coverage. It is the Company's responsibility to maintain all insurance of the business and facilities, including, but not limited to: fire, theft, flood, and liability insurance.

VI. Taxes, Worker's Compensation, and Unemployment Insurance
It is the responsibility of the Contractor to pay all his or her required taxes, including local, state, and federal withholding, Medicare, and Social Security Tax. The Company is not responsible for maintaining Workers' Compensation and Unemployment Insurance.

VII. Confidentiality
During and after the contractual period, the Contractor will not divulge or reveal any secret or confidential information or knowledge relating to the Company. After expiration or termination of this agreement, the Contractor agrees not to willingly enter into competition with the Company. Further, the Contractor also agrees not to appropriate confidential information, material resources, or Company clients for his or her own benefit. Confidential and proprietary information shall include but not be limited to: client lists, personal information of clients, client assessment and treatment documents, company marketing plans, company business plans, and company paperwork.

VIII. Ammendment and Termination of Agreement
This agreement may be amended by mutual agreement of both parties. As long as both parties are living, no persons other than the parties mentioned herein, shall have rights or responsibilities in this agreement. Without cause, either party may terminate this agreement at any time upon seven days of written notice. Immediate termination may be enacted by either party without mutual consent should the following events occur:

a. The Company's decision to terminate its business and liquidate assets.
b. Bankruptcy or Chapter 11 reorganization.

c. Contractor being convicted of any felony or criminal charge.
d. Loss of requisite certifications or licensure by the Contractor.
e. Material violations of the provisions included in this agreement and in the employee handbook.
f. Any activity that jeopardizes client or coworkers' health or safety.
g. Violation of ethical standards as defined by local and national associations or governments.
h. Contractor's abuse of any chemical substance that negatively affects performance and/or the well-being of clients and coworkers.
i. Contractor violating confidentiality or engaging in fraud, embezzlement, or similar behavior.

This constitutes the entirety of the Agreement between the two parties. This document takes precedence over all verbal or previously written agreements.

Signatures:

Contractor: ________________________ Date: ______________

Company: ________________________ Date: ______________

TOOLS FOR OPTIMIZING AND MANAGING TIME

Weekly Day Planner

	Mon	Tues	Wed	Thurs	Fri	Sat	Sun
6:00 am							
7:00 am							
8:00 am							
9:00 am							
10:00 am							
11:00 am							
12:00 am							
1:00 pm							
2:00 pm							
3:00 pm							
4:00 pm							
5:00 pm							
6:00 pm							
7:00 pm							
8:00 pm							
9:00 pm							
10:00 pm							

Notes ____

FIGURE B-1

Time Log

Today's Date____________

Today's Goal____________________

Time	Activity	Time Spent	Importance Level to My Goal (low, medium, high)

FIGURE B-2

Action Plan

Today's Date ________

Statement of Goals/Objectives

____

____

____

Implementation:

What needs to be done?	**By when?**	**Priority?**
1) ____________________	________	________
2) ____________________	________	________
3) ____________________	________	________
4) ____________________	________	________
5) ____________________	________	________

Assessment:

How will I know if the task is complete?

1) ____

2) ____

3) ____

4) ____

5) ____

To-Do List

Activity	**Priority (1–5)**

FIGURE B-3

HIPPOCRATIC OATH: MODERN VERSION

I swear to fulfill, to the best of my ability and judgment, this covenant:

I will respect the hard-won scientific gains of those physicians in whose steps I walk, and gladly share such knowledge as is mine with those who are to follow.

I will apply, for the benefit of the sick, all measures [that] are required, avoiding those twin traps of overtreatment and therapeutic nihilism.

I will remember that there is art to medicine as well as science, and that warmth, sympathy, and understanding may outweigh the surgeon's knife or the chemist's drug.

I will not be ashamed to say "I know not," nor will I fail to call in my colleagues when the skills of another are needed for a patient's recovery.

I will respect the privacy of my patients, for their problems are not disclosed to me that the world may know. Most especially must I tread with care in matters of life and death. If it is given me to save a life, all thanks. But it may also be within my power to take a life; this awesome responsibility must be faced with great humbleness and awareness of my own frailty. Above all, I must not play at God.

I will remember that I do not treat a fever chart, a cancerous growth, but a sick human being, whose illness may affect the person's family and economic stability. My responsibility includes these related problems, if I am to care adequately for the sick.

I will prevent disease whenever I can, for prevention is preferable to cure.

I will remember that I remain a member of society, with special obligations to all my fellow human beings, those sound of mind and body as well as the infirm.

If I do not violate this oath, may I enjoy life and art, respected while I live and remembered with affection thereafter. May I always act so as to preserve the finest traditions of my calling and may I long experience the joy of healing those who seek my help.

Source: Written in 1964 by Louis Lasagna, Academic Dean of the School of Medicine at Tufts University, and used in many medical schools today.

HIPPOCRATIC OATH: CLASSIC VERSION

I swear by Apollo Physician and Asclepius and Hygieia and Panaceia and all the gods and goddesses, making them my witnesses, that I will fulfill according to my ability and judgment this oath and this covenant:

To hold him who has taught me this art as equal to my parents and to live my life in partnership with him, and if he is in need of money to give him a share of mine, and to regard his offspring as equal to my brothers in male lineage and to teach them this art—if they desire to learn it—without fee and covenant; to give a share of precepts and oral instruction and all the other learning to my sons and to the sons of him who has instructed me and to pupils who have signed the covenant and have taken an oath according to the medical law, but no one else.

I will apply dietetic measures for the benefit of the sick according to my ability and judgment; I will keep them from harm and injustice.

I will neither give a deadly drug to anybody who asked for it, nor will I make a suggestion to this effect. Similarly I will not give to a woman an abortive remedy. In purity and holiness I will guard my life and my art.

I will not use the knife, not even on sufferers from stone, but will withdraw in favor of such men as are engaged in this work.

Whatever houses I may visit, I will come for the benefit of the sick, remaining free of all intentional injustice, of all mischief and in particular of sexual relations with both female and male persons, be they free or slaves.

What I may see or hear in the course of the treatment or even outside of the treatment in regard to the life of men, which on no account one must spread abroad, I will keep to myself, holding such things shameful to be spoken about.

If I fulfill this oath and do not violate it, may it be granted to me to enjoy life and art, being honored with fame among all men for all time to come; if I transgress it and swear falsely, may the opposite of all this be my lot.

Source: Translation from the Greek by Ludwig Edelstein. From *The Hippocratic Oath: Text, Translation, and Interpretation,* by Ludwig Edelstein. Baltimore: Johns Hopkins Press, 1943.

NCBTMB CODE OF ETHICS

NCBTMB certificants and applicants for certification shall act in a manner that justifies public trust and confidence, enhances the reputation of the profession, and safeguards the interest of individual clients. Certificants and applicants for certification will:

I. Have a sincere commitment to provide the highest quality of care to those who seek their professional services.
II. Represent their qualifications honestly, including education and professional affiliations, and provide only those services that they are qualified to perform.
III. Accurately inform clients, other health care practitioners, and the public of the scope and limitations of their discipline.
IV. Acknowledge the limitations of and contraindications for massage and bodywork and refer clients to appropriate health professionals.

V. Provide treatment only where there is reasonable expectation that it will be advantageous to the client.
VI. Consistently maintain and improve professional knowledge and competence, striving for professional excellence through regular assessment of personal and professional strengths and weaknesses and through continued education training.
VII. Conduct their business and professional activities with honesty and integrity, and respect the inherent worth of all persons.
VIII. Refuse to unjustly discriminate against clients and/or health professionals.
IX. Safeguard the confidentiality of all client information, unless disclosure is requested by the client in writing, is medically necessary, is required by law, or necessary for the protection of the public.
X. Respect the client's right to treatment with informed and voluntary consent. The certified practitioner will obtain and record the informed consent of the client, or client's advocate, before providing treatment. This consent may be written or verbal.
XI. Respect the client's right to refuse, modify or terminate treatment regardless of prior consent given.
XII. Provide draping and treatment in a way that ensures the safety, comfort and privacy of the client.
XIII. Exercise the right to refuse to treat any person or part of the body for just and reasonable cause.
XIV. Refrain, under all circumstances, from initiating or engaging in any sexual conduct, sexual activities, or sexualizing behavior involving a client, even if the client attempts to sexualize the relationship unless a pre-existing relationship exists between an applicant or a practitioner and the client prior to the applicant or practitioner applying to be certified by NCBTMB.
XV. Avoid any interest, activity or influence which might be in conflict with the practitioner's obligation to act in the best interests of the client or the profession.
XVI. Respect the client's boundaries with regard to privacy, disclosure, exposure, emotional expression, beliefs and the client's reasonable expectations of professional behavior. Practitioners will respect the client's autonomy.
XVII. Refuse any gifts or benefits that are intended to influence a referral, decision or treatment, or that are purely for personal gain and not for the good of the client.
XVIII. Follow the NCBTMB Standards of Practice, this Code of Ethics, and all policies, procedures, guidelines, regulations, codes, and requirements promulgated by the National Certification Board for Therapeutic Massage & Bodywork.

Source: Revised October 2008. National Certification Board for Therapeutic Massage and Bodywork. www.ncbtmb.org.

AMTA CODE OF ETHICS

This Code of Ethics is a summary statement of the standards by which massage therapists agree to conduct their practices and is a declaration of the general principles of acceptable, ethical, professional behavior.

Massage therapists shall:

1. Demonstrate commitment to provide the highest quality massage therapy/bodywork to those who seek their professional service.
2. Acknowledge the inherent worth and individuality of each person by not discriminating or behaving in any prejudicial manner with clients and/or colleagues.
3. Demonstrate professional excellence through regular self-assessment of strengths, limitations, and effectiveness by continued education and training.
4. Acknowledge the confidential nature of the professional relationship with clients and respect each client's right to privacy.
5. Conduct all business and professional activities within their scope of practice, the law of the land, and project a professional image.
6. Refrain from engaging in any sexual conduct or sexual activities involving their clients.
7. Accept responsibility to do no harm to the physical, mental and emotional well-being of self, clients, and associates.

Source: American Massage Therapy Association. www.amtamassage.org.

ABMP CODE OF ETHICS

As a member of Associated Bodywork & Massage Professionals, I hereby pledge to abide by the ABMP Code of Ethics as outlined below.

Client Relationships

- I shall endeavor to serve the best interests of my clients at all times and to provide the highest quality service possible.
- I shall maintain clear and honest communications with my clients and shall keep client communications confidential.

- I shall acknowledge the limitations of my skills and, when necessary, refer clients to the appropriate qualified health care professional.
- I shall in no way instigate or tolerate any kind of sexual advance while acting in the capacity of a massage, bodywork, somatic therapy or esthetic practitioner.

Professionalism

- I shall maintain the highest standards of professional conduct, providing services in an ethical and professional manner in relation to my clientele, business associates, health care professionals, and the general public.
- I shall respect the rights of all ethical practitioners and will cooperate with all health care professionals in a friendly and professional manner.
- I shall refrain from the use of any mind-altering drugs, alcohol, or intoxicants prior to or during professional sessions.
- I shall always dress in a professional manner, proper dress being defined as attire suitable and consistent with accepted business and professional practice.
- I shall not be affiliated with or employed by any business that utilizes any form of sexual suggestiveness or explicit sexuality in its advertising or promotion of services, or in the actual practice of its services.

Scope of Practice/Appropriate Techniques

- I shall provide services within the scope of the ABMP definition of massage, bodywork, somatic therapies and skin care, and the limits of my training. I will not employ those massage, bodywork or skin care techniques for which I have not had adequate training and shall represent my education, training, qualifications and abilities honestly.

TABLE B-1 Main Massage Therapy Organizations in the United States

Organization Name	Common Acronym	Type	Publication	Founded	Website
Associated Bodywork & Massage Professionals	ABMP	Professional Association and Member Services	*Massage & Bodywork Magazine*	1987	www.abmp.com
American Massage Therapy Association	AMTA	Professional Association and Member Services	*Massage Therapy Journal*	1943	www.amtamassage.org
International Massage Association	IMA	Professional Association and Member Services	None	1994	www.imagroup.com
Commission on Massage Therapy Accreditation	COMTA	Massage School Accreditation	*COMTA News*	1992/1997	www.comta.org
Council of Schools (AMTA)	COS	Massage School Membership	None	1982	www.amtamassage.org
Massage School Alliance (ABMP)	MSA	Massage School Membership	None	1992	www.abmp.com
Massage Therapy Foundation	MTF	Outreach, Research, Education	*International Journal of Therapeutic Massage & Bodywork (IJTMB)*	1990	www.massage therapyfoundation.org
National Certification Board for Therapeutic Massage and Bodywork	NCBTMB	National Certification	*Connection; InfoLine; Approved Provider News*	1992	www.ncbtmb.org
Federation of State Massage Therapy Boards	FSMTB	National Certification	None	2007	www.fsmtb.org

TABLE B-2 Professional Associations for Massage Therapy

Association	Address	Web/Email
Alexander Technique International	1692 Massachusetts Ave, 3rd floor, Cambridge, MA 02138 (888) 668-8996	www.ati-net.com/index.php ati-usa@ati-net.com
Alliance for Alternatives in Healthcare	PO Box 6279, Thousand Oaks, CA 91359 (805) 374-6003	www.alternativeinsurance.com
American Medical Massage Association	1845 Lakeshore Drive, Suite 7, Muskegon, MI 49441 (888) 375-7245	www.americanmedicalmassage.com info@americanmedicalmassage.com
American Association of Alternative Healing	PO Box 10026, Sedona, AZ 86339	www.cris.com/aaah/toc.htl
American CranioSacral Therapy Association/The Upledger Institute, Inc.	11211 Prosperity Farms Road, Suite D-325, Palm Beach Gardens, FL 33410-3487 (800) 311-9204	www.iahp.com iahp@iahp.com
American Polarity Therapy Association	PO Box 19858, Boulder, CO 80308 (303) 545-2080	www.polaritytherapy.org hq@polaritytherapy.org
American Society for the Alexander Technique	PO Box 60008, Florence, MA 01062 (800) 473-0620	info@amsat.ws
American Alliance of Aromatherapy	PO Box 309, Depoe Bay, OR 93741 (800) 809-9850	
American Association of Oriental Medicine	PO Box 162340, Sacramento, CA 95816 (866) 455-7999	www.aaom.org execdir@aaom.org
American Organization for Bodywork Therapies of Asia	1010 Haddonfield-Berlin Road, Suite 408, Voorhees, NJ 08043-3514 (856) 782-1616	www.aobta.org office@aobta.org
Ancient Healing Arts Association	PO Box 1785, Bensalem, PA 19020 (866) 843-2422	www.ancienthealingarts.org
Bowen Therapy Academy of Australia North American Registry	337 North Rush Street, Prescott, AZ 86301 (866) 862-6936	www.bowtech.com/welcome.do usbr@bowtech.com
The Day Spa Association	310 17th Street, Union City, NJ 07087 (201) 865-2065	www.dayspaassociation.com
Esalen Massage and Bodywork Association	55000 Highway 1, Big Sur, CA 93920 (831) 667-3018	www.esalenmassage.org info@esalen.org
The Feldenkrais Guild of North America	3611 SW Hood Avenue, Ste100, Portland, OR 97201 (800) 775-2118	www.feldenkrais.com
Guild for Structural Integration	3197 28th Street, Boulder, CO 80301 (800) 447-0122	www.rolfguild.org gsi@rolfguild.org
Hawaiian Lomilomi Association	15-156 Puni Kahakai Loop, Pahoa, HI 96778 (808) 965-8917	www.lomilomi.org
Healing Touch International	445 Union Blvd., Suite 105, Lakewood, CO 80228 (303) 989-7982	www.healingtouch.net HTIheal@aol.com
Hellerwork International	3435 M Street, Eureka, CA 95503 (707) 441-4949	www.hellerwork.com info@hellerwork.com
Hospital-Based Massage Network	612 S College Avenue, Ste 1, Fort Collins, CO 80524 (970) 407-9232	www.info4people.com
International Association of Animal Massage & Bodywork	3347 McGregor Lane, Toledo, OH 43623 (800) 903-9350	www.iaamb.org info@iaamb.org
International Association of Infant Massage	1891 Goodyear Avenue, Suite 622, Ventura, CA 93003 (805) 644-8524	www.iaim-us.com iaim4us@aol.com
International Association of Pfrimmer Deep Muscle Therapists	809 S. Harrison St, Alexandria, IN 46001 (877) 484-7773	www.pfrimmer.com
International Myotherapy Association	PO Box 65240, Tucson, Arizona 85728-5240 (800) 221-4634	www.bonnieprudden.com info@bonnieprudden.com

(Continued)

TABLE B-2 Professional Associations for Massage Therapy *(Continued)*

International Thai Therapists Association	PO Box 1048, Palm Springs, CA 92263 (773) 792-4121	www.thaimassage.com itta@core.com
International Spa Association	2365 Harrodsburg Rd, Ste A325, Lexington, KY 40504 (888) 651-ISPA	www.experienceispa.com/ISPA
National Association for Holistic Aromatherapy	3327 W. Indian Trail Road, PMB 144, Spokane, WA 99208 (509) 325-3419	www.naha.org
National Association of Nurse Massage Therapists	PO Box 24004-6749 Willow Creek Dr, Huber Hts, OH 45424 (800) 262-4017 or (937) 235-0872	www.nanmt.org nanmtadmin@nanmt.org
National Association of Rubenfeld Synergists	7 Kendall Road, Kendall Park, NJ 08824 (877) RSM-2468	www.rubenfeldsynergy.com jeannere@comcast.net
National Association of Bodyworkers in Religious Service	5 Big Stone Court, Baltimore, MD 21228-1018 (410) 455-0277	nabrs@aol.com
Nurse Healers-Professional Association, Inc.	PO Box 158, Warnerville, NY 12187-0158	www.therapeutic-touch.org nhpai@therapeutic-touch.org
The Spa Association	PO Box 273283, Fort Collins, CO 80527 (970) 207-4293	www.thespaassociation.com info@thespaassociation.com
Touch for Health Kinesiology Association	PO Box 392, New Carlisle, OH 45344 (800) 466-8342	www.touch4health.com
Trager Association	13801 W Center St, Suite C, Burton OH 44021	www.trager-us.org/usta.html
United States Association for Body Psychotherapy	PMB 294, 7831 Woodmont Avenue, Bethesda, MD 20814	www.usabp.org/index.cfm usabp@usabp.org
United States Medical Massage Association	PO Box 2394, Surf City, NC 28445 (910) 328-3323	www.usmedicalmassage.org info@usmedicalmassage.org
U.S. Sports Massage Federation/ International Sports Massage Federation	2156 Newport Blvd, Costa Mesa, CA 92627 (949) 642-0735	
Zero Balancing Health Association	Kings Contrivance Village Center, 8640 Guilford Road, Suite 240, Columbia. MD 21046 (410) 381-8956	www.zerobalancing.com zbaoffice@zerobalancing.com

- I shall be conscious of the intent of the services that I am providing and shall be aware of and practice good judgment regarding the application of massage, bodywork or somatic techniques utilized.
- I shall not perform manipulations or adjustments of the human skeletal structure, diagnose, prescribe or provide any other service, procedure or therapy which requires a license to practice chiropractic, osteopathy, physical therapy, podiatry, orthopedics, psychotherapy, acupuncture, dermatology, cosmetology, or any other profession or branch of medicine unless specifically licensed to do so.
- I shall be thoroughly educated and understand the physiological effects of the specific massage, bodywork, somatic or skin care techniques utilized in order to determine whether such application is contraindicated and/or to determine the most beneficial techniques to apply to a given individual. I shall not apply massage, bodywork, somatic or skin care techniques in those cases where they may be contraindicated without a written referral from the client's primary care provider.

Image/Advertising Claims

- I shall strive to project a professional image for myself, my business or place of employment, and the profession in general.
- I shall actively participate in educating the public regarding the actual benefits of massage, bodywork, somatic therapies and skin care.
- I shall practice honesty in advertising, promote my services ethically and in good taste, and practice and/or advertise only those techniques for which I have received adequate training and/or certification. I shall not make false claims regarding the potential benefits of the techniques rendered.

Source: Associated Bodywork and Massage Professionals. www.abmp.com.

SELF-CARE TEMPLATE

A. Mental (continuing education, read a book, take a class, write an article, learn something new, etc.)

	Pursuit	When	What I need	Completed
1.				
2.				
3.				
4.				
5.				

B. Physical (exercise, diet/nutrition, sleep, massage, health care, etc.)

	Pursuit	When	What I need	Completed
1.				
2.				
3.				
4.				
5.				

C. Social (time with spouse/partner, family occasions, book club, dinner with friends, networking events, etc.)

	Pursuit	When	What I need	Completed
1.				
2.				
3.				
4.				
5.				

D. Spiritual (prayer, meditation, religious groups, retreat, pilgrimage, etc.)

	Pursuit	When	What I need	Completed
1.				
2.				
3.				
4.				
5.				

SELF-CARE ACTIVITIES ON A BUDGET

You don't have to spend a fortune to take care of yourself, and you may find that most things that feed the body, mind, and spirit don't cost a dime. Here is a list of things that you can do for little or no money. Then, make a list of self-care things you can do for free.

- Exercise
- Soak in the tub
- Use a theracane to work your muscles
- Sit in the garden
- Watch a classic movie
- Give yourself a pedicure
- Give yourself a facial
- Call a long-distance friend
- Play with children
- Garden
- Clean out a closet
- Journal
- Do a jigsaw puzzle
- Bake cookies
- Write a letter to a loved one
- Write a gratitude list

- Blow bubbles
- Turn off the cell phone/computer/tv
- Drink plenty of water
- Breathe deeply
- Do yoga
- Meditate
- Watch the clouds
- Color
- Write a poem
- Laugh with your spouse or partner
- Write yourself a fan letter
- Make a scrapbook
- Dust off the boardgames
- Stargaze
- Make sock puppets
- Sip tea
- Make a paper airplane
- Go to an art gallery opening
- Read the comics
- Go for a long walk
- Light a candle

COMMON OBSTACLES IN FINANCIAL PLANNING

You have explored some of your very personal internal financial obstacles; now consider some of the most common mistakes and pitfalls that others make along the financial path. Fear not if you identify with one or all of these behaviors; they are the result of human nature and often evolutionary hardwiring. It behooved your ancestors to consume as much as possible. Acquiring is instinctual (just observe a two-year old); gathering ensured survival. According to Eric Tyson, one of the forefront authors on financial planning, there are several common financial problems, such as:

- *Not planning*: Many people put off things they know they should do. "I'll go to the gym tomorrow" or "It'll be a lot easier to quit smoking once I'm through this deadline/holiday/exam/relationship/etcetera ad nauseum" are very common maxims amongst us. After all, why plan when not planning is so much easier? The reason: in the long run, simple planning and small steps are MUCH easier than waiting for the eagle of procrastination to swoop down before you scramble to get it together. To paraphrase the old aphorism about prevention and cures, a speck of planning saves a world of hurt.
- *Overspending*: This is a huge one in today's culture. For years, Americans have been bombarded with easy credit and huge tantalizing advertisements: the average teenager will see over 360,000 television ads before they don a cap and gown at graduation. That's a whole lot of temptation to resist for any one organism, especially without a foundation of financial understanding. After the attacks on September 11, 2001, President Bush addressed the American people and urged them to show their patriotism by going shopping. The message: not only does consuming benefit you, it benefits everyone.
- *Consumer credit*: Hot on the heels of overspending, consumer credit debt has reached dizzying heights. And as the economic markets began collapsing in 2008, CNN and *Business Week* reported that outstanding consumer credit debt in the United States was approximately $2.6 trillion. Trillion. That's closing in on the national debt. The average U.S. household lays claim to 14 distinct credit cards. As the subprime mortgage crisis uncovered, credit had been readily and conveniently available to most everyone, and nothing promulgates spending more than you have or can afford like credit. Of course things have changed due to the global economy plunge, but the scars of easy credit run deep.
- *Delaying saving for the future*: Most people like the idea of early or at least comfortable retirement in the abstract, but when it comes to retiring at all, many do not actually save for this goal. Admittedly, for many in their 20s and 30s, actually reaching 65 seems like an inapplicable concept that floats out in the ether. Add to that the difficulty of slaloming through the day-to-day financial obligations, and it becomes all the more palatable to put off. Unfortunately, the longer you wait, the steeper the uphill battle becomes to reach retirement goals.
- *Not doing your homework*: As we mentioned earlier, it is imperative to educate yourself and take the time to really understand your options and the risks/rewards they carry before plunging in. There are many scams out there, and many unnecessary risks that could easily be avoided or at least minimized with a bit of foot work.
- *Focusing too much on money*: It is not just lip service to say that money cannot buy happiness. By fixating upon money, you lose perspective and miss out on the things that are really important. It takes great compassion, patience, and awareness to balance between extremes of keeping your financial head in the sand and your hands in the cookie jar. Aim instead for awareness, empowering action, and aligning your money behaviors with your values and goals.

Sources: Tyson, E. (2003). *Personal Finance for Dummies.* New York: Wiley; Glickman, M. (1999). *The Mindful Money Guide.* New York: Ballantine Wellspring; Bacevich, A. J. (2008, October 5). He Told Us to Go Shopping—Now the Bill is Due. *Washington Post;* and Hamm, S. (2008, October 10). The New Age of Frugality. *Business Week.*

LIST OF VALUES

Compassion	Acceptance	Autonomy
Learning	Loyalty	Fairness
Relationships	Health	Communication
Exploration/Openness	Family	Travel
Creativity	Sexuality	Community
Spirituality	Empowering Others	Education
Romance	Truth	Power
Diversity	Joy	Religion
Harmony	Adventure	

ALIGNING VALUES WITH FINANCIAL GOALS: FINANCIAL PLANNING EXERCISE

Values

1. Independence
2. Exploration and play
3. Time with friends, family and staying home with children
4. Connection
5. Having choices

Financial Goals

1. I will pay back all of my credit card debt by April 15, 2013.
2. I will have started an account that is just for having fun (my joy account) with automatic deposits of $50/month. I will open this account by February 6, 2013.
3. I will increase my massage income by 15 percent by July 15, 2013. By doing this, I will be able to save and invest money for when a baby comes.
4. I will join a Women's Financial Planning Group in my neighborhood by January 20, 2013.
5. I will meet with a certified financial planner by January 1, 2013 to discuss the options available to me.

Obstacles

1. It will be hard to pay off the old debt when I need to keep generating more debt to buy things like groceries.
2. The idea of committing $50 a month automatically is difficult. Besides, how would I even do that?
3. The economy has been really poor lately. Even if I manage to grow my business 15 percent, my investments could lose their value.
4. I am so busy and do not have to add another group into the mix.
5. I have a lot of fear around money, have always employed the "don't look" approach. Meeting with a financial planner is really scary.

Potential Strategies for Dealing with Obstacles

1. I don't need to use my credit card to buy everything as I usually do. I can start paying for groceries and entertainment with cash, which will help me to spend less.
2. I can consider the $50 one of my obligations, ensuring I pay myself first. Online research has shown me that nearly every bank has an easy automated set-up.
3. Businesses can grow even in bad economies. I will maximize my marketing plan in order to grow my practice. I will also research investments that are less risky, even FDIC insured.
4. I have been budgeting my time this long—is an hour or two a month really that difficult to add in?
5. Just doing the exercises and learning about this stuff has empowered me. I will find a financial planner who I feel comfortable with, and who is good at breaking things down. Also, if I get some of the financial planning books out there and read more, I will go into the meeting feeling confident.

FINANCIAL CLEARING EXERCISES

Exercise 1: Feeding It to the Fire

Write down all the beliefs you have about money that you feel might be holding you back. To get started, you might take a look back at the "Put it in Writing" exercise you did in Chapter 7 where you brainstormed all the phrases and quotes you could think of about money. If you see that any of them are limiting or especially charged for you, write these down on a piece of paper. If more come up as you are writing, jot these down as well. Take a pair of scissors, and cut each distinct idea away from the others, making small scraps.

You can do the next part of this exercise in two ways. In the first one, take one of the scraps in your hand and read what it says. Look at the phrase and acknowledge the belief you have been holding. Now close your eyes and imagine a big bonfire. See yourself dropping that slip of paper into the bonfire as you release the belief. The alternative, of course, is to drop the slips of paper into an actual fire, which has a much more kinetic impact. The way you do this exercise is entirely dependent on your physical situation, safety concerns, and your own comfort with fire. Regardless of whether you visualize yourself burning the slips or actually burn the slips, put each one into the fire until they are all gone.

Exercise 2: Money Jars

Did you ever keep a piggy bank when you were a kid? Then you will relate to this exercise. Sometimes the hardest part of creating a financial plan is getting started. If you are new to saving, give this one a try. This exercise will help you get used to allocating your money on a regular basis. Go back to the five values you chose in Chapter 2 and choose five places (accounts) that you would like to direct your money toward in alignment with those goals. One jar could be investing for retirement, another saving for a house for your family, still another for saving for your children's retirement. Or perhaps you'd like to have a fund for taking vacations with the person you love most. Write the desired purpose of each account on the jar. Commit to putting money in to each jar every day—even if it is only one penny. The benefit of this exercise is twofold. It gets you in the habit of making regular contributions to your goals, and you get a visual of your money growing in alignment with your values.

Exercise 3: Affirmations for Financial Health

Say the following affirmations every day for a week, and see how your relationship to money changes.

- I take full responsibility for all areas of my health, including finances.
- I acknowledge with compassion the financial blocks in my life, and I am happy to let them go.
- I release with empathy my old limiting beliefs about money.
- I forgive those who have given me negative money messages.
- I manifest abundance in everything I do.
- My financial health is in good order.
- Prosperity is my right.
- I free myself of any anxiety, stress, anger, or worry I have held about money in the past.
- I forgive myself for ways I have harmed others financially.
- I am a healthy, wealthy and wise person.
- I am capable of setting and achieving ALL my financial goals.
- I attract wealth.
- I manage my personal finances wisely and trust myself to manage my money successfully.
- There is enough for everyone to prosper.
- I am healthy in all areas of my life: physically, mentally, financially, spiritually, emotionally.
- It is all right for me to be rich.
- Money is a tool for me to express my purpose in life and live my values.

THRIFTY TIPS

There are so many ways to cut costs in your personal finances. This will allow you to consciously direct your money toward the things that are important to you. You will often find that many of the ways that you can conserve money are also beneficial in other ways—to your health, to your time with your family, to the environment. The possibilities for constructive thrift are endless, and the following is a mere spattering to help you get started:

- *Take your bike to work.* This will help you save money on both transportation costs and a gym membership! If this isn't feasible, consider alternatives like public transportation or carpooling to minimize costs.
- *Keep a money diary for a week.* Don't just list what you buy and how much it costs, but write down the reason you bought it. This will illustrate the where why and how your money goes, which can inspire you to be more conservative.
- *Pack a lunch.* Not only will this be better for your body, as prepackaged, restaurant, and fast food is typically higher in sugars, preservatives, and saturated fats—it will save you a lot of money!
- *Shop smart!* Every store has sales, coupons, and promotions that reduce selling prices. Do some comparative shopping to make sure you're getting the best price.

- *Unplug Your Appliances.* Most people leave all of their appliances plugged in throughout the day, not realizing the energy vampires that are running up their utility bills. According to the U.S. government's Energy Star Program, 40 percent of the electricity used in homes and businesses is consumed while the machine is off. Not only does it save you money, it's good for the planet!
- *Have a joy account.* Have some money set aside that is strictly for fun and for indulging yourself. This will help you stave off feelings of deprivation and sacrifice.
- *Call your credit cards and ask for a rate reduction.* Competition is tight in the credit card market, and they know you have a lot of options. If they can't give you a lower rate, another company might. Cutting your percentage even a few points can save you hundreds of dollars.
- *Weatherize your home.* A lot of energy is lost through drafty windows or leaky roofs. With utility prices ever on the rise, make sure you aren't paying to heat or cool the outside.
- *Make coffee and tea at home.* If you are a coffee or tea drinker, make it at home instead of paying the high prices in coffee shops.
- *Find the free stuff around town.* Check the local community calendar to find all the free events going on in your area. From concerts to plays to art shows to lectures, you can stay very active without spending money. If you can't find anything, take your family to the park or go on a bike ride with a friend.
- *Drink water instead.* Alcohol, beer, soda, even juice—all these things can be costly, not to mention high in sugars and calories. Water is free and fabulous for your health!
- *Make a list.* If you go to the grocery store with a plan, you are more likely to spend less. Having a list of the things you need will deter you from impulse buying.
- *Find a bank with lower fees and higher interest for your savings.* Many banks will hit you up with all kinds of fees to maintain your account. Online banks are often able to offer higher annual percentages by cutting their operational overhead.
- *Make your own gifts.* It isn't just your mom who appreciates your thoughtful handiwork—people are touched when they receive homemade gifts. Crochet a baby blanket, make pumpkin bread, cast candles, bead a bracelet—tap your creativity and save your money when giving a gift.
- *Invite your friends to your house.* Instead of meeting up at the fancy new restaurant in town, have friends over for a potluck game night instead. This keeps your costs down while allowing you to enjoy your time together.
- *Go to the library.* Heard about a great book? Save your $15 and check it out for free at your local library. Even if they don't have it at your branch, odds are good you can reserve it through an interlibrary loan.
- *Give a gift of beneficial service, not stuff.* When life gets harried, giving a gift of time or service can be the most meaningful (and least expensive). Give a friend a massage certificate for her birthday. Instead of buying your nephew that new Wii or iPad, take him to the museum. This will help you enrich and nurture your relationships while cutting your expenses at the same time.
- *Dig the lunch menu.* Love to go out to eat at restaurants but trying to cut your spending? Most restaurants have two distinct menus, one for lunch and one for dinner. You'll find that lunch menus often offer steep reductions of the dinner time prices. That way you can still enjoy a meal out while being easier on your wallet.
- *Install CFL light bulbs.* Quickly usurping Edison's incandescent bulbs in spite of their heftier up-front price, compact fluorescent light bulbs (CFLs) have longer lives and use less energy than traditional bulbs. Check out Energystar.com for other energy-saving appliances.

TABLE B-3 Personal Budget Worksheet

Category	Monthly Amount	Yearly Amount	Percentage of Income
Total income	$	$	$
Savings/investments	$	$	$
Rent/mortgage	$	$	$
Food	$	$	$
Transportation costs	$	$	$
Insurance	$	$	$
Debt repayment (loans, credit cards)	$	$	$
Entertainment	$	$	$
Clothing	$	$	$
School/childcare	$	$	$
Miscellaneous	$	$	$

THINKING VALUES WORKSHEET

In Table B-4 ■, place a **Y** next to those values you hold personally, and an **N** next to those that are not important to you. When you have finished, put numbers next to the top 10 **Ys** most important to you, and the top 5 **Ns** least important to you.

TABLE B-4 Thinking Values Worksheet

	Y	N	#		Y	N	#
Abundance				New Experiences			
Ambition				Optimism			
Authenticity				Organization			
Adventure				Open-mindedness			
Balance				Passion			
Belonging				Power			
Bravery				Playfulness			
Competition				Privacy			
Compassion				Prosperity			
Commitment				Respect			
Control				Religion			
Creativity				Recognition			
Dependability				Satisfaction			
Devotion				Security			
Diversity				Selflessness			
Education				Sexuality			
Efficiency				Simplicity			
Energy				Spirituality			
Faith				Spontaneity			
Family				Strength			
Financial Independence				Success			
Generosity				Tolerance			
Gratitude				Teamwork			
Growth				Thrift			
Harmony				Tradition			
Health				Trust			
Humor				Truth			
Intelligence				Transcendence			
Imagination				Understanding			
Intuition				Uniqueness			
Independence				Usefulness			
Joy				Unity			
Justice				Variety			
Kindness				Victory			
Love				Vivacity			
Loyalty				Wealth			
Leadership				Winning			
Making a Difference				Wisdom			
Mastery				Youth			
Mindfulness							

Now narrow these down to the top three:

The Values Most Important to Me:
1. ______________________
2. ______________________
3. ______________________

The Values Least Important to Me:
1. ______________________
2. ______________________
3. ______________________

Source: Adapted from Quality Media Resources. www.qmr.com.

TWO-YEAR PLAN TEMPLATE

Goals

Over the next two years, I intend to achieve the following large goals:

1. ______________________

2. ______________________

Each large goal has several supporting goals, or sub-goals. Write these below and in Figures B-4 ■ and B-5 ■.

Goal 1: ______________________
- Sub-goal 1: ______________________
  - Mini sub-goal 1.1 ______________________
  - Mini sub-goal 1.2 ______________________
- Sub-goal 2: ______________________
  - Mini sub-goal 2.1 ______________________
  - Mini sub-goal 2.2 ______________________
- Sub-goal 3: ______________________
  - Mini sub-goal 3.1 ______________________
  - Mini sub-goal 3.2 ______________________

Goal 2: ______________________
- Sub-goal 1: ______________________
  - Mini sub-goal 1.1 ______________________
  - Mini sub-goal 1.2 ______________________
- Sub-goal 2: ______________________
  - Mini sub-goal 2.1 ______________________
  - Mini sub-goal 2.2 ______________________
- Sub-goal 3: ______________________
  - Mini sub-goal 3.1 ______________________
  - Mini sub-goal 3.2 ______________________

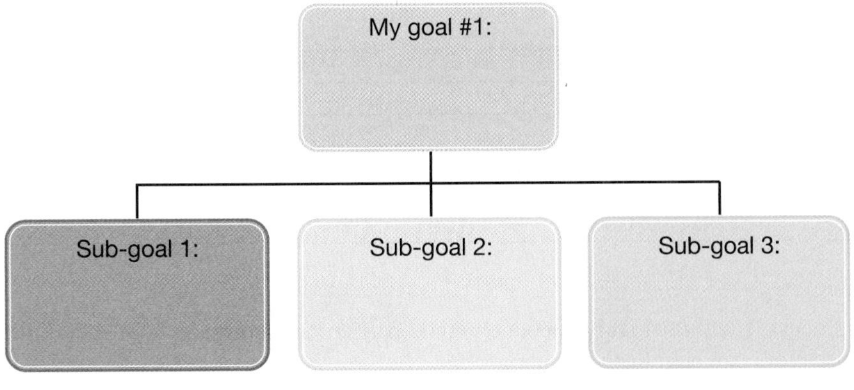

FIGURE B-4

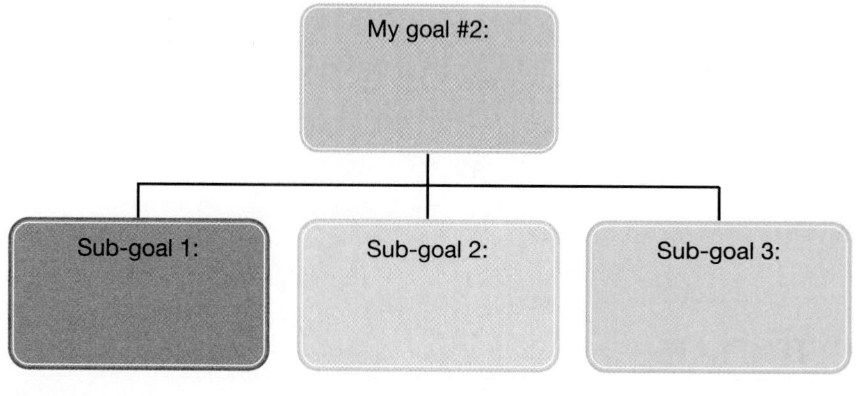

FIGURE B-5

Values

Throughout my life, I have, do and will continue to hold the following values.

1. ______________________________
____
____
2. ______________________________
____
____
3. ______________________________
____
____

How these values manifest in my life.

1. ______________________________
____
2. ______________________________
____
3. ______________________________
____

Purpose

The purpose of my life's career is to ____________ and to ____________ so that ____________.

Vision

____
____
____
____
____
____
____

Obstacles

As I go through this process, I will invariably encounter some barriers and contradictions, both internally and externally. Some of the largest obstacles I can anticipate include:

1. ______________________________
____

2. ____

____

3. ____

____

Solutions

For every obstacle that I identified above, there are many solutions I can think to counter the challenges and help me reach my goal.

1. ____

____

2. ____

____

3. ____

____

Timeline

TABLE B-5 Year One

Action	J	F	M	A	M	J	J	A	S	O	N	D

TABLE B-6 Year Two

Action	J	F	M	A	M	J	J	A	S	O	N	D

SAMPLE COMPLETED TWO-YEAR PLAN: COPIA FINANCIAL HEALTH

Goals

Over the next two years, I intend to achieve the following large goals:

1. Start a financial management company for women
2. Have a baby

Each large goal has several supporting goals, or sub-goals (see Figure B-6 ■).

Goal 1: Start a financial management company for women
- Sub-goal 1: finish MBA
- Sub-goal 2: finish one-year apprenticeship with financial planner
- Sub-goal 3: pass my Series 66 exam
  - Mini sub-goal 1: do exam prep courses
  - Mini sub-goal 2: register with exam administrator

Values

Throughout my life, I have, do, and will continue to hold the following values.

Compassion: The ability to empathize and relate to another just as they are with kindness.
Learning: To be enriching and cultivating my mind, body, and spirit in expansive ways throughout my life.
Exploration/Openness: A willingness to say yes to life.
Relationships: Surrounding myself with quality players and nurturing the bonds between us.

This is how these values manifest in my life.

Compassion: My desire and passion to attend to others' empowerment with the belief that everyone is inherently good and powerful.
Learning: Choosing education in everything, academic or not. Insatiable thirst for reading, lectures, and the lessons parlayed from others' wisdom.
Exploration: My first spoken word was "yes." My thirst for travel, new languages, new cultures, and new experiences is interminable. Whether hip-hop dancing in front of 500 people, traveling the world alone, or venturing deep within my own psyche, I revere the yes (while still appreciating it's balancing no).
Relationships: My relationships are inexplicably important to me, and the portal through which I have really made sense of my world. Interrelationships are my processing places, my challenges, and my spiritual connections. Though in times of great stress, it often easy to go slack on relational attention, I strive to put those I love at the forefront of my mindfulness.

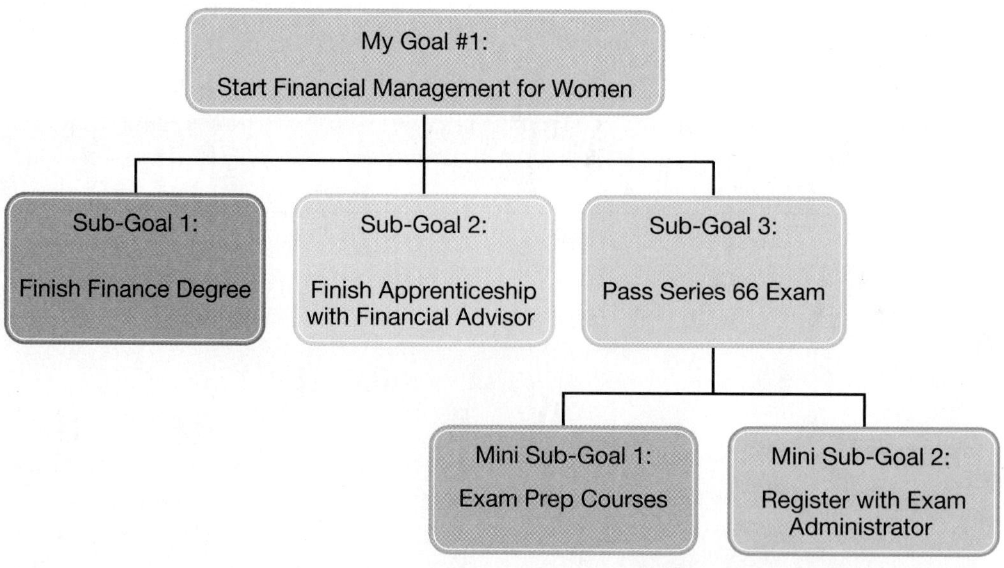

FIGURE B-6

Purpose

The purpose of my life's career is to make financial information accessible to communities that are underserved, and to utilize my compassion and skills to help the grounded discover their wings so that my children can live in an empowered world.

Vision

A short swift ride on my bicycle delivers me to work, and I enter the doors of my beloved financial business. I am the founder and director of Copia, a center devoted to the financial and spiritual abundance of women. Named for the Roman goddess of wealth and plenty, Copia is now in its second year of providing support to women in their quest for financial health and wellness through transformational education. My profession is empowerment, and I educate women from all walks of life on how to be strong financially, to grow strong roots and wings. We work together to blend their values, their spirits, their faith, their minds and ultimately land on financial strength. We work together to see financial health as equally as important as and intertwined with physical, emotional, mental, and spiritual health. I travel. I talk. I share.

My office is indeed a special place, and I have put a lot of attention into making it a warm, welcoming space for all who enter. It is bright, colorful, and cheery, balanced with a quiet sophistication but still very soft and convivial. On my walls, you'll find works by some of my favorite artists: Joan Miró, Alphonse Mucha, and my daughter Peyton. Upon my desk, I have pictures of my family and our adventures together: my husband and I parasailing in New Zealand, in Thailand on our honeymoon, the three of us hiking the beginning section of Napali Coast trail, Peyton papoosed upon my back. There is also one of me with my beautiful sister, father, and mother, and friends from around the world. Above my desk, in the place of honor, is an embroidered plaque made by my grandmother that bears my favorite mantra: "May that which comes to me as seed go on as flower. May that which comes to me as flower go on as fruit." These are words we take very seriously in this organization, and in our lives beyond.

Obstacles

As I go through this process, I will invariably encounter a bevy of barriers and contradictions, both internally and externally. Though they exist over a continuum of scale and severity, I will share a few of the most salient hurdles upon my path.

- *Fear and lack*: I did not grow up with a financial basis. Moreover, I grew up with a great deal of fear about money. Both my parents are wildly intelligent and well educated, and both very loving, compassionate, socially minded people. However, they habitually and vehemently fought over money, and the sense of lack was pervasive.
- *Background*: I do not have a financial background. This external barrier will indeed be an issue for me in the beginning, especially in the publishing realm, where it is incredibly hard to present nonfiction without heavyweight credentials.
- *Lack of follow through*: I've mentioned that one of my values is openness to life. This desire to say yes has resulted in what some might perceive as a scattered collection of accomplishments. I am actually proud of my life's diversity and I excel at all my undertakings, but I have found that I often avoid resolute commitment for fear of missing out on other opportunities.
- *Competition*: While the United States has had a very challenging financial experience, and many people have been seeking financial health in the aftermath, there are still so many people in the country who are not getting the information they need. In addition, the financial landscape has shifted so dramatically from that of even 30 years ago as we watch pensions and social securities dissipate for our generation. This has led to an influx of people flocking to the profession of financial planning, and an increase of self-help finance writers such as Suze Orman, David Bach, and T. Harv Ecker. Thus, I know there is a great deal of healthy competition out there. I also know that I'm not an inherently competitive person, but rather thrive in collaboration.

Solutions

For every obstacle that I identified above, there are many solutions I can think to counter the challenges and help me reach my goal.

- *Fear and lack*: I have done and will continue to do a lot of self-work to examine and shift these beliefs. And though I feel I've done well, fear and lack are still my default settings of which I must be ever-vigilant and aware. I continue to work on my own belief system and to work with my own spiritual mentors and psychological mentors around this area. I do that happily, though.
- *Background*: To counter my lack of financial background thus far, I will do everything I can to extend the depth of my ability and the breadth of my knowledge. I intend to do this by seeking the best post-MBA training, and through continued educational courses throughout my career. I have also found a few financial planning mentors. The support of the women around me and the ability to go forth as a team might also mitigate this issue. I will present less as myself and more of a representative of Copia, something larger than myself.

- *Lack of follow through*: At the heart of my lack of follow through is the fear that I will be trapped in something boring. However, because there is so much to learn and teach in this topic, I don't imagine that I will feel bored or trapped for long. Moreover, I will be accountable to something larger than myself, and that will compel me to follow through.
- *Competition*: The market that I am targeting and the approach that I am taking (psychospiritual finance) are not altogether common in today's financial planning sphere. I believe those two niche aspects will give me (us) a strong competitive edge. Finally, and I hate to sound broken record-ish here, but my own awareness and introspection on my own feelings and beliefs about competing will help me with this obstacle. My solid conviction that everyone CAN win will sustain me through the challenge.

Timeline

TABLE B-7 Year One 2012

Action	J	F	M	A	M	J	J	A	S	O	N	D
Finish MBA	X	X	X	X	X	X	X					
Literary research	X	X		X	X	X	X	X	X	X	X	X
Community networking		X		X	X	X	X	X	X	X	X	X
Vacation			X									X
Licensing												X
U-4 card and fingerprints for pre-step securities							X					
File application & fee for securities license exam								X				
Register for security exam									X			
Exam prep Series 66									X	X		
Informational interviews	X	X		X	X	X						
Seek financial mentor (Jake, LifePlanning- Kinder Institute?)	X	X		X	X	X						
6-month mentorship								X	X	X	X	X
Business license/register name								X				
Securities exams											X	
Pre-natal prep and conception attempts	X	X	X	X	X	X	X	X				
Pregnancy									X	X	X	X

TABLE B-8 Year Two 2013

Action	J	F	M	A	M	J	J	A	S	O	N	D
Mentorship	X											
Start looking for office space	X	X	X									
Rent office space			X									
Hire assistant		X	X									
Teach Women's Finance, Colo. Free University	X	X								X	X	X
Pregnancy	X	X	X	X	X	X						
Baby							X	X	X	X	X	X
Periodic newsletter, articles in women's publications	X		X		X							
Teach Women's Finance Class, Women's Bean Project			X	X								
Develop clientele	X	X	X	X	X	X	X	X	X	X	X	X
Website development (book sales, classes)			X	X	X							
First staff retreat												X
Community networking	X	X	X	X	X	X	X	X	X	X	X	X
Spiritual practice	X	X	X	X	X	X	X	X	X	X	X	X
Vacation					X							

MARKETING PLAN TEMPLATE

Marketing Plan

Therapist's Name:
Company Name:
Address:
Website:
Phone:

I. Executive Summary
Give a brief overview of your company.

II. Mission and Purpose
Why are you in the massage business? What are you setting out to do?

III. Industry Trends
What is happening in the local massage industry? Nationally?

IV. Target Market
Who are your potential customers? How many of them are there? How do they make purchasing decisions?

V. Company Analysis
What are my (our) goals? Culture? Budget? Experience?

VI. Competitor Analysis
With whom am I competing? Why do I consider them my competition? What do I have that they don't?

VII. Four Ps
How will I define my product/service and placement? How will I structure price? And what promotional tactics will I use?

Strengths, Weaknesses, Opportunities and Threats

	Helpful (supports goals)	*Harmful* (can hurt goals)
Internal (personal or professional aspects)	**Strengths:**	**Weaknesses:**
External (environmental conditions)	**Opportunities:**	**Threats:**

FIGURE B-7

VIII. SWOT Analysis (Figure B-7 ■)

IX. Implementation Tactics (Table B-9 ■)

X. Conclusion
Summarize your plan.

____
____
____
____
____

TABLE B-9 What are the steps to accomplish your goals? What are the deadlines?

Goal	Tactic	Description	Completion Date
Goal 1:	1.a		Completed_____
	1.b		Completed_____
	1.c		Completed_____
	1.d		Completed_____
Goal 2:	2.a		Completed_____
	2.b		Completed_____
	2.c		Completed_____
	2.d		Completed_____
Goal 3	3.a		Completed_____
	3.b		Completed_____
	3.c		Completed_____
	3.d		Completed_____

SAMPLE MARKETING PLAN

Marketing Plan

Therapist's Name: Lauren McGrew
Company Name: Healing Touch
Address: 951 E. 6th Ave, Denver, Colorado
Website: www.healingtouchmassage.net
Phone: 803.992.3744

I. Executive Summary
Healing Touch is Denver premier location to receive high-quality healing at an accessible value. We specialize in deep tissue, neuromuscular, and sport massage. We provide a welcoming venue for restorative therapy, and offer our clients a safe space to unwind and release pain and tension. Healing Touch responds to increased demand in the massage therapy industry, and anticipates the competition that typically arises in response to market growth. Our target market consists of active individuals with disposable income in the Metro Denver area who value their health and healing. The experience and education of Healing Touch's owner, Lauren McGrew, is an asset to the company. Internal attributes and external conditions will be examined to determine the optimal marketing ventures for the company.

II. Mission and Purpose
The mission of Healing Touch is to provide consistently superlative therapeutic massage so that clients can achieve and maintain optimal physical and emotional health. We reliably provide a warm, receptive, and serene environment that fosters true healing for all. We continually adhere to the highest of quality standards for all our products and services.

III. Industry Analysis
The massage industry has seen significant changes in the last two decades. For many years, individual massage therapists and collective massage organizations have fought for legitimacy and professional respect. It wasn't long ago that people used the term masseuse or masseur interchangeably for therapeutic and sexual work. But the differentiation from the massage parlor has not been the only area where legitimacy has been sought. Being recognized as a reputable member of the medical family has also been a challenge to the massage community. The United States has traditionally relied on allopathic, or conventional, medicine, and only in recent years have alternative modalities gained popularity.

The massage therapy market in Denver is currently thriving. In the last decade, the landscape has continued to shift. As demand grows and more people seek to join the industry, massage therapy training facilities are springing up rapidly. As an example of this, six years ago there were five massage schools in the greater Denver area; today there are 31 (see www.naturalhealers.com/denver). These 31 schools vary significantly in curricula and size of student body, but the obvious result of this is far more therapists competing in the market than ever before.

IV. Target Market
Denver is replete with members of the target market for Healing Touch. The target customer for Healing Touch is between 33 and 60 years of age. People in this age range are typically more established financially and thus have disposable income. In addition, the 33–60 age range is typically characterized with a preoccupation with health, particularly in Colorado. Denver is the baby boom capital of the country, so there is no lack of individuals in this 27-year age range. The target customer is also well educated, and values health. Because Denver is known as one of the healthiest cities in the country, massage is a valued part of a healthy routine and currently in demand. In addition, Denver has one of the most educated populations in the country, with over 39 percent of the population holding a college degree or higher. Men and women require massage in equal measure, so both genders are targeted by the company.

Although everyone is welcome at Healing Touch and discounts are available to those in need (see section VII of this plan), our target customer has a median income of $30,000 or greater. We believe that this is the breaking point for disposable income—massage is typically considered discretionary income and thus purchased typically from disposable income. Healing Touch is located in the 80218 zip code, where the per capita income is $33,412. In addition, 9192 individuals fall within the target age range in the 80218 area, and more than half (5148) hold a college degree or higher.

V. Company Analysis

Goals:

1. To market to 500 new potential clients from the target market by April 5, 2013.
  (a) To increase clientele by 20 percent by December 31, 2014.
  (b) To develop marketing campaign for new line of private label retail items by June 15, 2014.

Company Culture: Healing Touch is characterized by a tranquil and serene culture, just as the name indicates. Balance and harmony are emphasized and encouraged, as well as self-care for the therapist.
Experience: Lauren McGrew, sole owner of Healing Touch, LLC, has been practicing massage therapy for over seven years. She received her training from the Massage Therapy Institute of Colorado in 2002, and has continued her education throughout her practice. In addition, Ms. McGrew has obtained her Masters in Business Administration, and is working on her MS in Marketing. Her experience as a small business coach and consultant is an asset to Healing Touch, and a key element to its success.

VI. Competitor Analysis
The National Certification Board for Therapeutic Massage and Bodywork reports that there are currently 87,000 nationally certified practitioners serving consumers. The American Massage Therapy Association estimates that there are 300,000 licensed practitioners in the United States. Just as demand for massage has escalated, so has supply of massage therapists.

Locally, the boom in demand for massage has translated into ever-increasing competition for Healing Touch. There are 11 yoga studios, salons, and spas that offer massage therapy within a 2-mile radius of our location (see www.80218.net). Internet research and sidewalk pounding have uncovered over 40 private therapists in the area, 10 of whom practice a combination of deep tissue and sport massage. Due to geographic proximity, price points, and stylistic similarities, the five key competitors for Healing Touch are as follows: Indie 6 Salon (550 E. 6th Ave); NuGenesis Wellness Center (616 Washington Street #109); Wellspring Massage Center (616 Washington St. #103); The Woodhouse Day Spa (941 E. 17th Ave); Jenny Preuss, CMT (931 E. 6th Ave.)

In spite of the quantity of massage therapists in the area, Healing Touch maintains a strong competitive edge due to the following factors: experience in the industry, continued education, business strategies, loyal customer base, and a strong marketing plan with a multiprong approach to promotion.

VII. Four Ps

Product/Service: The services of Healing Touch include deep tissue massage, neuromuscular massage, and sports massage. Value-added services include hot stones and aromatherapy. The company also sells high quality aromatherapy oils, as well as private-label organic bath and body products.
Place: Healing Touch is located at 951 E. 6th Ave, in affiliation with Axis Chiropractic. Healing Touch includes a reception/waiting room, three treatment rooms, an office, a bathroom, and a changing area. Nearly all transactions of products and services occur at this location.
Price: Price has been structured in the mid to high end of the accepted range for massage therapy in the Denver area. Prices were adopted after an evaluation of local norms, and a valuation of the service due to experience, skill, and target market price thresholds. The new product line, *Sweet Serenity,* will be priced competitively with other private label products offered at competing salons and spas. Figure B-8 ■ is a current menu of products services offered by Healing Touch.

As part of the price structuring, Healing Touch offers discounts to retired individuals, students, and military personnel. This satisfies the inclusive philosophy of our mission.
Promotion: Healing Touch employs a combination of advertising, public relations, publicity, and word of mouth.

- Advertising: $250/month is budgeted for a recurring ad in *Wellness Colorado.* E-newsletters are sent monthly. $150 is budgeted for promotional mailings and special occasion cards to clients.
- Public Relations: Healing Touch volunteers chair massage at local fundraisers and sporting events, and donates massage to local charities.
- Publicity: Press releases are sent to local media whenever new classes are offered to the public. A press release will be sent to local media when Healing Touch begins manufacturing and distributing its new private label retail line, *Sweet Serenity* (projected May 2014).
- Word of mouth: this method is enhanced through the use of a referral program and free services to complimentary holistic practitioners who may be interested in reciprocal referral networks.

VIII. SWOT Analysis (Figure B-9 ■)

IX. Implementation Tactics (Table B-10 ■)
The three primary goals per this Marketing Plan (as of Feb. 1, 2008):

1. To advertise to 500 new potential clients from the target market by April 5, 2014.
   (a) To increase clientele by 20 percent by December 31, 2014.
   (b) To develop marketing campaign for new line of private label retail line (*Sweet Serenity)* by May 5, 2014.

Service Menu	
60-minute massage	$65
90-minute massage	$80
Hot stones included in massage	$+20
Aromatherapy add-on	$+15
Royal Package (includes 60-minute massage, hot stones, aromatherapy)	$95
Luxury Package (includes 90-minute massage, hot stones, aromatherapy)	$105
Product Menu	
Sweet Serenity Aromatherapy Lotion	$20
Sweet Serenity Bath Milk	$14
Sweet Serenity Energizing Shower Gel	$16
Sweet Serenity Oatmeal Face Mask	$16
Sweet Serenity Sugar Scrub	$14

FIGURE B-8

	Helpful (supports goals)	*Harmful* (can hurt goals)
Internal (personal or professional aspects)	**Strengths** -good reputation in community -strong professional network -ongoing massage education -marketing expertise	**Weaknesses** -high rent costs -organization skills -balancing many obligations outside of massage -currently underdeveloped web presence
External (environmental conditions)	**Opportunities** -growth in demand for sports massage -new athletic club four blocks away -increase in demand for private label and organic products like *Sweet Serenity* -old competitor has left area	**Threats** -increase in competition in area -massage prices trending down in Denver -new Massage Envy chain opened up in neighborhood -economy is slowing: people spend less on massage

FIGURE B-9

TABLE B-10

Goals	Tactic	Description	Completion Date
Goal 1: Advertise to 500 potential clients by April 5, 2008	1.a	Conduct an analysis of the types of media most likely to reach target market. Determine which one is most cost effective.	Completed 2/17 _____
	1.b	Design an ad for distribution or publication.	Completed 3/25 _____
	1.c	If distributing by mail/email: compile or purchase addresses and send out materials.	Completed 4/5 _____
	1.d	If publishing in a particular media, pay for and submit advertisement.	Completed 4/5 _____
Goal 2: Increase clientele by 20% by December 31, 2008	2.a	Complete Goal #1.	Completed 4/5 _____
	2.b	Compile and organize database for ongoing monthly e-newsletter distribution.	Completed 4/15 _____
	2.c	Design, write and submit first e-newsletter (repeat every 25th of the month).	Completed 4/25 _____
	2.d	Develop and submit curriculum for fall massage class at Colorado Free University.	Completed 5/15 ____
	2.e	Sign up to do massage for summer sports events and fundraisers.	Completed 5/20 _____
	2.f	Quantify client base and contrast against February 08 client numbers.	Completed 12/31 _____
Goal 3: Develop marketing campaign for private-label line	3.a	Take online course on private-label marketing.	Completed 3/5 _____
	3.b	Design and create labels for all *Sweet Serenity* products.	Completed 4/1 _____
	3.c	Design consistent marketing materials (brochure, potential advertisement). Include in newsletter.	Completed 4/25 _____
	3.d	Send press release to local media about the new *Sweet Serenity* line.	Completed 5/5 _____

X. Conclusion

Healing Touch is a value-driven business. Due to the positive demand trends in the Denver area and the proliferation of individuals in the target market, the company is confident of a wealth of opportunities for growth. In spite of a commensurate surge in competition due to the increased demand, the expertise, marketing stratagems, new product line, and attendant skill of the practitioner, Healing Touch has a competitive edge that its competitors do not. Products and services are competitively priced without compromising value, and the price structure highlights perceived value and value-added services. An awareness of the company's strengths, weaknesses, opportunities and threats, as well as a comprehensive tactical plan, ensure that the company is poised for highly effective marketing and continued success of operations.

Sources for Denver demographic information: U.S. Census Bureau, 1998 Census and American Community Survey 2007; www.80218.net/; www.hometodenver.com/Stats_Denver.htm#pop; Metro Denver Health and Wellness Commission, July 2007. See also Rogerson, P. (1999). *Migration Restructuring in the United States: A Geographic Perspective,* eds. Pandit, K. & Withers, S. D. New York: Rowman and Littlefield.

PRESS RELEASE TEMPLATE

Company Logo

Press Contact:

Contact Name
Company Name
Phone Number
Contact email
Website

FOR IMMEDIATE RELEASE

Main Headline of Press Release

Paragraph 1
Physical Location (Month, Day, Year)—A strong introductory paragraph that provides a "hook" that captures a reader's attention and compels him or her to read more. Contains the most important aspects of message and tells the media outlet why people will care about this topic. Also includes the who, what, where, when and why of the story.

Paragraphs 2, 3, 4
These expand on the information in the first paragraph, providing more detailed information. Start each paragraph with the most important information first, building on paragraph one. You might include quotes, testimonials, historical background, or other information that demonstrates value for the community. In the final paragraph, summarize key points.

Additional
Provide a call to action or a way for readers to learn more, such as a contact person and website.

(end all press releases with the following marks)

###

SAMPLE PRESS RELEASE

Press Contact:

Jamison Hamlin
Take Time Massage
709-219-4440
Jamison@taketimemassage.net
www.taketimemassage.net

FOR IMMEDIATE RELEASE

Take Time Massage Center brings convenient and affordable wellness services to Old Town Littleton

Littleton, MI (June 4, 2010)—Take Time Massage Center has opened its doors to Old Town Littleton, offering a wide range of affordable massage and wellness services. With a mission to bring wellness to consumers during difficult financial times, Take Time Massage Center is providing its services for 20 percent below market price through the end of 2012. Take Time Massage Center is conveniently located in the tastefully remodeled townhome at 109 S. Albert St. that also houses the personal training experts at Fitness Now. Take Time Massage Center is currently offering a wide range of massage styles, from familiar offerings such as Deep Tissue, Sport Massage, and Hot Stone, to the more exotic Thai and Balinese massage. Take Time will also offer signature services, such as Momssage™, which is custom-designed for new mothers whose bodies have unique post-delivery needs, and Mayan Abdominal Massage, which aids women with fertility and reproductive issues.

Owner Jamison Hamlin has a mission: to bring the expert therapy that our overtaxed bodies need together with the luxurious experience sophisticated clients expect at a price more people can realistically afford. The Center aims to create a physical space where people can retreat from the toxic effects of chronic stress.

"Our goal is to not only to offer a lavish but affordable escape for our clients in the midst of their breathless and harried lives, but also to help them release genuine physical pain and imbalance. And we aren't satisfied to have the therapeutic retreat experience end when our clients leave. We want to help support our clients in ongoing wellness, and provide them with the tools and resources for creating their own 'everyday escape.'"

Future offerings will include meditation classes, coaching, local and international retreats as well as other wellness modalities that support optimal health such as acupuncture and nutrition. Today, more and more people are turning to alternative health centers as a resource for preventative treatment, injury alleviation, chronic illness, and palliative care. The Journal of American Medical Association (JAMA) reported that Americans spent $40 billion out of pocket (not covered by insurance) on alternative therapies such as massage, yoga, and acupuncture in 2008. Take Time Massage Center is poised to help clients in the Littleton area who are ready to be a proactive participant in their own thriving health.

You can learn more about Take Time Massage Center, and get their free stress retreat kit, by visiting their website at www.taketimemassage.net.

###

TABLE B-11 Would Like versus Must Have Exercise

Item	Cost	Would Like	Must Have

TABLE B-12 Monthly Expense Worksheet

Expense	Estimated Monthly Cost	Cost for the Year (x 12)	Fixed	Variable
Rent/lease				
Accounting				
Marketing				
Licenses and permits				
Equipment (oils, etc)				
Laundry				
Insurance				
Taxes				
Professional fees				
Car expense (for business use only)				
Office supplies				
Postage				
Telephone				
Travel expenses				
Interest payments				
Loan payments				
Payroll				
Payroll taxes				
Repairs				
Inventory				
Other				
Monthly Total:				
	Annual Total (× 12):			

ASSETS		LIABILITIES		OWNERS' EQUITY	
Cash	$____	Accounts payable	$____	Capital	$____
Accounts receivable	____	Salaries payable	____		
Inventory	____	Loans	____		
Supplies	____	Total Liabilities	$____	Total Equity	$____
Total Assets	$____			Total Liab. + OE	$____

FIGURE B-10
Balance Sheet

Revenues:		$____
Expenses:		
Lease	$____	
Advertising	____	
Licenses	____	
Linen cleaning	____	
Professional fees		
Salary	____	
Supplies expense	____	
Interest expense	____	
Total Expenses		(__)
Net Income		$____

FIGURE B-11
Income Statement

Statement of Cash Flows	
Operating Activities	
Cash received from massage services	$________
Cash received from sale of products	________
Cash paid for lease expense	________
Cash paid for salaries	________
Cash paid for other operating items	________
Cash provided by operations	$________
Investing Activities	
Cash used to buy property (PPE)	________
Cash used to buy fixed assets	________
Cash provided by investing	$________
Financing Activities	
Cash paid for interest expense	________
Cash provided by investing	$________
Cash Increase/Decrease	$________
Cash at Beginning of Quarter	$________
Cash at End of Quarter	$________

FIGURE B-12
Statement of Cash Flows

THE IRS "TWENTY FACTORS" TEST

The following 20 factors have been developed by the Internal Revenue Service to determine the status of independent contractors and employees. There are three main groups of factors: behavioral control, financial control, and the nature of relationship between the parties. The extent of importance of each factor varies depending on professional context and service conditions. The more control a business owner has over a person's work, the more likely that person is to be considered an employee.

1. Instructions: A worker that must comply with directives on when, where, and how he or she is to work is generally an employee.
2. Training: Anyone provided training by a company in order for services to be performed in a specific manner is generally considered an employee.
3. Integration: If worker's services are integrated into business operations (and those services are critical to business functioning), that worker is generally an employee.
4. Services rendered personally: The worker must perform the services him or herself.
5. Hiring, supervising, and paying assistants: If the individual has control of assistants that the worker hires, supervises, or pays, and has control of the outcome of this work, this usually indicates independent contractor status.
6. Continuing relationship: An ongoing relationship between the worker and the business can indicate an employee–employer relationship.
7. Set hours of work: If the business or individual for whom services are performed establishes fixed hours of work, this indicates employer control.
8. Full time required: If the individual must work the equivalent of full time, the business or individual controls the schedule of the worker and implicitly restricts the worker from doing other gainful work. An independent contractor is free to work whenever and for whomever he or she chooses.
9. Doing work on employer's premises: If a business owner controls where services are to be performed, particularly if the work could be performed elsewhere, this can indicate an employee–employer relationship.
10. Order or sequence set: If work must be performed in the order, routines, or sequence established by the employer, this indicates employer control.
11. Oral or written reports: If a worker is required to submit regular written or oral reports to the person or business for whom services are done, this indicates employer control.
12. Payment by intervals: If an individual is paid by the hour, week, or month (as opposed to by the project or on commission), this can indicate an employee–employer relationship.
13. Payment of traveling and/or business expenses: If an individual is reimbursed for directed business expenses or travel activities, this typically suggests an employee–employer relationship.
14. Supplying of tools and materials: If an individual uses tools, materials, and equipment provided by the individual or business for whom services are performed, this suggests an employee–employer relationship.
15. Significant investment: An individual's lack of investment in the facilities or amenities used in providing services suggests an employee–employer relationship.
16. Profit or loss: The more a worker can realize a profit or loss as a result of his or her services (through investment or expenditures, etc.), the more likely he or she is to be an independent contractor. If a worker has no sufficient economic risk, he or she is more likely to be an employee.
17. Working for more than one entity at a time: If a worker performs services for multiple individuals or businesses at the same time, this indicates independent contractor status.
18. Making services available to the general public: If an individual renders his or her services available to the public on a consistent basis, this suggests an independent contractor relationship.
19. Right to discharge: If an individual or business for whom services are provided retains the right to discharge a worker, this is indicative of an employee–employer relationship.
20. Right to terminate: If a worker retains the right to end his or her relationship with the individual or business for whom services are performed at any time and without incurring liability, that is usually indicative of an employee-employer relationship.

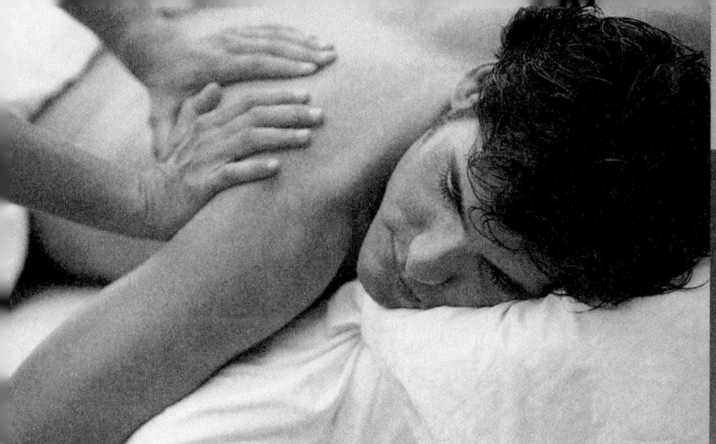

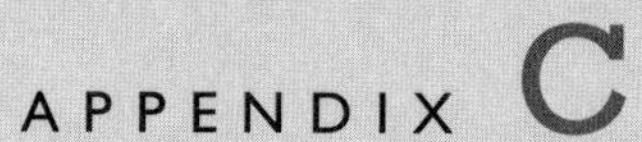

APPENDIX C

Endnotes

INTRODUCTION

1. Associated Bodywork and Massage Professionals. Retrieved from www.abmp.com.
2. Retrieved from www.massageandbodywork.com.

CHAPTER 1: IS A MASSAGE THERAPY CAREER RIGHT FOR YOU?

1. Calvert, R. N. (2002). *The History of Massage: An Illustrated Survey from Around the World.* Healing Arts Press.
2. Calvert.
3. Calvert.
4. Calvert.
5. Issel, C. (1996). *Reflexology: Art, Science and History.* New Frontier Publishing.
6. Lu, G. D. & Needham, J., (2002). *Celestial Lancets: A History and Rationale of Acupuncture and Moxa[bustion].* Routledge Curzon Press.
7. www.etymonline.com. *The Online Etymology Dictionary.* Retrieved April 30, 2010.
8. Greene, E. (2004). *Encyclopedia of Alternative Medicine: Massage Therapy.* Thomas Gale Publishing.
9. Greene.
10. Kellogg, J. H. (1929). *Art of Massage: A Practical Manual for the Nurse, the Student and the Practitioner.* Battle Creek, MI: Modern Medicine Publishing.
11. Greene.
12. www.ncbtmb.com. "Consumers". Retrieved April 30, 2010.
13. www.amtamassage.org "2009 Massage Therapy Industry Fact Sheet." Retrieved April 30, 2010.
14 Bureau of Labor Statistics, U.S. Department of Labor. *Occupational Outlook Handbook: Massage Therapists 2010–2011 Edition.*
15. *Occupational Outlook Handbook.*
16. *Occupational Outlook Handbook.*
17. Association of Bodywork and Massage Professionals.
18. www.massagetherapy.com. "Massage Therapy Fast Facts." Retrieved March 5, 2009.
19. *Merriam-Webster English Dictionary.* (2004). Merriam-Webster Publishing.
20. Brown, F. (n.d.) Spalutions. www.spalutions.com.
21. Sinetar, M. (1989). *Do What You Love and the Money Will Follow: Discovering Your Right Livelihood.* Dell Publishing.

CHAPTER 2: CAREER STRATEGIES AND PROFESSIONAL DEVELOPMENT

1. Bureau of Labor Statistics, U.S. Department of Labor. *Occupational Outlook Handbook: Massage Therapists 2008–2009 Edition.*
2. *Occupational Outlook Handbook.*
3. American Massage Therapy Association. www.amtamassage.org "2009 Massage Therapy Industry Fact Sheet." Retrieved April 30, 2010.
4. "Massage Makes a Global Impact." International Spa Association Study. (2007, August). *Massage Today,* 7(8).
5. "Massage Makes a Global Impact." International Spa Association Study. (2007, August). *Massage Today,* 7(8).
6. Kania, A. (2007, February/March). Building a Hospital-Based Massage Therapy Practice. *Massage and Bodywork Magazine.*
7. Hanlon, P. (2009, February). The Challenges and Rewards of Hospice Massage. *Massage Magazine.*
8. Johnson, R. (2003, October/November). Cruise Industry Employment: Pros and Cons. *Massage & Bodywork Magazine.*
9. Cassidy, K. (2003). Independent Contractor, Employee, Booth Renter: Which Piece Am I? *Associated Bodywork and Massage Professionals* and *Massage & Bodywork Magazine.* Retrieved March 15, 2009 from www.abmp.org.
10. Internal Revenue Service. www.irs.gov."Independent Contractor or Employee?" Retrieved March 30, 2009.
11. Benjamin, P. (2009). *Profession Foundations for Massage Therapists.* Upper Saddle River, NJ: Pearson/Prentice Hall.
12. Internal Revenue Service. www.irs.gov."Independent Contractor or Employee?" Retrieved March 30, 2009.

13. Internal Revenue Service. www.irs.gov."Independent Contractor or Employee?" Retrieved March 30, 2009.
14. Schmucker, P. (2007, June). Product Liability: Are You Covered? Retrieved March 20, 2009 from www.skininc.com.
15. Cassidy.
16. Cassidy.
17. Internal Revenue Service. www.irs.gov. 1099 Tax form. Retrieved April 30, 2010.
18. Cassidy.
19. Rosenberg, A. D. (2007). *The Resume Handbook: How To Write Outstanding Resumes and Cover Letters for Every Situation.* Avon, MA: Adams Media.
20. Pritchard, C. W. (2006). *101 Strategies for Recruiting Success: When, Where, and How to Find the Right People Every Time.* New York: AMACOM
21. Brown, M. & Reitman, A. (2005). *High-Level Resumes: High-Powered Tactics for High-Earning Professionals.* Franklin Lakes, NJ: Career Press.
22. Karsh, B. & Pike, C. (2009). *How to Say It On Your Resume: A Top Recruiting Director's Guide to Writing the Perfect Resume for Every Job.* New York: Prentice Hall.
23. Armstrong, S. & Mitchell, B. (2008). *The Essential HR Handbook: A Quick and Handy Resource for Any Manager or HR Professional.* Franklin Lakes, NJ: Career Press.
24. Johnson, T. (2006, March 16). Dusting Your Digital Dirt. Retrieved March 9, 2009 from ABCNews.com.
25. Johnson, T.
26. Armstrong & Mitchell.
27. Heathfield, S. (n.d.) Listen With Your Eyes: Tips for Understanding Nonverbal Communication. Retrieved March 3, 2009 from www.humanresources.about.com.
28. Beshara, T. (2008). *Acing the Interview: How to Ask and Answer the Questions that Will Get You the Job.* New York: AMACOM.
29. Fitzwater, T. L. (2001). *Preparing for the Behavior-Based Interview: How to Get the Job You Want.* Rochester, NY: Thomson West.
30. Cascio, W. (2006). *Managing Human Resources: Productivity, Quality of Work Life, Profits.* New York: Tata McGraw-Hill.
31. Schmidt, F. L., Hunter, J. E., McKenzie, R., & Muldrow, T. (1979). The Impact of Valid Selection Procedures on Workforce Productivity. *Journal of Applied Psychology,* 64, 609–26.
32. Kador, J. (2002). *201 Best Questions to Ask On Your Interview.* New York: McGraw-Hill.
33. Patterson, V. (2004, March 29). How to Negotiate Pay in a Tough Economy. *Wall Street Journal.* Retrieved April 5, 2009 from online.wsj.com.
34. Wellness Council of America. Negotiating the Right Salary: Seven Strategies for Securing a Comfortable Future. Retrieved April 5, 2009.
35. Leslie, D. L. (2008). *Labor Law in a Nutshell.* St. Paul, MN: Westlaw Publishing, Thomson West.
36. Leslie.
37. Leslie.
38. Peters, T. (1997, August 31). *The Brand Called You.* Retrieved April 7, 2009 from www.fastcompany.com/magazine/10/brandyou.html. See also Ventrella, S. W. *Me, Inc.: How to Master the Business of Being You.* Hoboken, NJ: John Wiley & Sons.

CHAPTER 3: TIME MANAGEMENT

1. Hofstede, G. (2001). *Culture's Consequences: Comparing Values, Behaviors, Institutions, and Organizations Across Nations.* Sage Publications.
2. Hofstede.
3. Hofstede.
4. Koch, R. (1998). *The 80/20 Principle: The Secret to Success by Achieving More with Less.* New York: Random House.
5. *Merriam-Webster English Dictionary.* (2004). Merriam-Webster Publishing.
6. U.S. Department of Labor, Bureau of Labor Statistics. (2007, May). *National Occupational Employment and Wage Estimates.*
7. Pollar, O. (1998). *Organizing Your Work Space: A Guide to Personal Productivity.* Rochester, NY: Thomson West.
8. Cressy, S. (2003). *Business Management for Hairdressers and Therapists.* Oxford, UK: Heinemann Educational Publishers.

CHAPTER 4: PROFESSIONAL ISSUES

1. Benjamin, P. J. (2009). *Professional Foundations for Massage Therapists.* Upper Saddle River, NJ: Pearson Prentice Hall.
2. Howard, R. A. & Korver, C. D. (2008). *Ethics for the Real World: Creating a Personal Code to Guide Decisions in Work and Life.* Boston: Harvard Business School Publishing.
3. Adapted from www.thebodyworker.com and Medical Ethics Quiz. Retrieved July 30, 2009 from www.thebodyworker.com.
4. Braun, M. B. & Simonson, S. J. (2007). *Introduction to Massage Therapy.* Philadelphia: Lippincott, Williams & Wilkins.
5. "I will use those dietary regimens which will benefit my patients according to my greatest ability and judgement, and I will do no harm or injustice to them." excerpt from the Hippocratic Oath. Retrieved July 27, 2009 from National Institutes of Health, www.nih.gov.
6. Benjamin, P. J.
7. Hippocratic Oath. Retrieved July 28, 2009 from www.hipaa.org.
8. Hippocratic Oath, www.hipaa.org.
9. Benjamin, P.J.

10. Onofrio, J. (n.d.) Ethics Principles for Massage Therapists. Retrieved July 28, 2009 from www.thebodyworker.com.
11. Onofrio.
12. Green, E. & Goodrich-Dunn, B. (2003). *The Psychology of the Body.* Philadelphia: Lippincott Williams & Wilkins.
13. Benjamin, P.J.
14. Onofrio.
15. Yardley-Nohr, T. (2006). *Ethics for Massage Therapists.* Philadelphia: Lippincott Williams & Wilkins.
16. Benjamin, B. (2004, January). Core Psychological Concepts. *Massage Today.* 4(0).
17. Henderson, S. Psychological Dynamics: Rules and Boundaries in Massage. Academic paper. Retrieved July 30, 2009.
18. Onofrio.
19. Benjamin, B. & Sohnen-Moe, C. (2003). *The Ethics of Touch.* Tucson, AZ: Sohnen-Moe Associates; see also Benjamin, P. J.
20. McIntosh, N. (2005). *The Educated Heart: Professional Boundaries for Massage Therapists, Bodyworkers, and Movement Teachers.* Philadelphia: Lippincott, Williams & Wilkins.
21. Green & Goodrich-Dunn.
22. Benjamin & Sohnen-Moe.
23. McIntosh.
24. Excerpt from the Hippocratic Oath, National Institutes of Health. See also Wall, D. (2009, May). Malpractice Claim: Sexual Misconduct. *Massage Today* 9(5).
25. Ashley, M. (2000). *Massage: A Career at Your Fingertips, 3rd Edition.* Carmel, NY: Enterprise Publishing.
26. Wall.
27. Retrieved July 27, 2009 from www.ncbtmb.com.
28. National Certification Board for Therapeutic Massage and Bodywork. *National Certification Examination Candidate Handbook.* Retrieved July 30, 2009.
29. Benjamin, P. J.
30. Bureau of Labor Statistics. *Occupational Outlook Handbook, 2010–2011 Edition: Massage Therapists.* Retrieved July 30, 2009 from www.bls.gov/oco/ocos295.htm.
31. Onofrio, J. (n.d.). Male Issues in Practicing Massage Therapy. Retrieved July 31, 2009 from www.thebodyworker.com.
32. Ashley.
33. Ashley.
34. Allen, L. (2009). *One Year to a Successful Massage Therapy Practice.* Philadelphia: Lippincott Williams & Wilkins.
35. State Board Requirements. Retrieved July 31, 2009 from www.massagetherapy.com.
36. AMTA Glossary of Massage Terms. Retrieved July 31, 2009 from www.amta.com.
37. Benjamin, P. J.
38. O'Leary, M. DC Holistic Business Directories. Alexandria, VA: Holistic Business Development.

CHAPTER 5: SELF-CARE

1. Brunner, N. (n.d.). Massage Profession Metrics. Retrieved November 30, 2008 from MassageTherapy.com (publication of Associated Bodywork and Massage Professionals).
2. Guthrie, J. (n.d.). Retrieved November 30, 2008 from www.healersinbalance.com.
3. The Compassion Fatigue Awareness Project. (n.d.). Retrieved November 13, 2008 from www.compassionfatigue.org.
4. Al Madeed, N. May, 2007. Stress and Stressors in House. Retrieved April 3, 2009 from thebusinessofamericaisbusiness.blogspot.com.
5. Lesch Kelly, A. (2002, November). The 4 Biggest Job Stressors. *Shape Magazine.*
6. Sollis, A. (2007, February 22). Enjoying the Benefits of Stress. *Globe.*
7. Palmer, S. (2000). *Physiology of the Stress Response.* London: Centre for Stress Management, City University.
8. Creamer, M., O'Donnell, M.L., & Pattison, P. (2004). Acute Stress Disorder Is of Limited Benefit in Predicting Post-Traumatic Stress Disorder in People Surviving Traumatic Injury. *Behavior, Research and Therapy 42,* 315–28.
9. Stocker, S. (1999, April). Studies Link Stress and Drug Addiction. *National Institute on Drug Abuse* 14(1).
10. Mandel, D. (2008). *Addicted to Stress: A Woman's 7 Step Program.* San Francisco: Jossey-Bass.
11. Mandel.
12. Hellmich, N. (2008, January 7). Friends Help Carry the Burden of Dieting. *USA Today.*

CHAPTER 6: NETWORKING

1. www.thefreedictionary.com. Retrieved January 13, 2009.
2. Olsen Laney, M. (2002). *The Introvert Advantage: How to Thrive in an Extrovert World.* New York: Workman Publishing.
3. Media Awareness Network. 2004 report: "Kids, Alchohol, and Advertising: Understanding Brands." Retrieved October 21, 2008 from www.mediaawareness.ca.
4. Gallo, C. (2006, March 2). You: The Brand. *Business Week.* Retrieved January 13, 2009 from businessweek.com.
5. McGahan, A. M. & Ghemawat, P. (1994, Spring). Competition to Retain Customers. *Marketing Science* 13(2).
6. Mullins, J., Walker, O. C., & Boyd, H. W. (2005). *Marketing Management: A Strategic Decision Making Approach.* New York: McGraw-Hill Publishers.

7. Rubin, G. C. "Seven Tips for Making Good Conversations with a Stranger". Posted May 20, 2009. Retrieved June 29, 2009. www.thehappinessproject.com.
8. Savar, S. (2008). *The Power of Networking.* Reston, VA: BAMA Press; Gitomer, J. (2003). *The Sales Bible.* Hoboken, NJ: Wiley Press.
9. O'Leary, M. "5 Common Mistakes Holistic Entrepreneurs Make." Posted March 3, 2009. Retrieved March 12, 2009. www.holisticbusinessnetworkdevelopment .com.
10. Halpern, N. (2000, April 28). E-Networking. Riley Guide. Retrieved April 13, 2009 from www.rileyguide .com/enetwork.html.
11. Crowder, D. A. *Building a Website for Dummies. 3rd Edition.* Indianapolis: Wiley Publishing.
12. Flynn, N. & Kahn, R. (2003). *E-mail Rules: A Business Guide to Managing Policies, Security, and Legal Issues For E-mail and Digital Communication.* New York: AMACOM.
13. Strawbridge, M. (2006). *Netiquette: Internet Etiquette in the Age of the Blog.* Cambridgeshire, UK: Software Reference LTD.
14. Hansen, K. (n.d.). The Value of a Mentor. Quintessential Careers. Retrieved March 20, 2009 from www .quintcareers.com/mentor_value.html.
15. Eaton, G. Finding A Mentor is Key to a Successful Massage Career. March 25, 2009. Retrieved March 29, 2009 from Massageschoolsguide.com.
16. National Certification Board for Therapeutic Massage & Bodywork. (n.d.). Fraud Alert. Retrievied March 20, 2009 from www.ncbtmb.org/certificants_scam_ alert.php.

CHAPTER 7: ABUNDANCE FROM WITHIN: PERSONAL FINANCIAL MANAGEMENT

1. McLaughlin, C. (2004). *Money as Spiritual Asset.* Center for Visionary Leadership. www.visionarylead .org/articles/money_asset.htm.
2. Williams, R. (2001). *A Woman's Book of Money and Spiritual Vision.* Philadelphia: Inisfree Press.
3. Stanny, B. (1997). *Prince Charming Isn't Coming: How Women Get Smart About Money.* New York: Penguin Putnam, Inc.
4. International Accounting Standards Board. Retrieved October 10, 2008 from www.iasb.com.
5. CNNMoney.com. "Money 101: Controlling Debt." Retrieved October 10, 2008 from money.cnn..com.
6. Financial Literacy and Education Commission. (2006). *Taking Ownership of the Future: The National Strategy for Financial Literacy.* www.mymoney.gov/ pdfs/owndership.pdf.
7. Bach, D. (2004). *The Automatic Millionaire: A Powerful One-Step Plan to Live and Finish Rich.* New York: Broadway Books.
8. Bach.
9. Kiyosaki, R. & Lichter, S. (2000). *Rich Dad, Poor Dad: What the Rich teach their Kids About Money that the Poor and Middle Class Do Not.* Warner Business Books.
10. Shipman, W. G. (2001, December 10). Is the Stock Market Too Risky for Retirement? National Center for Policy Analysis. Retrieved October 6, 2008 from www.ncpa.org/pub/ba382/.
11. Adapted from Investopedia. "Understanding the Time Value of Money." Retrieved October 7, 2008 from www.investopedia.com.
12. Caruso, D. (2007, October 7). Securing Very Important Data: Your Own. *New York Times.* Retrieved October 3, 2009 from www.nytimes.com. See also Eldon, E. (2007, September 18) Mint: The Easiest Way to Manage Your Personal Finances. *Venture Beat.* Retrieved October 3, 2008 from www.venturebeat.com.
13. Comcast.net. (2008, August 11) How Much Auto Insurance Do You Need? Retrieved October 7, 2008 from finance.comcast.net.
14. National Coalition of Health Care. "Quick Facts." Data retrieved October 7, 2008 from www.nchc.org.
15. Baker, S. A. (2007). *The Complete Guide to Planning Your Estate: A Step-by-Step Plan to Protect Your Assets, Limit Your Taxes, And Ensure Your Wishes are Fulfilled.* Ocala, FL: Atlantic Publishing.
16. Cope, S. (1999). *Yoga and the Quest for the True Self.* New York: Bantam Books.
17. Azar-Ruckquoi, A. (2002). *Money as Sacrament: Finding the Sacred in Money.* Berkeley, CA: Celestial Arts.

CHAPTER 8: YOUR OWN PRACTICE: GETTING STARTED

1. Hay, L. (1999). *You Can Heal Your Life.* Carlsbad, CA. Louise Hay, Inc.
2. From O'Connor, E. J. (2006). *Visionary Leadership: Creating the Consensus You Need to Succeed.* Denver: Implementation Institute.
3. McCormack, M. H. (1986). *What They Don't Teach You at Harvard Business School.* New York: Bantam Books.
4. McCormack.
5. O'Connor.
6. Adapted from O'Connor.

CHAPTER 9: LOCATION LOCATION LOCATION

1. Spaeder, K. (n.d.). How to Find the Best Location. Entrepreneur.com. Retrieved March 6, 2009 from www.entrepreneur.com/startingabusiness/startupbasics/ index.html.
2. Spaeder.

3. Officespace.com Frequently Asked Questions—Commercial Real Estate Leasing. Retrieved May 11, 2010 from Officespace.com.
4. Hendricks, R. B. (2006). *Strategic Decisions for Small Business.* iUniverse Inc.
5. Runion, S. How to Choose a Great Massage Business Location. Alternative Health Business. Retrieved November 4, 2008 from www.alternativehealthbusiness.com.
6. Benjamin, P. J. (2009). *Professional Foundations for Massage Therapists.* Upper Saddle River, NJ: Pearson Prentice Hall.
7. McCall, K. (2000, March). Home-Based Business: Is It for You? *Inc.* Retrieved November 4, 2008 from www.inc.com.
8. Farrell, M. (2006, October 13). Top Five Tax Breaks for At-Home Entrepreneurs. *Forbes.* Retrieved November 2, 2008 from www.forbes.com.
9. LaPlant, C. (2005, Spring). Guide To Starting Your Own Business. *Massage Therapy Journal* 44(1).
10. Benjamin.
11. Mullick-Kanwar, M. (2004, May). The Evolution of Private Label Branding. brandchannel. Retrieved March 10, 2009 from www.brandchannel.com.

CHAPTER 10: ORGANIZING AND LEGAL STRUCTURE

1. Bagley, C. & Savage, D. W. (2006). *Managers and the Legal Environment: Strategies for the 21st Century.* Mason, OH: Thomson Higher Education.
2. U.S. Small Business Administration. Choose a Structure: Forms of Ownership. Retrieved June 2, 2009 from www.sba.gov.
3. U.S. Small Business Administration.
4. U.S. Small Business Administration.
5. Bagley & Savage.
6. Bagley & Savage.
7. Bagley & Savage.
8. Braun, M. B. & Simonson, S. J. (2008). *Introduction to Massage Therapy.* Philadelphia: Lippincott Williams & Wilkins.
9. Business.gov. Corporations. Retrieved June 2, 2009 from www.business.gov.
10. Business.gov.
11. Daily, F. W. (2006). *Tax Savvy for Small Business, 10th Edition.* Berkeley, CA: Nolo Publishing.
12. Daily.
13. Adapted from Business.gov. Retrieved June 26, 2009 from www.business.gov.
14. Daily.
15. Business.gov. Bartering. Retrieved June 26, 2009 from www.business.gov.
16. Business.gov.
17. Business.gov.
18. Internal Revenue Service. Hiring Employees (updated December 17, 2008.) Retrieved June 26, 2009 from www.irs.gov.
19. Internal Revenue Service.
20. US Department of Health and Human Services. (September, 1996). The Personal Responsibility and Work Opportunity Reconciliation Act of 1996. Washington, DC. HHS Press.
21. Greenhouse, S. (2010, February 17). U.S. Cracks Down on 'Contractors' as a Tax Dodge. *The New York Times.*
22. Wall, D. (2006, March). Success with the IRS. *Massage Today,* 6(3).
23. Sohnen-Moe, C. (2004). *Business Mastery, 3rd Edition.* Tuscon, AZ: Sohnen-Moe Associates Inc.
24. Schmucker, P. (2007, July). Product Liability: Are you Covered? *Skin Inc.*
25. U.S. Department of Labor. Unemployment Insurance. Retrieved June 29, 2010 from www.dol.gov.
26. Business.gov. Insurance Requirement for Employers. Retrieved June 30, 2009 from www.business.gov.
27. Business.gov.
28. Cutler, N. (2007, June 2). Insurance Billing for the Massage Therapist. *Institute for Integrative Healthcare Studies.* Retrieved July 1, 2009 from www.integrative-healthcare.org.
29. Benjamin, P. J. (2009). *Professional Foundations for Massage Therapists.* Upper Saddle River, NJ: Pearson Education, Inc.
30. Internal Revenue Service. Instruction W-9. Retrieved July 1, 2009 from www.irs.gov.
31. Allen, L. (2009). *One Year to a Successful Massage Therapy Practice.* Philadelphia: Lippincott Williams & Wilkins.
32. Cutler.
33. Federal Trade Commission. (2002, May 22). The Integrity and Accuracy of the "WHOIS" Database. Retrieved July 1, 2009 from www.ftc.gov.
34. Federal Trade Commission.

CHAPTER 11: MARKETING FUNDAMENTALS

1. Capellini, S. (1999). *Massage Therapy Career Guide for Hands-On Success.* Thomson Learning.
2. Tallim, J. (2004). Kids, Alcohol and Advertising: Understanding Brands. *Media Awareness Network.* Retrieved May 13, 2010 from www.media-awareness.ca.
3. Ware, L. (2002). *Selling It: The Incredible Shrinking Package and Other Modern Marvels of Marketing.* Consumer's Union of United States, Inc.
4. Mullins, et al. (2005). *Marketing Management: A Strategic Decision-Making Approach, 5th Edition.* McGraw-Hill.
5. Marn, et al. (2004). *The Price Advantage.* Hoboken, NJ: McKinsey & Company, Inc.

6. Shutes, J. & Weaver, C. (2008). *Aromatherapy for Bodyworkers.* Upper Saddle River, NJ: Pearson Education.
7. Sohnen-Moe, C. M. (1997). *Business Mastery 3: A Guide for Creating a Fulfilling, Thriving Business and Keeping it Successful.* Tucson, AZ: Sohnen-Moe Associates, Inc.
8. Sohnen-Moe.
9. Trout, J. (2006, March 6). Tales from the Marketing Wars: Is Word of Mouth All That It's Cracked Up to Be? *Forbes.*
10. Silverman, G. (2001). *Secrets of Word of Mouth Marketing.* Amacom Books.
11. Silverman.
12. Trout.
13. Zahorsky, D. (n.d.). *Low-Budget, High-Impact Marketing Plan.* Small Business Information Newsletter. Retrieved April 14, 2009 from www.sbinformation.about.com
14. Mullins, et al.
15. Barringer, B.R. & Ireland, R. D. (2008). *Entrepreneurship: Successfully Launching New Ventures.* Upper Saddle River, NJ: Prentice Hall/Pearson.
16. Retrieved April 14, 2009 from www.starbucks.com/aboutus/environment.asp.
17. Retrieved April 14, 2009 from www.tomsofmaine.com/about/reason.asp.
18. Retrieved April 14, 2009 from www.southwest.com/about_swa/mission.html.
19. Sohnen-Moe.
20. Denver-Boulder Metro Area Population Projections. Retrieved April 19, 2009 from www.colorado.gov/demog.
21. Freiberg, J. & Freiberg, K. (2004). *Guts!: Companies That Blow the Doors Off Business As Usual.* New York: Random House.
22. Porter, M. (1998). *Competitive Advantage: Creating and Sustaining Superior Performance.* New York: Free Press.
23. Harper, M. (2005). *Operations Management.* Thomson Custom Publishing.
24. Kerin, R. et al. (2004). *Marketing: The Core.* McGraw-Hill.

CHAPTER 12: MORE MARKETING FOR MASSAGE

1. McKenzie, R. B. & Lee, D. R. (2006). *Microeconomics for MBAs: The Economic Way of Thinking for Managers.* Cambridge: Cambridge University Press.
2. McKenzie & Lee.
3. Austin, P. & Austin, B. (2007). *How to Get Free Publicity: A Handbook for Small Businesses, Clubs, Schools, or Charities.* Oxford: How To Books Ltd.
4. Jackson, E. (n.d.). Does My Small Business Really Need a Press Kit? Business Know-How. Retrieved July 2, 2009 from www.businessknowhow.com.
5. Sohnen-Moe, C. (1997). *Business Mastery: A Guide for Creating a Fulfilling, Thriving Business and Keeping it Successful.* Tucson, AZ: Sohnen-Moe Associates, Inc.
6. Mullins, et al. (2005). *Marketing Management: A Strategic Decision-Making Approach.* McGraw-Hill.
7. Benjamin, P. J. (2009). *Professional Foundations for Massage Therapists.* Upper Saddle River, NJ: Pearson Education, Inc. See also National Certification Board for Therapeutic Massage and Bodywork *Code of Ethics* (October, 2008). Retrieved July 3, 2009 from www.ncbtmb.org.
8. O'Leary, M. (2009). *The Mindfulpreneur Training Program.* Alexandria, VA: Holistic Business Development.
9. O'Leary, C. (2008). *Elevator Pitch Essentials: How to Create an Effective Elevator Pitch.* The Limb Press.
10. O'Leary, M.
11. Sohnen-Moe.
12. McKenzie & Lee.
13. Shultis, K. (2008). How to Recession-Proof Your Massage Business. Retrieved July 15, 2009 from www.riverrockmassage.com/recession.html.
14. Shultis.
15. Streicher, M. (2009, July 2). Sifting Through Billions and Billions of Bytes. *Linux Magazine.*

CHAPTER 13: ABUNDANCE FROM WITHOUT: FINANCIAL MANAGEMENT FOR YOUR BUSINESS

1. Mui, Y. Q. (2008, October 24). The Starter Life: Want to Start Your Business? The Timing Is Always Right. *Washington Post Express.* Retrieved October 24, 2008 from www.expressnightout.com.
2. Burstiner, I. (1997). *The Small Business Handbook: A Comprehensive Guide to Starting and Running Your Own Business, 3rd Edition.* New York: Fireside Books.
3. Burstiner.
4. Rocky Mountain Microfinance Institute. www.rmmfi.org
5. McAleese, Tama. (2004). *Get Rich Slow: Build a Firm Financial Foundation a Dollar at a Time, 4th Edition.* Franklin Lakes, NJ: Career Press.
6. Sohnen-Moe, C. (1997). *Business Mastery: A Guide for Creating a Fulfilling, Thriving Business and Keeping it Successful.* Tucson, AZ: Sohnen-Moe Associates, Inc. Adapted from Sohnen-Moe's Monthly Business Expense Worksheet.
7. Burstiner.

8. Gompers, P. & Lerner, J. (2004). *The Venture Capital Cycle, 2nd Edition.* Cambridge, MA: MIT Press.
9. Tyson, E. and Schell, J. (2008). *Small Business for Dummies, 3rd Edition.* Hoboken, NJ: Wiley Publishing; Worrell, D. (2002, October). Bootstrapping Your Startup. *Entrepreneur.* Retrieved October 29, 2008 from Entrepreneur.com.
10. Whitaker, B. (2007, May 2). Small Business 101: How to Get Started. *New York Times.*
11. Rogers, S. (2009). *Entrepreneurial Finance: Finance and Business Strategies for the Serious Entrepreneur.* Syracuse, NY: McGraw-Hill Companies.
12. Rogers.
13. Mariotti, S. (2006). *Entrepreneurship: How to Start and Operate a Small Business.* New York: The National Foundation for Teaching Entrepreneurship.
14. Brigham, E. F. & Ehrhardt, M. C. (2005). *Financial Management Theory and Practice.* Mason, OH: Thomson-Southwestern.
15. La Plante, C. (2005, Spring). A Guide To Starting Your Own Business. *Massage Therapy Journal.*
16. International Reciprocal Trade Association. Retrieved April 1, 2009 from www.irta.com.
17. Bandyk, M. (2009, March 4). U Exchange and Other Bartering Sites Benefit from Recession. *US News and World Report: Money.*
18. Sohnen-Moe, C. (1997). *Business Mastery.* Tucson, AZ: Sohnen-Moe Associates.
19. Adapted from *Financial Bingo* by Christopher Yukna. Business Emporium, Ecole Nationale Superieure des Mines. Retrieved March 16, 2009 from www.emse.fr .~yukna/business/businessemporium.html.

CHAPTER 14: MANAGING YOURSELF AND OTHERS

1. Benfari, R. (1999). *Understanding and Changing Your Management Style.* San Francisco: Jossey-Bass, Inc.
2. Melchior, D. (n.d.). 5 Common Management Styles. Article Click. Retrieved July 16, 2009 from www .articleclick.com.
3. Melchior.
4. Benfari.
5. Freiberg, J. & Freiberg, K. (2004). *Guts!: Companies that Blow the Doors Off of Business-as-Usual.* New York: Random House.
6. Freiberg & Freiberg.
7. Brown, F. (2003, April/May). Employees and Independent Contractors. *Massage & Bodywork Magazine.*
8. Sohnen-Moe, C. (1997). *Business Mastery, 3rd Edition.* Tuscon, AZ: Sohnen-Moe Associates, Inc.
9. Cascio, W. (2006). *Managing Human Resources: Productivity, Quality of Work Life, Profits.* New York: McGraw Hill.
10. Zimmerer, T. & Scarborough. (2008). *Essentials of Entrepreneurship and Small Business Management.* Upper Saddle River, NJ: Pearson Prentice Hall.
11. Krames, J. A. (2003). *What the Best CEOs Know.* New York: McGraw-Hill.
12. Cascio.
13. Cascio.
14. Society for Human Resource Management. Joinson, Carla. (2000, July). "In-depth analysis of your organization's turnover may help gain support." *HR Magazine.* Retrieved July 24, 2009 from www.shrm.org.
15. Fields, B. (2008, June 24). Recruiting Generation Y: 15 Questions You Will Probably be Asked in a Gen Y Interview. Fast Company. Retrieved July 23, 2009 from www.fastcompany.com.
16. Accelerated Training Solutions. (n.d.). What Factors Lead to Employee Turnover. Cited July 23, 2009 from www.accelerateyourtraining.com.
17. Freiberg & Freiberg.
18. Harkins, P. & Hollihan, K. (2005). *Everybody Wins: The Story and Lessons Behind RE/MAX.* Hoboken, NJ: John Wiley & Sons, Inc.
19. Cascio.
20. Zimmerer & Scarborough.
21. Conner, M. J. & Clawson, J. G. (2004). *Creating a Learning Culture: Strategy, Technology, and Practice.* New York: Cambridge University Press.
22. Presley, A. (n.d.). Scheduling Employees Must Obey Applicable Laws and Account For Employee Shortages. Retrieved July 27, 2009 from www.timeforge.com.
23. Zimmerer & Scarborough. See also Pfeffer, J. (2002, December). The Face of Your Business. *Business 2.0;* and Amdocs, Inc. (2004, June 15). Two Strikes and You're Out . . . for Poor Customer Service. Retrieved July 27, 2009 from www.amdocs.com/News.

CHAPTER 15: LEVERAGING THE INTERNET

1. Ghosemajumder, S. (2002). *Advanced Peer-Based Technology Business Models.* Cambridge, MA: MIT Sloan School of Management.
2. Passarelli, K. H. (2008, October 30). Summary of 9-Month 2008 Results. BIA/Kelsey. Retrieved November 21, 2008 from www.kelseygroup.com.
3. DoubleClick Touchpoints. (2005, July). The Internet's Role in the Modern Purchase Process. Retrieved November 15, 2008 from emea.doubleclick.com/UK/ downloads pdfs/.
4. Horrigan, J. (2007, June). Home Broadband Adoption 2007. Washington, DC: Pew Internet & American Life Project.
5. Horrigan.

6. Brown, E. (n.d.). Create Your Massage Website in a Week. Massage Therapy Radio. Retrieved November 7, 2008 from www.massagetherapyradio.com.
7. Castro, E. (2006). *HTML, XHTML, and CSS, 6th Edition.* Berkeley, CA: Peachpit Press.
8. Langer, M. (2000). *Putting Your Small Business on the Web.* Berkeley, CA: Peachpit Press.
9. Langer.
10. DoubleClick Touchpoints.
11. Internet History: Search Engines (from Search Engine Watch). (2001, September). www.leidenuniv.nl/letteren/internethistory/.
12. Tahmincioglu, E. (2008, June 20). Search Engine Optimization for Small Businesses. *Business Week.* Retrieved November 7, 2008 from www.businessweek.com.
13. Chakrabarti, S. (2003). *Mining the Web: Discovering Knowledge from Hypertext Data.* San Francisco: Morgan Kaufmann Publishers.
14. Thackston, K. (n.d.). Your Site Map. Spider Food or Just a Light Snack? Retrieved November 24, 2008 from www.theallineed.com.
15. Kent, P. (2004). *Search Engine Optimization for Dummies.* Indianapolis: Wiley Publishing, Inc.
16. Jensen, M. (2003, September) Emerging Alternatives: A Brief History of Web Logs. *Columbia Journalism Review,* 5.
17. Jensen.
18. Brown, B. C. (2007). *The Complete Guide to Email Marketing: How to Create Successful, Spam-Free Campaigns to Reach your Target Audience and Increase Sales.* Ocala, FL: Atlantic Publishing Group.
19. Various authors. Technorati's State of the Blogosphere 2009. Retrieved January 10, 2009 from www.technorati.com.
20. Hammersley, B. (2005). *Developing Feeds with RSS and Atom.* Sebastopol, CA: O'Reilly Media.
21. 8 Best Open Source Shopping Carts. (2008, December 4). WebTecker. Retrieved January 8, 2009 from www.webtecker.com.
22. Kent.
23. Bradbury-Haehl, N. (2008, August 17). When It's Online, It's There Forever: Protecting Your Reputation and Your Future Job Prospects. Busted Halo. Retrieved January 8, 2009 from www.bustedhalo.com/features.
24. Alexander, P. (2005, July 5). Is Your Biz Safe from Internet Security Threats? *Entrepreneur Magazine.*
25. Federal Trade Commission. Protecting Personal Information: A Guide for Businesses. Retrieved January 15, 2009 from www.ftc.gov.
26. Harding, K. (2009, September 17). "Mommy Blogger" Heather Armstrong Monetizes the Hate. Retrieved May 18, 2010 from www.jezebel.com.

Glossary

Accountability partner A trusted friend, family member, or colleague who helps you stay responsible to the self-nurturing goals that you have set for yourself. Similar to coaches and mentors, accountability partners check in with one another often to ensure that they are fulfilling all of the tasks and goals to which each person has committed.

Accountant A professional who helps individuals, groups, and businesses to track and accurately report financial information. Accountants are highly versed in the often complex tax codes, and can help you clarify and demystify your tax liabilities.

Accounting The consistent recordkeeping, verification, interpretation, and reporting of a business's assets, liabilities, expenses, cash inflows, cash outflows, and financial activities.

Accounts payable Money that a business owes to vendors, suppliers, or creditors for goods or services that were extended on credit rather than cash.

Accounts receivable Money that is owed a company in exchange for goods or services that were extended on credit rather than on a cash basis.

Action plan Like a business plan or a marketing plan, an action plan is a time management tool that helps break goals into actionable steps on a monthly, weekly, daily, or even hourly basis.

Advertising The public paid promotion of your good or service; there are several different advertising media available from which to choose.

Affiliate programs When one company pays another company a commission of sales to promote its products and hyperlink to its website.

Affirmations Positive assertions about the way things are that can help manifest a positive reality.

Asset An item of value that is owned by an individual.

At-will employment An American edict that outlines an employee–employer relationship with the understanding that either party can break the relationship at any time without legal liability.

Automobile insurance Required in most states, this insurance covers your vehicle and ranges from basic liability to full coverage.

Bad debt Money that is borrowed to purchase things that do not appreciate in value or contribute to your financial health.

Balance The ability to evenly distribute your energy to the things you value, while maintaining physical, emotional, and mental equanimity.

Balance sheet A document that gives details of a company's liabilities, assets, and equity in order to understand its financial condition at a specific point in time.

Bartering The exchange of goods or service without the use of money.

Beneficiary A person to whom money, assets, or other benefits pass.

Blog A contraction of the original "web log," a blog is a site devoted to an individual or company's thoughts, reflections, commentary, or news. Blogs are kept updated with fresh original content on an ongoing basis.

Booth renter A business owner who leases space within an existing company and operates his or her business out of that space. Although the term comes from salon booths, it is often used to describe massage therapists that pay a flat rate for use of a massage room within an established business. Booth renters are responsible for booking clients, setting their own service fees, and managing all the aspects of their small business.

Boundaries Limits that define and clarify personal and professional space and maintain areas of comfort while upholding integrity between individuals. The emotional, mental, and physical space that are placed between yourself and others.

Brand loyalty A consumer's propensity to purchase repeatedly the goods or services of another.

Breakeven The "just scraping by" point where profits and expenses are the same and there is neither profit nor loss.

Brick-and-mortar business Any business that operates out of a physical location and offers face-to-face contact with clients and customers.

Capital Resources (typically financial) available to create new resources.

Career stressors Job-related conditions that often have an adverse effect on employees, such as job insecurity, insufficient income, an overwhelming or unrealistic workload, or unpleasant working conditions.

Certified financial advisor A financial professional who has been certified with a reputable national organization such as the National Association of Personal Financial Planners, Certified Financial Planner Board of Standards, and the Financial Planning Association.

Chronological résumé A resume style that begins by listing work experience in sequential order, starting with current or most recent position and working backward in time. This is a good résumé choice for individuals with a strong professional background in the field for which they are applying.

Collateral An asset that is held as a guarantee for repayment of a loan by the lending institution to insure against potential loss.

Combination résumé A résumé that merges the attributes of a functional résumé with a chronological résumé, typically listing skills first and professional timelines second. Combination résumés allow the job seeker to emphasize the skills that he or she feels are most relevant to the job, while still highlighting work history that employers may want to see.

Commercial real estate agent A professional who helps broker the lease and sale of commercial property. Agents are often hired by commercial real estate owners to lease or sell property on their behalf, although they can be hired as a representative of the tenant to scout out a prime location.

Community relations Activities that develop and strengthen relationships with the community, often through philanthropic activities.

Company analysis An assessment of internal conditions, strengths, and weaknesses within a company.

Company culture Refers to the shared values, practices, and behaviors in a company. Even if you're the only person in your massage business, you still have a company culture, usually defined by your personality and the experience you create for your clients.

Compassion fatigue An affliction induced by constant exposure to the pain and suffering of others, which can result in a decreased ability to care effectively for oneself. This term is used interchangeably with secondary post-traumatic disorder, and is a common affliction of those in healing professions.

Competitive analysis An assessment of external conditions, opportunities, and threats posed by other competitors within a market. Competitors can also be collaborators.

Competitive edge Anything that sets an individual or company apart from the competition. This edge, or advantage, could be due to geography, technical skill, price differentiation, or myriad of other factors.

Consistency As a professional, you will want to do what you say you are going to every time. Consistency is the foundation of successful marketing. With your marketing materials, you will want to keep things looking the same.

Continuing education The ongoing participation in classes, workshops, apprenticeships, or anything else that deepens your knowledge and skill base as a professional practitioner.

Cookies Little packages of Internet information sent between the server and the client browser that help sites track user preferences, behaviors, and information.

Cooperative marketing The practice of jointly promoting distinctive businesses, and leveraging relationships of practitioners across disciplines for collective benefit.

Copyright The legal right to protect your original work; it is automatic as soon as the work is created.

Countertrade The exchange of goods or services paid for in whole or in part with other goods and services.

Cover letter The letter of introduction and intent that typically accompanies a résumé. Cover letters provide an overview of the information in a résumé, and compel the employer to take the time to read the rest of a job seeker's information.

Craniosacral therapy A gentle, subtle treatment technique that evaluates and corrects the craniosacral system. During a treatment, a therapist detects and corrects cerebral and spinal imbalance or impasses that could be causing physical dysfunction.

Creative visualization The practice of envisioning and manifesting desired outcomes.

Customer service The client care activities, both material and intangible, that support the delivery of a business's core product or service. Customer service also helps to build loyalty by meeting and exceeding client expectations.

Day planner A time management tool that helps organize your schedule. Planners can be electronic or paper-based depending on your preference.

Debt financing Funding a business with money borrowed from an outside source, with the promise to return the principal sum and the interest on it.

Deep tissue massage Focuses on the interior core muscles beneath the superficial ones. This is typically quite focused work, and the therapist accesses deep layers of soft tissue to release chronic adhesions, tension, and pain.

Determination The commitment to a goal or outcome regardless of external or internal circumstances.

Differential pricing Occurs when different classes of customers are charged different rates. Also known as discriminatory pricing.

Digital dirt Any information about an individual available online that could be viewed unfavorably by employers or other web users.

Discounting Temporarily reducing the set price for a good or service as an incentive for purchase.

Discretionary spending Money spent on nonessential items.

Due diligence The process of gathering relevant information, assessing risks, researching opportunities and threats, and thoroughly investigating potential investments or acquisitions for a business.

E-commerce The buying and selling of products and/or services over the Internet.

Elevator pitch A brief overview of a product or service that an entrepreneur uses to sell an idea to a potential customer.

E-mail marketing A marketing campaign in which a business promotes its products and services in electronic mailings to a target market.

Emergency fund The foundation of a financial house, this account is dedicated only to emergencies such as unexpected loss of income or unanticipated expenses.

Employee Someone who performs activities and services for an organization that controls what, when, and how those activities and services will be done.

Employee agreement A document that serves as a contract between a company and an employee that outlines rights and obligations of each party.

Employee fit The degree to which a person matches the company culture in which he or she works. Career experts agree that fit is an integral part of overall career success, as it effects performance, motivation longevity, and income over time.

Employee manual A handbook that outlines expectations, operating procedures, and guidelines that are unique to the company and to which all employees must adhere.

E-networking Leveraging the tremendous possibilities of the Internet into the techniques and goals of traditional networking.

Entrepreneur A person who creates a new business venture and assumes the financial, personal, and professional risks involved.

Equipment Any tangible materials used to perform or produce a product or service and run a business.

Equity Total assets minus total liabilities.

Estate planning A plan that designates how your assets will be distributed before or after your death.

Executive summary The introduction for a business, marketing, financial, or any other kind of plan that gives a brief synopsis of what is to come in the plan.

Exit strategy An agreement about what will happen in the event that anyone in a partnership decides to leave the business for any reason. Exit strategies outline transition of ownership between parties and help to plan ways for individuals to sell their interest, recoup their investment, or reclaim their assets in the business.

Exposure In networking, the frequency of contact with others.

Extrovert An individual who is energized or nourished by contact with others. The word comes from *extra,* the Latin word for "outside of," and *vertere,* the Latin word for "to turn."

E-zine A virtual magazine, article, or newsletter disseminated to a target market, typically via mass e-mailings. E-zines are a key component of e-mail marketing.

Fear A powerful component of self-sabotage that undermines the achieving of goals.

Financial community A network of people who come together for the common goal of financial health.

Financial health One of the components of overall balance, financial health involves a positive relationship to money and the development of constructive financial practices and management.

Financial literacy The ability to understand and manage your financial health and plan for your financial present and future.

Financial plan A written plan that outlines your goals and objectives and delineates your strategy for achieving your financial ambitions.

Financial statements Documents that provide a more thorough outline of your business's financial health over a short- and long-term view. Financial statements include a balance sheet, income statement, and statement of cash flows.

Firewall A group of security devices that assess the Internet traffic passing through your computer and prevent unauthorized access to it.

Fixed costs Expenses that must be paid regardless of business productivity.

Follow-up The proactive post-interview behavior that keeps you active in the candidate selection process through assertive and professional communication. Follow-up can give you the competitive edge in the job seeking process and make you stand out from other interviewers.

Forecast A researched, calculated, and carefully formulated projection of the expected financial situation of a business. Forecasts are generally based on the current understanding and future expectations of many internal and external conditions.

Form 1099 A form from the Internal Revenue Service that an independent contractor receives at the end of the year from any business that has paid him or her in excess of $600 for services performed.

Functional résumé A résumé that provides a summary of skills rather than your specific work history and timeline; this style of resume is typically useful for individuals who are just beginning their careers, are changing professions, or have long periods out of the workforce.

Goal setting The intentional positioning of an ambition and the implementation of actionable steps towards actualizing that aim.

Good debt Money that is borrowed in order to obtain something that will ultimately increase in value. Examples of this include taking out a school loan to pay for college, a home mortgage, or a business loan.

Grant A form of financial endowment that is typically given to a recipient by a foundation, a corporation, an individual, or the government.

Gratitude list Based on the holistic principle that what you focus on tends to expand, these lists are a written compilation of all the positive aspects of your life.

Healer A practitioner who works with a body's natural restorative and curative properties to optimize another's health.

Healthy selfishness The practice of systematically ensuring your own needs are cared for before attending to the needs of another.

Healthy touch The use of physical contact that is noninvasive, and has as its focus the intent of healing.

Home page The primary HTML document and the URL that all users will see when they visit a site, whether through direct access or through a link from another site. This is a website's reception area and often the place where first impressions are made for a business.

Hot stone massage Massage that incorporates heated stones into a treatment. The stones used are typically basalt, a black volcanic rock that absorbs and retains heat well.

HTML (HyperText Markup Language) The basic and original language of the Internet. It is what formats your website so that it looks and behaves the way that it does.

Hyperlink Electronically embedded connection in a website that navigates to another location. Hyperlinks can connect a user to other pages within a contained site, or redirect them to another website altogether.

Identity theft When someone uses another individual's identifying information (social security number, birthdate, address) for his or her own benefit or profit.

Image The combination of aspects you present to others that becomes instrumental in their perception of you. Personal appearance, body language, and confidence are some of the many factors that contribute to your overall image.

Implementation tactics The way in which goals are broken down into small, manageable pieces. Implementation tactics are actionable steps towards accomplishing those goals.

Income statement Summarizes a business's revenues, expenses, and profits over a period of time (usually an accounting quarter). Income statements are also known as Profit & Loss Statements, or PNLs.

Industry analysis An examination of the market conditions within an industry. Industry analysis facilitates understanding of a business's position in the market.

Inflow Money that comes into the business as a result of operating, financial, or investment activities. Product sales, services rendered, rent income, or investment dividends are all examples of inflows.

Informational interview A less formal interview in which a person seeks advice and gathers information rather than employment. Here, a student or job seeker is gathering useful knowledge about a particular company or profession while building a professional network.

Insurance A way to guarantee your financial protection against possible losses.

Insurance policy A contract in which an individual or business receives financial protection or compensation against loss from an insurance provider.

Intellectual property An asset that is usually intangible and has been produced by human creativity. Examples include music, writing, copyrights, trademarks, and patents.

Interest The money paid on borrowed resources as a fee to use those resources.

Internet A global system of interconnected computer networks by which individuals, governments, academics, and businesses all come together to share information and resources, and conduct commerce.

Interview A formal meeting that is designed to gauge the qualifications, skills, and fit of a potential employee by an employer, and vice versa. Interviews can be conducted either in person or over the phone.

Introvert A person who is sapped being around others yet feels energized by being alone.

Key words Words or phrases that relate to your business, and typically the words that people looking for businesses like yours are likely to type into a search engine to find what they are looking for.

Labor law Federal and state regulations on the rights of employees in both public and private employ. Employees across industries have many of the same basic rights: the right to not be harassed or discriminated against, the right to a safe work place, the right to be paid minimum wage, the right to be paid for overtime, and so forth.

Lead generation Generating interest in products or services and developing an ongoing marketing relationship with someone via the contact information they provide.

Leasing agent A professional who typically works for landlords to identify, attract, and retain quality tenants to occupy commercial space.

Liabilities Financial obligations that you owe to another person or company in exchange for capital, products, or services you have used or consumed.

Libel A written defamation of another's character that falsely and harmfully impact his or her reputation.

Limited Liability Company (LLC) A business structure that provides limited personal liability for the debts and actions of the business. Often referred to as a hybrid of partnerships, sole proprietorships, and corporations, LLCs can provide the benefit of pass-through taxation while allowing relative flexibility in management.

Liquidity The degree to which an asset is convertible to cash.

Location mix The combination of all the factors that clients interact with sensorially at every direct point of contact with a business: locality, exterior, design, layout, aesthetics, retail sales offerings, even scents and sounds. It is the blend of factors that go into creating the experience for clients.

Logo A symbol or design that acts as a means of identification for a company or brand. Logos are important aspects of branding a business.

Long-term orientation Time orientation marked by patience, perseverance, and thrift.

Low-cost/no-cost marketing Creative, innovative, and effective techniques to market a business for little or no money.

Marketing Any activity that serves to let your market know about you, attract customers to your product or service, and keep them coming back for more. Marketing is how you match your capabilities to the needs of your potential and actual customers; it is the consistent experience you create for your market. Marketing is not one single activity, but rather a merging of the four marketing activities in the marketing mix.

Marketing mix Also known as the four Ps of marketing, the marketing mix includes product, placement, price, and promotion.

Marketing plan A document that details your marketing goals and the detailed steps you will take to achieve them. It is a blueprint for action and, done properly, a roadmap to success. With clear objectives and realistic steps, your marketing plan should be a reference to use as the basis for all marketing endeavors.

Massage therapy An umbrella term that refers to various types and modalities of soft tissue manipulation.

Mentee A person who is mentored, and is generally a novice in a profession or organization.

Mentor An experienced individual who imparts knowledge, skills, and wisdom to someone less seasoned. A mentor can be a teacher, an advisor, a sponsor, or a colleague.

Mission statement A mission statement reflects a person or company's raison d'etre, and should help guide and influence daily decisions. It encapsulates goals and purpose in a concise and straightforward way.

Monochronistic The belief that time is fixed. Punctuality, linearity, and timeliness are very important.

Myofascial release A treatment to realign the body and clear up restrictions in a client's fascia, the strong connective tissue that surrounds the muscle and provides structural support throughout the body. The therapist begins myofascial release treatments with a visual analysis of a client's upright body, whereby physical imbalances can be observed.

Narcisurfing The act of searching for yourself on various search engines to see what you can find out about yourself and what your personal brand is saying about you.

Netiquette The collective standards for interactions online, and the expectation for well-mannered comportment by Internet users.

Network A collection of all the people that you know, consisting of personal, professional, educational, and community contacts.

Networking The art of connecting with other people and building strategic alliances that are mutually beneficial and promote you, your career, and your business.

Non-compete clause (or agreement) Part of a contractual relationship between an employer and an employee or independent contractor. In a non-compete clause, the employee/contractor agrees to not pursue a similar trade in competition with the employer. This is to dissuade people from "stealing" clients or business from the employer.

Nonverbal communication The sending and receiving of messages without any words exchanged. It can include gestures, posture, facial expressions, and eye contact. Studies have shown that at least 55 percent of human communication is nonverbal.

Objectives The small steps that support the overarching goal.

Obstacles Internal or external conditions that can arise and challenge the achievement of goals.

Online forums A virtual platform where individuals can come together to ask questions, share knowledge, and discuss various topics. Also known as discussion boards.

On-site page optimization A way that a web creator influences directly a website's "findability." This is typically done by creating all web pages in such a way as to make them key word rich and search engine friendly.

Open source shopping carts Online systems that anyone can use and access for retailing products on their sites, often for little or no cost.

Organic search results A search engine result for a website that has gained priority naturally and by its own merit, and is not a paid advertisement.

Outflows All the money that goes out of a business to sustain operating, financing, or investment activities. Examples of outflows include utilities, mortgage payments, or loan payments.

Overhead Refers to the continual operating costs associated with running any business, such as rent, electricity, wages, and so forth.

Pareto Principle Named for Italian economist Vilfredo Pareto, this principle states that 80 percent of outcomes are typically generated from 20 percent of input. Also known as the 80–20 rule.

Partnership A business relationship between two or more individuals by shared risk, labor, cooperation, and responsibility. Typically all parties agree to provide financial, material, or knowledge capital for the business.

Passion The compelling excitement for, belief in, and devotion to your chosen focus.

Pay-per-click advertising (PPCA) A promotion technique in which an advertiser places an ad link on a given website, but only has to pay for it when users actually click on the link to the advertiser's own website.

Pay yourself first The financial planning and wealth-building precept that maintains that the first bill you pay is always to yourself.

Personal balance sheet A summary of an individual's financial position, or net worth, subtracting debts from assets.

Personal brand The unique combination of the components that make up who you are and what you have to offer others.

Personal budget The plan for how much money from your earnings you will allocate for your personal expenses and outlays.

Personal financial planning The application of financial principles towards your goals and the crafting of a workable plan to achieve those goals.

Placement The location where a product or service can be purchased, and one of the four Ps of marketing. Placement is also referred to as a "distribution channel." As a massage therapist, your placement will be wherever you perform your massages.

Polychronistic The belief that time is flexible, where schedules are approached in a more circuitous fashion.

Premium pricing Occurs when prices are set above those of the competitors to enhance the perceived value of the service and to attract luxury-seeking clients.

Pre/post-natal massage This technique aims to support women during their pregnancies, as well as during and after labor. It can help to alleviate discomfort, as well as reduce stress and physiological imbalances. Benefits extend to both mother and baby.

Pre-tax income Money earned by an individual from a company or investment before income tax deductions are applied.

Price One of the four Ps of marketing, price is the amount a customer pays for a product or service.

Principal The original amount invested or borrowed, unaffected by interest.

Prioritizing Choosing the things that are the most important and giving energy and attention to those things. Prioritizing ensures that the most essential things get done.

Private-label retail Products that are either created by a company for its own sales or manufactured by one company but sold under another company's brand.

Procrastination Deferring important activities until a later time. When done habitually, procrastination can become a saboteur of success and goal achievement.

Product One of the four Ps of marketing, product refers to the good or service being marketed.

Profits The money that is left after all costs are paid. The simple equation for profits is revenue minus expenses.

Promotion One of the four Ps of marketing, communication put into the market about goods and/or services. Elements of promotion include word of mouth, advertising, public relations, and publicity.

Publicity Attention that is garnered for an individual or for a company, usually in the form of feature articles, online mentions, radio or television appearances, giving a speech or talk, press releases, sponsorship deals, seminars, trade fairs, and so forth. Some advantages of publicity are that it is typically free or low-cost, and can lend an air of credibility to you and your service.

Public relations How an individual or business projects itself and interacts with the surrounding public. Anything you do to promote interest in your products/services and promote a favorable impression of yourself and your business is public relations. Public relations are aimed less at directly boosting sales, and more at promoting your overall image within your community.

Purpose The overarching culmination of values. Your purpose is not a destination or something that you ever complete, but rather something that gives your life perspective and meaning.

Reciprocal links Hyperlinks that mutually connect websites to one another.

Recurring expenses Ongoing costs that require repeated commitment and fulfillment, whether weekly, monthly, annually, or every few years. Recurring costs include rent expense, marketing collateral, insurance, loan payments, taxes, professional fees, and payroll expenses.

Reflexology In this technique, pressure points on the feet and hands are stimulated with a therapist's thumb, finger and hands. Reflexologists maintain that the pressure points follow the body's energy meridians and correlate with different internal organs and muscle groups. Oil and lotion are typically not used.

Résumé A document that succinctly demonstrates ones abilities and provides a synopsis of professional and academic credentials, as well as any relevant accomplishments and skills.

Revenue The total amount of money generated by a company for all goods and services sold.

RSS (Rich Site Summary) A series of web feeds that are used to publish web content that is frequently updated, such as blogs, news stories, or videos.

RSS reader A web-based or desk-based software that acts as a home for all the RSS feeds that a user subscribes to from favorite websites.

Salary negotiation The process of discussing and arriving at a compensation package that is mutually beneficial to you and your employer. Factors affecting a salary negotiation include aspects such as experience and skills, company guidelines, and industry standards.

Scale The size of a business.

Scam An intentional deception of an individual or group that aims to develop trust and confidence in order to defraud.

Scope The breadth of service and product offerings.

Search engine A system that mines and retrieves desired data, information, and resources found online.

Search engine optimization A way of getting a website priority in the listings of search engines in order to improve visitor traffic. A large part of successful Internet marketing strategies.

Search engine results page (SERP) The list of ranked web results that are based on key words or phrases entered by a user and generated by the search engine.

Self-care The practice of putting your needs first and nourishing your own spiritual, emotional, mental, and physical health before another's.

Self-care mission statement A written declaration of the purpose of self-care in your career. Often the cornerstone of a self-care plan, a self-care mission statement can help you connect to the underlying principle of self-care, define what it means for you, and keep you grounded in your commitment to putting yourself first.

Self-care plan A blueprint for your self-care goals, the reasons you want to achieve them, and how you are going to go about implementing actionable steps to achieve those goals. A self-care plan is driven by your self-care mission statement.

Self-sabotage Behavior, both conscious and unconscious, that subverts your goals and impedes your own success. Self-sabotage is the antithesis of self-care.

Shiatsu Known as the Japanese art of finger pressure, in which the therapist uses fingers, knuckles, elbows, feet, and the palm of the hand to apply pressure to a series of points along a muscle group. The goal is to restore "qi," or proper balance. Shiatsu incorporates traction, passive stretching, and acupressure.

Short-term orientation Time orientation that is focused primarily on the present. Someone with this orientation is more interested in instant gratification over sacrificing for future gain.

Simple interest Interest that is calculated only upon principal and does not account for compounding.

Site map An overview of all the content on a website that helps users connect to useful information if a site contains more than one page.

Skill The unique talents that a person has that generates value for another.

Slack labor market Occurs when there are more job seekers than jobs available, and competition between job hunters can be very fierce. Slack labor markets can be good for employers, however, as they have very talented pools to choose from.

SMART goals A helpful acronym for effective and concise goal setting, SMART stands for Specific, Measurable, Attainable, Realistic, and Timely goals.

Social networking The use of online sites to connect with other individuals through virtual communities. Social networks provide outlets for people to come together, associate, and communicate around shared ideas and interests.

Solutions Ways to overcome foreseeable obstacles when setting goals.

Spa consultants Industry experts who advise spa owners on all operational aspects of their business. Typically, these professionals have years of experience in creating, designing, marketing, and maintaining spas.

Spam Unsolicited e-mail advertisements.

Sports massage A technique focusing on muscle systems appropriate for particular sports, sports massage can be used before, during, and after athletic events. The goal is to help the athlete reach peak performance by increasing circulation, reducing swelling, elongating muscles, reducing tension, reducing lactic acid accumulation, and preventing injuries.

STAR technique An interviewing technique for job seekers, STAR is an acronym for Situation, Task, Action, Result. Using this technique helps the interviewee convey all the relevant and valuable information that interviewers are seeking.

Start-up costs The initial expenses associated with starting a new business.

Statement of cash flows An account of a company's cash activities, particularly as they relate to operations, investing, or financing. A statement of cash flows usually gives a snapshot of a period in time (usually a quarterly accounting period), similar to a balance sheet.

Strategic partners Individuals or businesses that come together in alliance to enhance one another's success.

Strategy A plan or series of methods to obtain a specific objective.

Stress A mental or physical reaction to the people and situations in life, and the perceived pressure that these things can bring to an individual.

Stressor Any event, person, situation, or change that provokes a stress reaction in the body and mind. Stressors can be anything that an individual perceives as a threat, irritation, or obstacle in achieving a desired goal.

Subscriber list A collection of names and physical or e-mail addresses obtained for the purpose of distributing information and communication to target markets. Also known as a user list.

Success A person, group, project, or event that carries out its intended purpose. Success is a very fluid concept, and can mean very different things to different people. Its ultimate definition is relative to the individual's own goals and values.

Support system A network of resources and people who offer mutual assistance to one another, and help sustain one another through the highs and lows of life.

Sweat equity The unpaid physical and mental labor of the owner of a business that increases the business's worth.

Swedish massage A technique using kneading and gliding strokes to increase blood flow. It focuses attention on the more superficial muscles of the body, and fosters healthy oxygen flow and toxin release from muscles. Petrissage, effleurage, and tapotement are some Swedish techniques.

SWOT analysis An examination of a company's Strengths, Weaknesses, Opportunities, and Threats. SWOT provides an exploration and description of the internal and external business, and can be applied as a strategic tool in marketing or for any business decision.

Tactic The steps taken to a execute a strategy piece by piece.

Targeted résumés Customized for specific jobs, highlighting different strengths and skills than those emphasized in other résumés.

Target market Those identified as actual or potential customers based on what the company has to offer.

Tax-deductible contributions The money put into a tax-deferred investment plan, taken out of pay before taxes are withheld.

Thank-you card Generally a handwritten or typed note that expresses your gratitude, highlights your interest in a company, and helps to solidify a professional relationship.

Thank-you letter Like a thank-you card, a letter is a form of follow-up after an informational or formal interview. It allows you to recap highlights from the interview, to clarify any areas of concern, and to address the ways in which problems will be solved for the interviewer.

Third-party merchant sites Usually the major e-commerce websites that, whether by auction or direct sale, act as retail clearinghouses for every kind of product imaginable. Examples include eBay, Half.com, and Amazon.

Tight labor market Occurs when there are more jobs than there are job seekers, resulting in competition between employers to recruit and retain quality talent. In this market, job seekers are in a better position, as they have many job opportunities from which to choose.

Time line A timetable or schedule of events; a graphic representation of the chronology of goals, objectives, strategies, and tactics.

Time log A time management tool to help track and analyze the way time is currently being spent. Also called a time journal.

Time management The art of maximizing the hours in a day to be more efficient in achieving your goals.

Time orientation The relationship and regard one has to a timetable; focus is typically short term or long term. Time orientation has many cultural implications.

Time wasters Activities that are not only nonessential to immediate goals, but superfluous altogether.

To-do list A catalog of the accomplishments and activities that need to be done to accomplish a goal.

URL (Uniform Resource Locator) The encoded address that denotes where information is available online and gives the proper Internet protocol for retrieving it.

Value-added Generating a perceived value to customers in addition to the standard product or service.

Values Your core beliefs that give meaning and direction in life.

Variable costs Expenses that fluctuate based on the volume of productivity and output activities of the business.

Vendor The company that provides the products to another company for resale or for general operations. Also known as a supplier.

Venture capitalist An individual or investment firm that manages the pooled money of others, and can provide a huge financial infusion to a start-up company.

Vision The blueprint for your own goals or the goals of a business.

Web authoring software A program that allows you to create your own web pages and interconnect them into a viable website.

Web crawlers Automated programs that seek out information on the web. Crawlers scour through websites for data to use in search engines indices. Also known as spiders, bots, and ants.

Web developer A professional who designs, develops, and maintains websites for others. Also known as webmasters or web architects.

Web hosting The housing, data storing, maintaining, and servicing of a website, and what needs to happen to facilitate and connect your website online.

Website An interconnected set of web pages that are furnished and supported by a host. It typically includes a home page and several other pages of interest that visitors can navigate.

Website templates Mass-produced site layouts that can be purchased, downloaded, and used for any type of business.

Wellness center Any location where multiple wellness services are offered for clients looking to reduce their risk of illness, increase their level of health and fitness, and improve their overall quality of life. Examples of services offered in wellness centers include things such as massage, personal training, nutrition counseling, acupuncture, yoga classes, health education classes, mental health counseling, and pre/post-natal care.

Word of mouth Informal communications by those who have experienced a product or service, including recommendations and referrals that clients make on your behalf. Word of mouth marketing is also known by its other aliases: viral marketing, grassroots, buzz marketing, product seeding, and referral programs.

Work-life balance The equilibrium achieved when one is able to strike an accord between professional and personal obligations.

Zoning The designation for use of different areas by local governments. Zoning laws or ordinances dictate what types of businesses can and cannot be conducted in various neighborhoods and locations.

Zoning variance An exception to an existing zoning law for which businesses can apply.

Index

Note: Page numbers with "f" indicate figures; those with "t" indicate tables.

C

D

E

I

N

O

P